Update in Dermatopathology

Guest Editor

TAMMIE FERRINGER, MD

DERMATOLOGIC CLINICS

www.derm.theclinics.com

Consulting Editor

BRUCE H. THIERS, MD

October 2012 • Volume 30 • Number 4

SAUNDERS an imprint of ELSEVIER, Inc.

W.B. SAUNDERS COMPANY
A Division of Elsevier Inc.

1600 John F. Kennedy Boulevard • Suite 1800 • Philadelphia, PA 19103-2899

http://www.theclinics.com

DERMATOLOGIC CLINICS Volume 30, Number 4
October 2012 ISSN 0733-8635, ISBN-13: 978-1-4557-4897-6

Editor: Stephanie Donley

Dermatologic Clinics (ISSN 0733-8635) is published quarterly by Elsevier Inc., 360 Park Avenue South, New York, NY 10010-1710. Months of publication are January, April, July, and October. Business and editorial offices: 1600 John F. Kennedy Blvd., Suite 1800, Philadelphia, PA 19103-2899. Customer service office: 11830 Westline Drive, St. Louis, MO 63146. Periodicals postage paid at New York, NY, and additional mailing offices. Subscription prices are USD 346.00 per year for US individuals, USD 512.00 per year for US institutions, USD 404.00 per year for Canadian individuals, USD 613.00 per year for Canadian institutions, USD 473.00 per year for international individuals, USD 613.00 per year for international institutions, USD 161.00 per year for US students/residents, and USD 233.00 per year for Canadian and international students/residents. International air speed delivery is included in all *Clinics* subscription prices. All prices are subject to change without notice. **POSTMASTER:** Send address changes to *Dermatologic Clinics*, Elsevier Health Sciences Division, Subscription Customer Service, 3251 Riverport Lane, Maryland Heights, MO 63043. **Customer Service: 1-800-654-2452 (U.S. and Canada); 314-447-8871 (outside U.S. and Canada). Fax: 314-447-8029. E-mail: journalscustomerservice-usa@elsevier.com (for print support); journalsonlinesupport-usa@elsevier.com (for online support).**

Reprints. For copies of 100 or more, of articles in this publication, please contact the Commercial Reprints Department, Elsevier Inc., 360 Park Avenue South, New York, New York 10010-1710. Tel.: (212) 633-3813; Fax: (212) 462-1935; Email: reprints@elsevier.com.

The *Dermatologic Clinics* is covered in *MEDLINE/PubMed (Index Medicus), Current Contents/Clinical Medicine, Excerpta Medica, Chemical Abstracts,* and *ISI/BIOMED.*

Printed and bound by CPI Group (UK) Ltd, Croydon, CR0 4YY

Transferred to digital print 2012

Contributors

CONSULTING EDITOR

BRUCE H. THIERS, MD
Professor and Chairman, Department of
Dermatology and Dermatologic Surgery,
Medical University of South Carolina,
Charleston, South Carolina

GUEST EDITOR

TAMMIE FERRINGER, MD
Section Head and Fellowship Director,
Dermatopathology, Department of Pathology;
Department of Dermatology, Geisinger
Medical Center, Danville, Pennsylvania

AUTHORS

GIUSEPPE ARGENZIANO
Dermatology and Skin Cancer Unit,
Arcispedale Santa Maria Nuova-IRCCS,
Reggio Emilia, Italy

KEIRA L. BARR, MD
Assistant Professor of Clinical Dermatology
and Pathology, University of California Davis
School of Medicine, Sacramento, California

KLAUS J. BUSAM, MD
Professor of Pathology and Laboratory
Medicine, Weill Medical College of Cornell
University; Director of Dermatopathology,
Memorial Sloan-Kettering Cancer Center,
New York, New York

LORENZO CERRONI, MD
Department of Dermatology, Medical
University of Graz, Graz, Austria

WANG L. CHEUNG, MD, PhD
Department of Pathology, Orlando Health,
Orlando, Florida

LOREN E. CLARKE, MD
Associate Professor, Departments of Pathology
and Dermatology, Penn State Hershey Medical
Center, Hershey, Pennsylvania

A. NEIL CROWSON
Clinical Professor, Departments of
Dermatology, Pathology, and Surgery, St John
Medical Center, University of Oklahoma;
Regional Medical Laboratory, St John Medical
Center, Tulsa, Oklahoma

JANYANA M.D. DEONIZIO, MD
Clinical Research Associate, Department of
Dermatology, Northwestern University,
Chicago, Illinois

LYN M. DUNCAN, MD
Associate Professor of Pathology, Harvard
Medical School; Director, Dermatopathology
Unit, Pathology Service, Massachusetts
General Hospital, Harvard Medical School,
Boston, Massachusetts

DIRK M. ELSTON, MD
Director, Ackerman Academy of
Dermatopathology, New York, New York

TAMMIE FERRINGER, MD
Section Head and Fellowship Director,
Dermatopathology, Department of Pathology;
Department of Dermatology, Geisinger
Medical Center, Danville, Pennsylvania

MAXWELL A. FUNG, MD
Professor of Clinical Dermatology and
Pathology; and Director, UC Davis
Dermatopathology Service, Department of
Dermatology, University of California Davis
School of Medicine, Sacramento, California

PEDRAM GERAMI, MD
Professor, Weill Medical College, Cornell
University, New York, New York

GARY GOLDENBERG, MD
Assistant Professor of Dermatology and
Pathology, Medical Director of the
Dermatology Faculty Practice, Mount Sinai
School of Medicine, New York, New York

JOAN GUITART, MD
Professor of Dermatology and Pathology,
Director of Dermatopathology, Department of
Dermatology, Unit and Cutaneous Lymphoma
Clinic, Northwestern University, Chicago,
Illinois

JOSHUA W. HAGEN
Tri-Institutional MD-PhD Program, Weill
Medical College of Cornell University,
New York, New York

WHITNEY A. HIGH, MD, JD, MEng
Vice Chair of Clinical Affairs, Dermatology,
Department of Dermatology, University of
Illinois at Chicago, Chicago, IL, USA;
Department of Pathology, University of
Colorado School of Medicine, Denver,
Colorado

MOLLY A. HINSHAW, MD
Dermpath Diagnostics, Brookfield, Wisconsin;
Clinical Associate Professor of Dermatology,
Department of Dermatology, University of
Wisconsin School of Medicine and Public
Health, Madison, Wisconsin; Clinical Assistant
Professor of Dermatology, Department of
Dermatology, Medical College of Wisconsin,
Milwaukee, Wisconsin

HEINZ KUTZNER, MD
Dermatopathologie Friedrichshafen,
Friedrichshafen, Germany

ALICE COELHO LOBO, MD
Department of Dermatology, Hospital das
Clinicas, University of Sao Paulo, Sao Paulo,
Brazil

CATERINA LONGO
Dermatology and Skin Cancer Unit,
Arcispedale Santa Maria Nuova-IRCCS,
Reggio Emilia, Italy

CYNTHIA M. MAGRO
Professor, Department of Pathology and
Laboratory Medicine, Weill Medical College of
Cornell University, New York, New York

AMANDA MARSCH, MD
Department of Dermatology, University of
Illinois at Chicago, Chicago, Illinois

RITA V. PATEL, MD
Resident in Dermatology, Department of
Dermatology, Mount Sinai School of Medicine,
New York, New York

GIOVANNI PELLACANI
Dermatology Unit, University of Modena and
Reggio Emilia, Reggio Emilia, Italy

ADRIANO PIRIS, MD
Instructor in Pathology, Harvard Medical
School, Dermatopathology Unit, Pathology
Service, Massachusetts General Hospital,
Harvard Medical School, Boston,
Massachusetts

LUIS REQUENA, MD
Department of Dermatology, Fundación
Jiménez Díaz, Universidad Autónoma, Madrid,
Spain

JENNIFER ROBERTS-BARNES
Department of Dermatology, St John Medical
Center, Tulsa, Oklahoma

OMAR P. SANGÜEZA, MD
Professor and Director of Dermatopathology,
Wake Forest University School of Medicine,
Winston Salem, North Carolina

HARLEEN K. SIDHU, MD
Fellow in Dermatopathology, Department of
Pathology, Mount Sinai School of Medicine,
New York, New York

BRUCE R. SMOLLER, MD
Executive Vice President, United States and
Canadian Academy of Pathologist, Augusta,
Georgia

IRIS ZALAUDEK
Department of Dermatology, University of
Graz, Graz, Austria

Contents

Analyses of genetic and genomic alterations of melanocytic tumors have not only led to a better understanding of the pathogenesis of melanocytic tumors but also created new opportunities for improvements in diagnostic accuracy in distinguishing nevus from melanoma, and more effective treatments for patients affected by melanoma. Cytogenetic tests have emerged as a promising ancillary method for the workup of diagnostically problematic melanocytic tumors with ambiguous light microscopic features. Mutation analysis not only is important in treatment decision making but also can be used for improved diagnostic accuracy, staging, and prognosis.

This article is an up-to-date overview of the potential uses and limitations of immunohistochemistry (IHC) in melanocytic lesions. The information is intended to assist dermatopathologists and dermatologists who read slides to appropriately use IHC in this setting. In addition, dermatologists who do not review microscopic slides will better understand the rationale of the pathologist when reading and interpreting the pathology report.

The seventh version of the American Joint Committee on Cancer (AJCC) Melanoma Staging guidelines, published in 2009, has significant revisions compared with the previous version. The current schema was based on the largest melanoma patient cohort analyzed to date and is the result of a multivariate analysis of 30,946 patients with stages I, II, and III melanoma and 7972 patients with stage IV melanoma. This article summarizes the findings and the new definitions included in the 2009 AJCC Melanoma Staging and Classification. The TNM categories and the stage groupings are defined. Changes in the melanoma staging system are summarized.

Understanding malpractice risk and practicing risk management strategies results in better care and a less stressful environment of practice. Errors in diagnosis are most commonly related to melanoma and neoplasms of the skin. To offset the threat of malpractice litigation, malpractice data can be used to focus safety efforts on common diagnostic errors. Recognition of sources of error in the analysis of pigmented lesions by dermatopathologists, and the development of new immunohistochemical

The complex and fascinating spectrum of inflammatory skin disease, and the comprehension of it, is ever expanding and evolving. During the first decade of the 21st century, numerous advances in the understanding of inflammatory disease mechanisms have occurred, particularly in psoriasis and atopic dermatitis. Continuation of this trend will assure a future in which molecular tests for biomarkers of immediate clinical relevance are used in routine patient care, not only for diagnosis but also for prognosis and management. This article focuses on selected recent or noteworthy developments that are clinically relevant for the histologic diagnosis of inflammatory skin diseases.

The diagnosis of alopecia and other hair-related disorders can be challenging. An appreciation of the newest diagnostic techniques and newly described entities can help clinicians to provide the best care for patients. This article focuses on advances in the histologic evaluation of alopecia. Also discussed are recent advances in the understanding of hair-related disorders that do not result in alopecia. Advances in the understanding of disease mechanisms can help in treating hair disorders that proved refractory in the past.

The past several decades have seen the advent and rapidly expanding use of biological agents in the treatment of chronic disease states. As increasingly large pools of patients have been enrolled in treatment protocols using these agents, physicians have become acquainted with both desired and adverse events associated with their use. Dermatologists frequently encounter patients affected by cutaneous drug reactions associated with the use of biological agents, thereby becoming familiar with the full range of side effects reported in the literature. This review discusses these adverse cutaneous effects, their underlying mechanisms, and efforts to predict and minimize their occurrence.

A large number of foreign substances may penetrate the skin for both voluntary and involuntary reasons. The voluntary group includes the particulate materials used in tattoos and cosmetic fillers, whereas the involuntary group is almost always caused by accidental inclusion of external substances secondary to cutaneous trauma. This article focuses on the histopathologic findings seen in cutaneous reactions to exogenous agents, with special emphasis on the microscopic morphology of the external particles in recognizing specifically the involved substance (something that is becoming increasingly important in the event of litigation).

Recent epidemiology studies have identified a steady increase in the incidence of cutaneous lymphomas over the past few decades. Although possible explanations for this increased incidence include heightened awareness of these conditions as well as a more refined diagnostic acuity by dermatologists and pathologists, an increase secondary to environmental factors cannot be discounted. Our understanding of cutaneous lymphomas keeps evolving. Consequently, our knowledge and understanding of cutaneous lymphomas requires reconsideration of past dogma and critical revision of the new proposals. In this article, some hot topics and important new findings in the field are reviewed.

Direct and indirect immunofluorescence (IF) plays a role in the evaluation of immunobullous diseases and their mimics, and in the investigation of vascular injury syndromes and autoimmune connective tissue disease (CTD). IF mapping may be an important adjunct in the assessment of congenital epidermolysis bullosa syndromes and in Alport disease, in which antibodies are directed at certain components of the basement membrane zone to assay for their deficiency. In many cases of immunobullous and autoimmune CTDs, correlation with direct IF results is useful and often decisive in lesional evaluation and thus in patient management.

In vivo confocal microscopy represents a new device that generates a virtual skin biopsy at cytologic resolution. This article describes the most relevant confocal findings and their histopathologic correlates in skin oncology and inflammatory diseases. The light and dark of confocal microscopy are briefly discussed in relation with its clinical applications.

Dermatopathology (DP) education is critical to the comprehensive training of dermatology and pathology residents and to the accurate diagnosis and management of cutaneous disease. DP has seen tremendous growth, and its success depends on our ability to effectively educate future leaders, teachers, and researchers who will continue to advance the field. This article focuses on DP education in the United States, although specific components, such as assessment of medical education and the future of DP education, are relevant to the larger DP community. It is hoped that this review will aid in discussions of direction and collaboration.

DERMATOLOGIC CLINICS

Preface

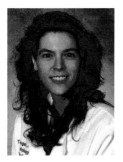

Tammie Ferringer, MD
Guest Editor

Do what you can where you are with what you have.

— *Theodore Roosevelt*

Remember when communication was by postal mail and rotary phone? These once routine components of daily life have nearly been replaced by an explosion of faster and more amazing technology including electronic mail, smartphones, and Internet voice/video calling. The microscope was a revolutionary invention that provided the first glimpse of the "invisible," but as we advance, this instrument is becoming old-fashioned, and the way dermatopathology is practiced is being reshaped by virtual slides with digital pathology and novel noninvasive in vivo diagnostic microscopy. However, it remains to be seen what will have persistent significance and what will simply be passing vogue.

Herein we hope to provide a review of the advances and recent contributions in dermatopathology, as they apply to clinical dermatology. I would like to thank the contributors of this issue for their expertise and willingness to share their experience and knowledge.

Since the last *Dermatologic Clinics* update in dermatopathology in 1999, a number of cutaneous lymphomas have been recategorized based on morphology, immunophenotype, and molecular data. Similarly, staging of melanoma has been restructured to reflect our growing knowledge of prognostic factors. In addition, our enhanced understanding of molecular alterations in melanoma has improved diagnostic and prognostic accuracy and created opportunities for therapeutic targets, such as the new BRAF inhibitor. In the late 1980s, immunohistochemistry was just beginning

to be incorporated into diagnostic dermatopathology. With each successive year new markers were identified and our experience has led to an awareness of their complexities and limitations. Over the last few decades there has been an explosion in biologic agents for the treatment of cancer and inflammatory disorders and with this comes numerous cutaneous effects that dermatologists will iatrogenically induce or see in consultation. These current developments are particularly addressed in this issue, as well as the resurfacing of outdated agents such as with levamisole and its induction of vasculopathy. Other topics include the latest in nonmelanocytic neoplasms (including fibrous/fibrohistiocytic and vascular tumors), inflammatory dermatopathology, alopecia, and other hair-related disorders, reactions to cosmetic fillers and other external agents, direct immunofluorescence, relevant medicolegal issues, and educating future generations about clinicopathologic correlation.

Dermatopathology is a challenging and forever evolving field of medicine. We have made enormous strides; however, much remains to be discovered. I can hardly wait to see where we will be in another 15 years.

Tammie Ferringer, MD
Dermatopathology
Geisinger Medical Center
100 North Academy Avenue
Danville, PA 17822-0131, USA

E-mail address:
tferringer@geisinger.edu

Cytogenetic and Mutational Analyses of Melanocytic Tumors

Pedram Gerami, MD[a], Klaus J. Busam, MD[b],*

KEYWORDS

• Melanoma • Mutation • Fluorescence in situ hybridization • Nevus

KEY POINTS

- Analyses of genetic and genomic alterations of melanocytic tumors have not only led to a better understanding of the pathogenesis of melanocytic tumors but also created new opportunities for improvements in diagnostic accuracy in distinguishing nevus from melanoma, and more effective treatments for patients affected by melanoma.
- Fluorescence in situ hybridization is the preferred assay for limited amounts of tissue targeting specific chromosomes commonly altered in melanoma, but not in nevi.
- Histopathologic analysis of hematoxylin-eosin–stained tissue sections and correlation with the clinical context remains the gold standard for diagnosing melanoma.

INTRODUCTION

Histopathologic analysis of hematoxylin-eosin–stained tissue sections and correlation with the clinical context remains the gold standard for diagnosing melanoma. In most cases, experienced dermatopathologists can make a definitive, reliable, and reproducible distinction between a melanocytic nevus and malignant melanoma. However, this distinction is not always straightforward. A subset of lesions has unusual or atypical histopathologic features. The difficulty in classifying them is reflected in terms such as *minimal deviation melanoma*,[1] *borderline melanocytic tumor*,[2] *prognostically indeterminate melanocytic tumor*,[3] *atypical Spitz tumor*,[4,5] *atypical spitzoid melanocytic tumor*,[6,7] *atypical Spitz tumor of uncertain malignant potential*,[8–10] and *atypical blue melanocytic neoplasms*.[11,12]

When pathologists disagree with each other or acknowledge the inability to render a definitive diagnosis based on routine sections, this poses a dilemma for clinicians and patients and leads to concerns and confusion about prognosis and further management.[13] Therefore, pathologists have explored the use of ancillary techniques to improve diagnostic accuracy for problematic melanocytic tumors. Cytogenetic methods have recently gained popularity for distinguishing nevi from melanoma, including fluorescence in situ hybridization (FISH) analysis and comparative genomic hybridization (CGH).[14–17]

Even when the diagnosis of melanoma has been established, it has become apparent that not all melanomas are the same. Different mutational subtypes have been identified.[18] This subclassification has become relevant in the optimal treatment selection for patients.

CYTOGENETIC STUDIES

CGH

Technical aspects

CGH is a method to detect copy number changes throughout the genome.[14,18–20] Total genomic DNA is isolated from tissue samples (tumor and

[a] Department of Dermatology, Northwestern University; [b] Department of Dermatopathology, Memorial Sloan-Kettering Cancer Center, 1275 York Avenue, New York, NY 10065, USA
* Corresponding author.
E-mail address: busamk@mskcc.org

Dermatol Clin 30 (2012) 555–566
http://dx.doi.org/10.1016/j.det.2012.06.015
0733-8635/12/$ – see front matter © 2012 Published by Elsevier Inc

normal control) and labeled with different fluoro-chromes. The mixture is then hybridized onto normal metaphase spreads from a healthy donor (classic CGH) or a microarray of mapped clones or genomic DNA (array CGH). Copy number gains or losses are identified based on differences in fluorescence intensities. CGH permits assessment of copy number changes of all chromosomes. However, tumor cell heterogeneity can be a problem. If copy number changes are present only in a minor subpopulation of the total tumor from which DNA is extracted for CGH, they may escape detection.[21] In general, approximately one-third of the tumor should harbor copy number changes for them to be clearly identifiable on CGH.

Clinical utility

Analysis of melanocytic tumors with CGH revealed that nevi and melanoma differ cytogeneti-cally.[14,15,22,23] Most melanomas show recurrent patterns of chromosomal aberrations, such as los-ses of chromosomes 6q, 8p, 9p, and 10q, along with copy number gains of 1q, 6p, 7, 8q, 17q, and 20q.[15,16,18] In contrast, CGH has shown that most melanocytic nevi lack copy number changes (**Fig. 1**). Exceptions are rare and include subtypes of Spitz nevus/tumor characterized by gains of 11p or loss of chromosome 3.[14,22,24] The lack of significant overlap in the patterns of chromosomal aberrations in melanoma and nevi provides the rationale for using CGH (or FISH; see later discus-sion) as an ancillary diagnostic tool for diagnosti-cally problematic melanocytic tumors.[17]

CGH has been and is currently most widely used clinically for the workup of diagnostically ambig-uous/problematic spitzoid melanocytic prolifera-tions. It can be applied to archival material (formalin-fixed and paraffin-embedded tissue). If

a Spitz tumor harbors a copy number gain of 11p, for example, the diagnosis of Spitz nevus can be made with reasonable confidence.[17,22] However, the detection of multiple copy number changes represents strong evidence in favor of malignant melanoma.

CGH can be applied similarly for ambiguous melanocytic tumors lacking spitzoid features, such as atypical cellular blue nevi or blue nevus–like melanomas. In general, the detection of chro-mosomal aberrations commonly associated with melanoma, particularly the presence of multiple aberrations, supports a diagnosis of melanoma.

Pitfalls of CGH

CGH-negative malignant melanomas Although most melanomas show chromosomal aberrations detectable on CGH, not all do. A rare melanoma may be CGH-negative. This finding may be related to test sensitivity or intrinsic biologic reasons. Test sensitivity is an issue when, for example, the quality or amount of extracted DNA is insufficient, or mela-nocytes with chromosomal aberrations represents only a minor component of the entire tissue used for DNA extraction. Admixed precursor nevomelano-cytes and/or stromal/inflammatory cells may dilute the cytogenetically aberrant melanoma, leading to a false-negative CGH result. However, on rare occasions even a uniform malignant tumor cell population may be CGH-negative because of the lack of chromosomal copy number changes.

Benign or indolent melanocytic proliferations with cytogenetic abnormalities Aberrations of specific chromosomal loci may have much greater significance in diagnosing melanoma. The pres-ence of a single copy number change in just any chromosome *per se* does not constitute proof of

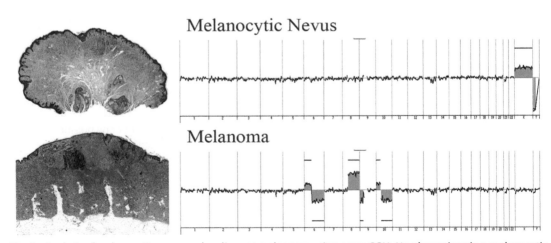

Melanocytic Nevus

Melanoma

Fig. 1. Analysis of melanocytic nevus and malignant melanoma using array CGH. No aberrations in a melanocytic nevus are seen. Several copy number gains and losses are found in the melanoma. (*Courtesy of* T. Wiesner, MD.)

malignancy. A Spitz nevus or tumor, for example, may harbor a gain in 11p[22] or loss of chromosome 3.[24,25] Other isolated rare copy number changes have also been found in spitzoid melanocytic proliferations lacking overt malignant features and behaving clinically in an indolent fashion. Thus, caution is necessary when confronted with an isolated chromosomal aberration, especially with regard to spitzoid tumors in children. The cytogenetic aberrations of these lesions must be evaluated on an individual basis, taking into account the specific alteration present, the clinical setting, and light microscopic and at times also immunohistochemical findings.

A further limitation of CGH is differentiating heterozygous from homozygous deletions. For example, a loss of a single copy of 9p21 can be seen not only in melanoma but also occasionally in some atypical Spitz tumors with indolent behavior. Alternatively, a homozygous deletion in 9p21 tends to be a much more specific finding for melanoma.[26] This distinction is not always readily apparent on CGH. Hence, the detection of a single copy number aberration including loss of 9p21 should be interpreted with caution and investigated further with FISH.[26]

FISH ANALYSIS
Technical Aspects

In contrast to CGH, FISH targets individual chromosomes or specific regions within a chromosome. Fluorescence-labeled oligonucleotide probes bind to their complementary DNA sequence and label that region, which can then be visualized under a fluorescence microscope (**Fig. 2**). Two types of probes are currently relevant for the workup of melanocytic tumors. Centromeric probes identify the centromeric region of a specific chromosome and thus help enumerate the number of copies of that chromosome, and allele-specific probes adhere to a specific target sequence such as cyclin D1 on chromosome 11q or *CDKN2A* (ie, p16 by its protein name) on 9p21.[23]

Unlike CGH, FISH permits detection of abnormal subpopulations within a heterogeneous tissue mix.[21] Hence, identification of much smaller populations of emerging clones of chromosomally aberrant cells is possible. Visual correlation between a cell nucleus with an abnormal number of chromosomes and cytologic features is possible to verify the identity of an affected cell. Much smaller amounts of tissue are necessary for FISH compared with CGH. For skin biopsies, 1 or 2 unstained 5-μm thin sections of formalin-fixed and paraffin-embedded material usually suffices to perform FISH. The FISH test has 2 major

drawbacks. First, it only tests for aberrations in the targeted areas, which is usually limited to 4 chromosomal loci (ie, it does not analyze the entire set of chromosomes as does CGH). Second, depending on the probe set used, the enumeration requires some level of expertise.[21] For example, with the current commercially available melanoma probe set, which targets 3 loci on chromosome 6 and 1 on chromosome 11, tetraploidy can often result in the false impression of copy number gains (**Fig. 3**). Newer probe sets testing a broader number of chromosomal loci may help diminish this problem.

Several FISH assays are currently available for use in dermatopathology. The so-called melanoma FISH test uses 4 probes, targeting *Ras* responsive element-binding protein 1 (Vysis LSI RREB1 SpectrumRed), myeloblastosis (Vysis LSI MYB SpectrumGold), cyclin D1 or chromosome 11q13 (Vysis LSI CCND1 SpectrumGreen), and centromeric enumeration probe control for chromosome 6 (Vysis LSI CEP 6 SpectrumAqua), from Abbott Molecular (Des Plaines, IL).[23] The enumeration protocol requires that a total of 30 lesional melanocytes be analyzed per case. A lesion is considered as having a positive FISH result if any of the following criteria are met: (1) gain in 6p25 (*RREB1*) relative to CEP 6 greater than 55%, (2) gain in 6p25 (*RREB1*) greater than 29%, (3) loss in 6q23 (*MYB*) relative to CEP 6 greater than 42%, or (4) gain in 11q13 (*CCND1*) greater than 38%.[23] Additional probes are currently being incorporated into clinical utility, such as those targeting 9p21, which are useful for diagnosing both conventional and spitzoid melanomas,[26] and those targeting 8q24,[27] which are useful for nodular amelanotic and nevoid melanomas.

Other FISH probes of interest for diagnosing melanoma include those targeting chromosome 3 (centromeric probe and *bcl2*) for diagnosing uveal melanoma,[28] and 22q21 (*EWSR1*) for diagnosing cutaneous clear cell sarcoma (CCS),[29] a soft tissue tumor with melanocytic differentiation, which can be confused with cellular blue nevus, primary nodular or metastatic melanoma (see below).

Utility of the FISH Assay

Distinction of nevus from melanoma
Because conventional nevi tend to lack chromosomal aberrations, but most melanomas harbor copy number changes, a FISH test using probes for chromosomes commonly altered in melanoma should have potential value as an ancillary diagnostic method. Gerami and colleagues[16] documented that such a test could be established and introduced it to the pathology community for

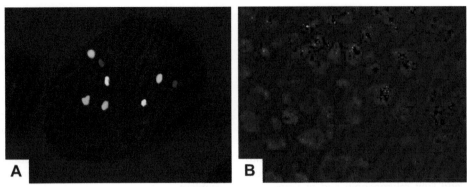

Fig. 2. Analysis of melanocytic nevus and malignant melanoma using FISH. The probes include (1) RREB1 (*Ras* responsive element-binding protein 1) on 6p25 (Vysis LSI RREB1 SpectrumRed), (2) MYB (V-myb myeloblastosis viral oncogene homolog) on 6q23 (Vysis LSI MYB SpectrumGold), (3) CCND1 (cyclin D1) on 11q13 (Vysis LSI CCND1 SpectrumGreen), and (4) the centromeric enumeration probe control for chromosome 6 (Vysis LSI CEP 6 SpectrumAqua). (*A*) There are 2 signals per probe in the cell nucleus of a nevomelanocyte indicating a normal diploid set of chromosomes. (*B*) Multiple copy number changes are seen in most melanoma cells.

diagnosing melanocytic tumors. Using probes targeting loci on 6p, 6q, 6cent, and 11q, they determined cutoff values (see earlier discussion), which permitted a test sensitivity of 85% and specificity of 95% for histopathologically obvious/noncontroversial benign and malignant lesions. Other investigators have reported similar results.

Vergier and colleagues'[30] FISH analysis of 43 non-equivocal melanomas and nevi showed a sensitivity of 85% and specificity of 90%. In a review of 500 cases from a commercial laboratory, 83.8% of melanomas were FISH-positive.[31] Another commercial laboratory analyzed 32 nevi and 31 melanomas using FISH and reported an

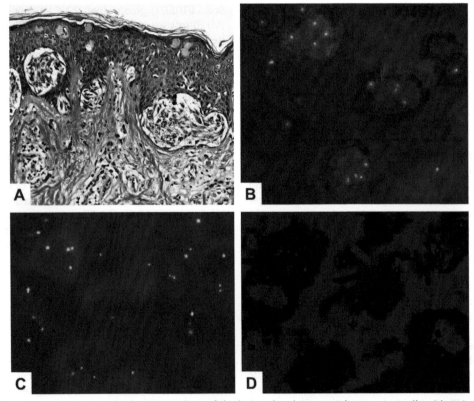

Fig. 3. Spitz nevus with tetraploidy. FISH analysis of the lesional melanocytes shows many cells with 4 signals per nucleus. (*A*) Hematoxylin-eosin of Spitz nevus. (*B*) *CCND1*. (*C*) Centromeric probe of chromosome 6. (*D*) RREB1.

overall sensitivity of 94% and specificity of 94%.[32] In a recent study from Memorial Sloan-Kettering Cancer Center, test specificity was 98% and sensitivity was 82%.[33]

Several studies confirmed that the FISH test correlates well with consensus diagnoses distinguishing conjunctival nevus from conjunctival melanoma,[34] sclerosing nevus from desmoplastic melanoma,[35] and blue nevus from blue nevus–like melanoma.[36] The test has also been used for diagnosing Spitz nevi.[37,38] Although Spitz nevi are usually negative, a significant subset of Spitz nevi is tetraploid,[38] which may lead to a false-positive enumeration (see later discussion). For distinguishing Spitz nevus from spitzoid melanoma, the addition of a probe for 9p21 (CDKN2A) has been shown to increase sensitivity and specificity.[26] In fact, a more recently validated probe set targeting 6p25, 11q13, 8q24, and 9p21 has been shown to have an overall improved sensitivity and specificity in distinguishing melanoma from benign nevi, with the probe targeting 9p21 being particularly helpful in identifying spitzoid neoplasms.[26]

Microstaging of primary melanoma

When a melanoma arises in association with a melanocytic nevus, precise assessment of tumor thickness can be problematic. If melanoma cells are distinctly different in appearance from adjacent nevus cells, measurement of Breslow thickness is straightforward. However, thickness may be wrongly measured if the melanoma does not contrast well cytologically with the nevus and the pathologist is uncertain how much of the intradermal melanocytic proliferation is nevus versus invasive melanoma. This possible inaccuracy not only affects the patient's overall prognosis but also may impact immediate surgical management and staging, such as eligibility for sentinel lymph node biopsy. Using the FISH assay may help in this regard through identifying intradermal melanoma cells with chromosomal gains.[39]

Primary nevus versus nevus-like metastatic melanoma

Metastatic melanoma can occasionally simulate the appearance of a melanocytic nevus. A notorious example is a blue nevus–like melanoma metastasis from primary cutaneous or ocular melanoma. Using the 4-color FISH test, Pouryazdanparast et al[36] documented that chromosomal changes were detected in 9 of 10 blue nevus–like melanoma metastases, but not in a single case of conventional blue nevus. Thus, a positive FISH test can confirm a suspected diagnosis of metastatic blue nevus–like cutaneous melanoma. A different probe set is needed for detecting blue nevus–like uveal melanoma. Because monosomy 3 and amplifications of MYC are common findings in metastasizing uveal melanoma, FISH probes targeting chromosomes 3 and 8 may be useful in diagnosing metastatic blue nevus–like uveal melanoma (**Fig. 4**). Caution is necessary, however, because cutaneous melanoma and a subtype of Spitz tumor may be associated with loss of chromosome 3 (see later discussion). Furthermore cutaneous

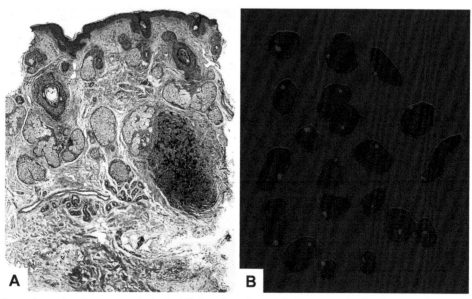

Fig. 4. Dermal uveal melanoma metastasis. (*A*) A melanotic nodule is present in the dermis. (*B*) The tumor cells carry only 1 copy of chromosome 3 (monosomy 3).

melanomas may also have 8q24 gains, particularly amelanotic nodular melanomas in areas of non-chronically sun-damaged skin. Although most metastatic melanomas will show copy number changes detectable on the FISH test, not all do.[33]

Nodal nevus versus metastatic melanoma

Melanoma may also be confused with a melanocytic nevus in the lymph node, with serious implications for prognosis (stage) and further management.[40] Although conventional microscopic analysis and immunohistochemical findings usually suffice to distinguish a nodal nevus from metastatic melanoma, the FISH test has been shown to have value for this diagnostic problem.

Histopathologically ambiguous melanocytic tumors

When the FISH test was developed, the main purpose was to use it eventually as an ancillary tool for cases that are difficult to solve through morphologic analysis alone, such as cases with unusual or conflicting morphologic features, when some features (eg, circumscribed wedge-shaped silhouette) favor a nevus, whereas others (eg, mitotic figures, incomplete maturation, and cytologic atypia) suggest a possible melanoma. This group of melanocytic tumors is generally referred to as "melanocytic tumors of uncertain malignant potential,"[41] "borderline tumors," or, referring to more specific findings, "atypical Spitz tumors"[9,42] or "atypical cellular blue tumors."[11] Most of the ambiguous lesions for which the FISH test has been used fall into the category of "atypical Spitz tumors."

The experience of various investigators in using the current commercially available melanoma FISH test for diagnostically ambiguous melanocytic neoplasms has been variable. Gerami and colleagues[16] examined a set of 27 ambiguous melanocytic tumors. FISH test results correlated well with outcome: all 6 tumors, which metastasized, were FISH-positive. Groups led by Massi[7] and Vergier[30] found similar utility in the test. In contrast, Raskin and colleagues[42] and Gaiser and colleagues[43] had a less successful experience in their use of the FISH test. Gaiser and colleagues[43] reported a specificity of only 50% for metastasis and a sensitivity of 60%. However, their FISH methodology differed significantly from that of Gerami and colleagues.[16] Furthermore, when evaluating the specificity of the FISH test, one must take into account what parameter the test result is compared with (histopathologic consensus diagnosis vs adverse event). For example, metastasis is not the only valid parameter of malignancy. A melanoma may be unequivocally malignant but

may be cured by surgical removal. Thus, failure to metastasize during a given follow-up period does not imply that a tumor is benign. Otherwise, histopathologic analysis would need to be said to have low specificity, because most melanomas judged clinically and according to conventional light microscopic criteria as malignant do not metastasize.

A major limitation of the studies assessing the diagnostic value of the FISH assay is the limited number of documented patients with ambiguous melanocytic neoplasms resulting in distant metastasis or death. For years it has been recognized that isolated lymph node involvement without disease progression could be seen in Spitz tumors. More recently, Ludgate and colleagues[9] showed in their experience of 67 cases of ambiguous Spitz tumors with follow-up that lymph node involvement was seen in 47% of their cases and that none of these developed distant metastasis or death. Hence, a paramount objective of any FISH assay for diagnosing ambiguous melanocytic neoplasms is to be able to successfully identify and discriminate the cases that are capable of and most likely to result in distant metastasis or death and determine whether it can do this better than light microscopic analysis alone.

Further improvements in the efficiency and diagnostic utility of FISH may develop as tailored probe sets emerge. For example, it has been recently recognized that, in cases with a concern for nodular amelanotic/nevoid melanoma in areas of nonchronically sun-damaged skin, a probe targeting 8q24 is highly useful, whereas in spitzoid neoplasms 9p21 is highly pertinent.[26,27]

Prognosis of melanoma

Preliminary evidence also has been presented that the FISH status of a melanoma is prognostically relevant. North and colleagues[44] analyzed 144 primary melanomas with a minimal tumor thickness of 2 mm and compared the development of metastatic disease versus melanoma-specific mortality and relapse-free versus disease-specific survival between FISH-positive and FISH-negative cases. The risk of metastasis or melanoma-related death was higher for patients with FISH-positive primary tumors compared with FISH-negative cases. The FISH status remained prognostically significant even after adjustment for other known prognostic parameters. In another case control study of 97 melanomas (55 metastasizing and 43 nonmetastasizing tumors), Gerami and colleagues[27] documented that copy number gains in 11q13 and 8q24 were predictive of metastatic disease. Independent studies have shown that 8q24 also has prognostic value in uveal melanomas. Thus, as in uveal melanomas, cytogenetic analysis of cutaneous melanomas may assist in a more accurate identification of tumors with metastatic potential. However, further studies are needed to determine whether any of these prognostic refinements impact on current clinical management. Moreover, limitations in the prognostic value of the FISH test are already apparent. Patients with a FISH-negative melanoma may die of metastatic disease, whereas others with FISH-positive melanoma may survive their melanoma for 5 years or longer.[33]

Diagnosis and prognosis of uveal melanoma

Uveal melanoma is the most common extracutaneous melanoma. Nearly half of all patients with uveal melanoma eventually die of metastatic disease. Nonrandom chromosomal alterations are present in most cases.[45,46] The most characteristic and prognostically powerful aberration is monosomy 3, which is seen in approximately half of the cases of uveal melanoma.[28,47] Copy number gains of 8q (MYC) are also not uncommon and seem prognostically relevant.[48] Accordingly, FISH analysis of uveal melanomas for monosomy 3 has become part of the workup of patients at tertiary care centers. Although the presence of monosomy 3 is typical of uveal melanoma, it is not specific. Correlation with clinical and other histopathologic findings is needed to distinguish uveal from cutaneous melanoma or nevi; occasional cutaneous melanomas or rare nevi may also show loss of chromosome 3.[25]

Diagnosis of melanoma of soft parts (CCS)

CCS, also known as melanoma of soft parts, is a unique malignant neoplasm initially described by Enzinger[49] in 1975. It is generally classified as sarcoma because of its typical presentation as a tumor nodule in association with tendons and aponeuroses of distal extremities. However, the tumor shows evidence of melanocytic differentiation on light and electron microscopy and immunohistochemically.[50] Cytogenetic studies have shown that most tumors harbor a characteristic reciprocal translocation, t(12;22)(q13;q12), which to date has not yet been found in cutaneous or mucosal melanomas. In most cases of CCS, the gene fusion product involves the EWS (22q12) and ATF1 (12q13) genes. However, another fusion product of EWS to CREB1 on 2q13 was recently found in a subset of CCS that preferentially affects the gastrointestinal tract.[51]

Although the deep location of the tumor, its predilection for adolescents and young adults, and some fairly characteristic histopathologic features (eg, the presence of multinucleate wreath-like giant cells, cells with clear cytoplasm,

sclerotic stroma) usually suffice to distinguish it from primary nodular or metastatic melanoma, a rare tumor of CCS may involve or even be centered in the dermis, thereby leading to possible diagnostic confusion. In problematic cases, FISH analysis using a 22q12 (EWS) probe documenting the presence of a translocation can provide a decisive diagnostic result.[29]

Pitfalls and Limitations of the FISH Test

FISH-negative malignant melanomas

As apparent from all reported studies, not all malignant melanomas are positive on FISH.[33] A negative FISH test result, despite the presence of unequivocally malignant tumor, may be because the melanoma might have copy number changes of chromosomes other than those targeted by the assay. It may also imply that not all melanomas are associated with copy number changes. Thus, one must be cautious when cytogenetic results are used for interpreting difficult melanocytic lesions. A negative FISH result does not exclude the diagnosis of malignant melanoma. The inclusion of additional probes, such as 9p21, increases the sensitivity of the test.[26,52]

FISH-positive melanocytic nevi

The less-than-perfect specificity of the FISH test implies that some nevi are reported as positive.[16,33] This result is likely most often from incorrect interpretation of the test, with a smaller percentage of cases reflecting a true biologic phenomenon. One pitfall with regard to a false-positive FISH result is polyploidy. For example, it has been documented that a minority of Spitz's nevi are tetraploid.[37,38] Thus, corrections for tetraploidy are needed when enumerating FISH results. Tetraploidy is apparent in the presence of 4 copies per nucleus of any chromosome tested. The issue of whether to discount tetraploid nuclei, however, is not always straightforward, especially when confronted with a mix of signals, including gains of 3 and 4 copies, and when outside material is sent with no specifications on how thick the sections are (truncated tetraploid nuclei may falsely appear to have only 3 copies of a chromosome). Although tetraploidy may be the most common reason for false-positive FISH results of melanocytic nevi, it does not explain all cases of melanocytic nevi with copy number changes meeting FISH criteria for melanoma.[33] Another interpretative error leading to a (false) positive FISH result of a nevus is related to "cherry-picking" of abnormal nuclei (ie, large nuclei at different foci in a lesion are selectively counted, instead of counting all nuclei in a given area). In some lesions, a false-positive FISH result is documented without any methodological flaw.[33] This case simply reflects the fact that some numerical chromosomal aberrations do occur in benign lesions, thereby setting inherent biologic limits to the specificity of empiric threshold or cutoff values. The basic principle that a chromosomal copy number gain can be found in a benign melanocytic proliferation is already well accepted; it is known that a subtype of Spitz nevus may have an isolated copy number increase of chromosome 11p where the HRAS gene is located, and most of these cases will also have an activating mutation in HRAS.[14,53] Another Spitz nevus/tumor composed of large epithelioid cell melanocytes has been found to be associated with loss of BAP1.[24]

MUTATIONAL ANALYSIS OF MELANOCYTIC NEVI AND MELANOMA

Genetic mutations and genomic aberrations are a hallmark of cancer cells. In melanoma, several driving genetic changes have been identified.[54–58] Most of them are point mutations. Somatic and genomic aberrations have been found in genes such as BRAF, NRAS, KIT, GNAQ/GNA11, PTEN, and MAP2K1/2. Most of these mutations are not restricted to malignant melanoma, but can also be detected in melanocytic nevi (see later discussion) (Table 1).

Testing for Genetic Changes

Gene mutations are detected using DNA sequence analysis (ie, determination of the order of the nucleotides adenine, guanine, cytosine, and thymine). Different analytical methods are available for sequencing. A technical discussion of different methods is beyond the scope of this review. Current commonly used methods for mutation analysis in solid tumors such as melanoma include direct sequencing (traditional chain termination, also known as Sanger sequencing),

pyrosequencing, or single nucleotide extension assays.[58] The advantage of direct sequencing is that it can identify all point mutations in a given stretch of DNA. However, it is less sensitive than other methods. For Sanger sequencing, for example, the mutant DNA must amount on average to at least 25% of the sample DNA, whereas in pyrosequencing, mutations can be detected even when the mutant DNA constitutes only 5% of the total DNA. Pyrosequencing uses an enzymatic assay to detect pyrophosphate after nucleotide incorporation into a growing DNA chain. It permits mutation analysis in a read length of 300 to 500 nucleotides. Single nucleotide extension assays are used for detecting a specific point mutation. Two commonly used techniques include iPlex (Sequenom, Inc, San Diego, CA) and SNaPshot (Applied Biopsystems, Inc, Foster City, CA). Roche has a real-time polymerase chain reaction (PCR)–based assay for detecting $BRAF^{V600E}$ mutations, known as the Cobas 4800, which is the only test approved by the U.S. Food and Drug Administration (FDA) and is the companion test to their FDA-approved BRAF inhibitor drug, vemurafenib.[59]

Common Genetic Mutations in Melanoma

BRAF
BRAF encodes a serine/threonine protein kinase downstream of the epidermal growth factor receptor (EGFR) and the RAS family of small G-proteins. It is mutated in 8% to 10% of human tumors and 40% to 60% of melanomas.[56,59] More than 90% of the mutated melanomas have a V600E point mutation. In this mutation, a thymidine at nucleotide 1799 on exon 15 is replaced by adenine, resulting in the substitution of glutamic acid for valine at residue 600. This mutation leads to greater than 10-fold activity of the kinase domain and subsequent downstream activation of the

Table 1
Mutations in melanocytic nevi and malignant melanoma

Mutation	Nevus Type	Melanoma Type
BRAF	Acquired nevi (ordinary and atypical/dysplastic)	Common in superficial spreading melanoma; rare in other types
NRAS	Congenital nevi	Common in nodular melanoma; can be found in other types
HRAS	Spitz nevi	
GNAQ/GNA11	Blue nevi	Blue nevus-like melanoma; Uveal melanoma
BAP1	Epithelioid Spitz nevi, often in the setting of a combined lesion	Uveal melanoma; rare cutaneous melanoma
KIT		Subset of acral and mucosal melanomas and melanomas of sun-damaged skin

mitogen-activated protein (MAP) kinase pathway. BRAF mutations among primary tumors tend to be associated with melanomas occurring in areas of intermittently sun-damaged skin, such as on the trunk or extremities. Pyrosequencing, nucleotide extension assays, and the Cobas 4800 real-time PCR assay are among the most commonly used methods to test for BRAF mutations.

NRAS mutations
NRAS is an isoform of the RAS family of GTPase proteins involved in cell growth and differentiation. NRAS affects several different pathways, including MAP kinase. Activating mutations of NRAS have been identified in 15% to 20% of melanoma samples.[58] The most common mutations are located in exon 2 at codon 61. NRAS mutations tend to occur in nodular melanomas and melanomas of sun-damaged skin.[60] They are usually mutually exclusive of BRAF mutations. NRAS mutations are also the predominant mutation identified in large congenital nevi.[61] Pyrosequencing and nucleotide extension assays are most commonly used to test for NRAS mutations.

GNAQ/GNA11 mutations
GNAQ and GNA11 encode for α subunits of G-protein–coupled receptors. Mutations result in constitutive activation. Downstream pathways include MAP kinase and PLC/PKC. Van Raamsdonk and colleagues[62] found somatic mutations in GNAQ or GNA11 in 83% of uveal melanomas. They are mutually exclusive. The most common mutation affects exon 5 (Q209). GNAQ and GNA11 mutations have also been identified in blue nevi and blue nevus–like melanomas.[54,63]

KIT mutations
KIT is a cell surface receptor tyrosine kinase that is involved in several intracellular signaling pathways, including MAP kinase and phosphoinositide kinase-3 (PI3K). KIT mutations tend to occur in approximately one-third of acral and mucosal melanomas,[64] but can also be found in a minor subset of melanomas arising on chronically sun-damaged skin. Mutations have been found in exons 9, 11, 13, and 17. There is no predominant mutation. Therefore, molecular testing for KIT mutations must evaluate multiple regions of the gene. Traditional Sanger sequencing is often used for this purpose.

Mutations in Melanocytic Nevi

Except for KIT mutations, all of the earlier-mentioned mutations can also be found in melanocytic nevi.[65] BRAF^{V600E} mutations predominantly occur in acquired melanocytic nevi, but have also been reported in a subset of congenital, Spitz, and blue nevi. NRAS mutations are predominantly found in congenital melanocytic nevi, especially medium and large congenital nevi.[61,66] GNAQ/GNA11 mutations have been found in blue nevi of various types (common, cellular, sclerosing, plaque type) and nevus of Ota.[54] Other mutations that have been reported to occur in nevi include HRAS, another member of the RAS family.[53] The most common mutation involves Q61 of exon 3, with replacement of glutamine by lysine. HRAS mutations predominantly affect Spitz nevi.[14] However, fewer than 20% of Spitz nevi carry HRAS mutations, and this tends to be limited to large bulky Spitz nevi with sclerosis of the deep dermal component.[53] Additionally, a HRAS mutation occasionally may be found in melanoma.

Clinical utility of mutation analysis
The identification of distinct genetic changes has led to the development of targeted therapies. The main clinical role of mutation analysis is to select patients for treatment to which they are most likely to respond. Vemurafenib, for example, is a targeted therapy against BRAF^{V600E} mutant melanomas.[59] It has been approved by the FDA for the treatment of patients with metastatic melanoma known to have the V600E mutation.[59] In limited studies, patients with KIT-mutated melanomas have shown responses to treatment with imatinib and other tyrosine kinase inhibitors.

However, mutation analysis is not only relevant for treatment selection but also useful for diagnostic purposes. For example, the detection of a GNAQ/GNA11 mutation in a sclerosing melanocytic tumor with a differential diagnosis of amelanotic sclerosing blue nevus versus desmoplastic melanoma would support the diagnosis of a blue nevus.[63] Mutation analysis may also be helpful for staging purposes, such as in a patient with a history of acral melanoma and new tumor with a differential diagnosis of epidermotropic metastasis versus second primary superficial spreading melanoma. If the primary acral melanoma was KIT-mutated and the new tumor was KIT-wild type but BRAF-mutated, this would be clinically valuable information.

Mutation analysis may also have prognostic value. NRAS mutation status has recently been suggested to predict shorter survival after a diagnosis of stage IV melanoma.[57]

SUMMARY

Cytogenetic and mutation analysis have led to improved understanding of the biology of melanocytic tumors and the development of new diagnostic and therapeutic opportunities. Some of the tests, such as the documentation of *EWS* rearrangement for CCS, have become diagnostic gold standard, or others, such as *BRAF* mutation analysis, routine workup for patients with advanced melanoma for treatment selection. CGH and FISH analysis are increasingly being used at specialized centers as ancillary tools for the workup of diagnostically problematic melanocytic tumors. The field is rapidly advancing. Issues remain concerning test sensitivity and specificity for diagnostically ambiguous tumors as more experience is gained with these novel techniques. An important issue also relates to the cost/benefit ratio, and determining to what extent the added cost from using these tests can be justified in a health care system with limited resources and conflicting needs.

REFERENCES

1. Reed RJ. Minimal deviation melanoma. Borderline and intermediate melanocytic neoplasia. Clin Lab Med 2000;20(4):745–58.
2. Magro CM, Crowson AN, Mihm MC Jr, et al. The dermal-based borderline melanocytic tumor: a categorical approach. J Am Acad Dermatol 2010;62(3):469–79.
3. Kim JC, Murphy GF. Dysplastic melanocytic nevi and prognostically indeterminate nevomelanomatoid proliferations. Clin Lab Med 2000;20(4):691–712.
4. Reed RJ. Atypical Spitz nevus/tumor. Hum Pathol 1999;30(12):1523–6.
5. Barnhill RL, Argenyi ZB, From L, et al. Atypical Spitz nevi/tumors: lack of consensus for diagnosis, discrimination from melanoma, and prediction of outcome. Hum Pathol 1999;30(5):513–20.
6. Busam KJ, Murali R, Pulitzer M, et al. Atypical Spitzoid melanocytic tumors with positive sentinel lymph nodes in children and teenagers, and comparison with histologically unambiguous and lethal melanomas. Am J Surg Pathol 2009;33(9):1386–95.
7. Massi D, Cesinaro AM, Tomasini C, et al. Atypical Spitzoid melanocytic tumors: a morphological, mutational, and FISH analysis. J Am Acad Dermatol 2011;64(5):919–35.
8. Urso C. The atypical Spitz tumor of uncertain biologic potential: a series of 67 patients from a single institution. Cancer 2010;116(1):258 [author reply: 258–9].
9. Ludgate MW, Fullen DR, Lee J, et al. The atypical Spitz tumor of uncertain biologic potential: a series of 67 patients from a single institution. Cancer 2009;115(3):631–41.
10. Tom WL, Hsu JW, Eichenfield LF, et al. Pediatric "STUMP" lesions: evaluation and management of difficult atypical Spitzoid lesions in children. J Am Acad Dermatol 2011;64(3):559–72.
11. Barnhill RL, Argenyi Z, Berwick M, et al. Atypical cellular blue nevi (cellular blue nevi with atypical features): lack of consensus for diagnosis and distinction from cellular blue nevi and malignant melanoma ("malignant blue nevus"). Am J Surg Pathol 2008;32(1):36–44.
12. Mones JM, Ackerman AB. "Atypical" blue nevus, "malignant" blue nevus, and "metastasizing" blue nevus: a critique in historical perspective of three concepts flawed fatally. Am J Dermatopathol 2004;26(5):407–30.
13. Busam KJ, Pulitzer M. Sentinel lymph node biopsy for patients with diagnostically controversial Spitzoid melanocytic tumors? Adv Anat Pathol 2008;15(5):253–62.
14. Bastian BC, LeBoit PE, Pinkel D. Mutations and copy number increase of HRAS in Spitz nevi with distinctive histopathological features. Am J Pathol 2000;157(3):967–72.
15. Bauer J, Bastian BC. Distinguishing melanocytic nevi from melanoma by DNA copy number changes: comparative genomic hybridization as a research and diagnostic tool. Dermatol Ther 2006;19(1):40–9.
16. Gerami P, Jewell SS, Morrison LE, et al. Fluorescence in situ hybridization (FISH) as an ancillary diagnostic tool in the diagnosis of melanoma. Am J Surg Pathol 2009;33(8):1146–56.
17. McCalmont TH, Vemula S, Sands P, et al. Molecular-microscopical correlation in dermatopathology. J Cutan Pathol 2011;38(4):324–6, 323.
18. Bastian BC, Olshen AB, LeBoit PE, et al. Classifying melanocytic tumors based on DNA copy number changes. Am J Pathol 2003;163(5):1765–70.
19. Kallioniemi A, Kallioniemi OP, Sudar D, et al. Comparative genomic hybridization for molecular cytogenetic analysis of solid tumors. Science 1992;258(5083):818–21.
20. Bauer J, Bastian BC. DNA copy number changes in the diagnosis of melanocytic tumors [in German]. Pathologe 2007;28(6):464–73.
21. Gerami P, Zembowicz A. Update on fluorescence in situ hybridization in melanoma: state of the art. Arch Pathol Lab Med 2011;135(7):830–7.
22. Bastian BC, Wesselmann U, Pinkel D, et al. Molecular cytogenetic analysis of Spitz nevi shows clear differences to melanoma. J Invest Dermatol 1999;113(6):1065–9.
23. Gerami P, Wass A, Mafee M, et al. Fluorescence in situ hybridization for distinguishing nevoid melanomas from mitotically active nevi. Am J Surg Pathol 2009;33(12):1783–8.
24. Wiesner T, Murali R, Fried I, et al. A distinct subset of atypical Spitz tumors is characterized by BRAF mutation and loss of BAP1 expression. Am J Surg Pathol 2012;36(6):818–30.

25. Wiesner T, Obenauf AC, Murali R, et al. Germline mutations in BAP1 predispose to melanocytic tumors. Nat Genet 2011;43(10):1018–21.

26. Gammon B, Beilfuss B, Guitart J, et al. Enhanced detection of Spitzoid melanomas using fluorescence in situ hybridization with 9p21 as an adjunctive probe. Am J Surg Pathol 2012;36(1):81–8.

27. Gerami P, Jewell SS, Pouryazdanparast P, et al. Copy number gains in 11q13 and 8q24 [corrected] are highly linked to prognosis in cutaneous malignant melanoma. J Mol Diagn 2011;13(3):352–8.

28. Fang Y, Wang X, Dusza S, et al. Use of fluorescence in situ hybridization to distinguish metastatic uveal from cutaneous melanoma. Int J Surg Pathol 2012; 20(3):246–51.

29. Hantschke M, Mentzel T, Rutten A, et al. Cutaneous clear cell sarcoma: a clinicopathologic, immunohistochemical, and molecular analysis of 12 cases emphasizing its distinction from dermal melanoma. Am J Surg Pathol 2010;34(2):216–22.

30. Vergier B, Prochazkova-Carlotti M, de la Fouchardiere A, et al. Fluorescence in situ hybridization, a diagnostic aid in ambiguous melanocytic tumors: European study of 113 cases. Mod Pathol 2011;24(5):613–23.

31. Moore MW, Gasparini R. FISH as an effective diagnostic tool for the management of challenging melanocytic lesions. Diagn Pathol 2011;6:76.

32. Hossain D, Qian J, Adupe J, et al. Differentiation of melanoma and benign nevi by fluorescence in-situ hybridization. Melanoma Res 2011;21(5): 426–30.

33. Fang Y, Dusza S, Jhanwar S, et-al. Fluorescence in situ hybridization (FISH) analysis of melanocytic nevi and melanomas: sensitivity, specificity, and lack of association with sentinel node status. Int J Surg Pathol, in press.

34. Busam KJ, Fang Y, Jhanwar SC, et al. Distinction of conjunctival melanocytic nevi from melanomas by fluorescence in situ hybridization. J Cutan Pathol 2010;37(2):196–203.

35. Gerami P, Beilfuss B, Haghighat Z, et al. Fluorescence in situ hybridization as an ancillary method for the distinction of desmoplastic melanomas from sclerosing melanocytic nevi. J Cutan Pathol 2011; 38(4):329–34.

36. Pouryazdanparast P, Newman M, Mafee M, et al. Distinguishing epithelioid blue nevus from blue nevus-like cutaneous melanoma metastasis using fluorescence in situ hybridization. Am J Surg Pathol 2009;33(9):1396–400.

37. Boone SL, Busam KJ, Marghoob AA, et al. Two cases of multiple Spitz nevi: correlating clinical, histologic, and fluorescence in situ hybridization findings. Arch Dermatol 2011;147(2):227–31.

38. Isaac AK, Lertsburapa T, Pathria Mundi J, et al. Polyploidy in Spitz nevi: a not uncommon karyotypic abnormality identifiable by fluorescence in situ hybridization. Am J Dermatopathol 2010;32(2): 144–8.

39. Newman MD, Lertsburapa T, Mirzabeigi M, et al. Fluorescence in situ hybridization as a tool for microstaging in malignant melanoma. Mod Pathol 2009; 22(8):989–95.

40. Dalton SR, Gerami P, Kolaitis NA, et al. Use of fluorescence in situ hybridization (FISH) to distinguish intranodal nevus from metastatic melanoma. Am J Surg Pathol 2010;34(2):231–7.

41. Cerroni L, Barnhill R, Elder D, et al. Melanocytic tumors of uncertain malignant potential: results of a tutorial held at the XXIX Symposium of the International Society of Dermatopathology in Graz, October 2008. Am J Surg Pathol 2010;34(3):314–26.

42. Raskin L, Ludgate M, Iyer RK, et al. Copy number variations and clinical outcome in atypical Spitz tumors. Am J Surg Pathol 2011;35(2):243–52.

43. Gaiser T, Kutzner H, Palmedo G, et al. Classifying ambiguous melanocytic lesions with FISH and correlation with clinical long-term follow up. Mod Pathol 2010;23(3):413–9.

44. North JP, Vetto JT, Murali R, et al. Assessment of copy number status of chromosomes 6 and 11 by FISH provides independent prognostic information in primary melanoma. Am J Surg Pathol 2011; 35(8):1146–50.

45. Hoglund M, Gisselsson D, Hansen GB, et al. Dissecting karyotypic patterns in malignant melanomas: temporal clustering of losses and gains in melanoma karyotypic evolution. Int J Cancer 2004; 108(1):57–65.

46. Harbour JW. The genetics of uveal melanoma: an emerging framework for targeted therapy. Pigment Cell Melanoma Res 2012;25(2):171–81.

47. Shields CL, Ganguly A, Bianciotto CG, et al. Prognosis of uveal melanoma in 500 cases using genetic testing of fine-needle aspiration biopsy specimens. Ophthalmology 2011;118(2):396–401.

48. Parrella P, Caballero OL, Sidransky D, et al. Detection of c-myc amplification in uveal melanoma by fluorescent in situ hybridization. Invest Ophthalmol Vis Sci 2001;42(8):1679–84.

49. Enzinger FM. Clear-cell sarcoma of tendons and aponeuroses. An analysis of 21 cases. Cancer 1965;18:1163–74.

50. Meis-Kindblom JM. Clear cell sarcoma of tendons and aponeuroses: a historical perspective and tribute to the man behind the entity. Adv Anat Pathol 2006;13(6):286–92.

51. Thway K, Fisher C. Tumors with EWSR1-CREB1 and EWSR1-ATF1 fusions: the current status. Am J Surg Pathol 2012;36(7):e1–11.

52. Gerami P, Mafee M, Lurtsbarapa T, et al. Sensitivity of fluorescence in situ hybridization for melanoma diagnosis using RREB1, MYB, Cep6, and 11q13

probes in melanoma subtypes. Arch Dermatol 2010; 146(3):273–8.

53. van Engen-van Grunsven AC, van Dijk MC, Ruiter DJ, et al. HRAS-mutated Spitz tumors: a subtype of Spitz tumors with distinct features. Am J Surg Pathol 2010;34(10):1436–41.

54. Van Raamsdonk CD, Griewank KG, Crosby MB, et al. Mutations in GNA11 in uveal melanoma. N Engl J Med 2010;363(23):2191–9.

55. Brose MS, Volpe P, Feldman M, et al. BRAF and RAS mutations in human lung cancer and melanoma. Cancer Res 2002;62(23):6997–7000.

56. Davies H, Bignell GR, Cox C, et al. Mutations of the BRAF gene in human cancer. Nature 2002; 417(6892):949–54.

57. Jakob JA, Bassett RL Jr, Ng CS, et al. NRAS mutation status is an independent prognostic factor in metastatic melanoma. Cancer, in press. doi: 10.1002/cncr.26724.

58. Wilson MA, Nathanson KL. Molecular testing in melanoma. Cancer J 2012;18(2):117–23.

59. Chapman PB, Hauschild A, Robert C, et al. Improved survival with vemurafenib in melanoma with BRAF V600E mutation. N Engl J Med 2011; 364(26):2507–16.

60. Lee JH, Choi JW, Kim YS. Frequencies of BRAF and NRAS mutations are different in histological types and sites of origin of cutaneous melanoma: a meta-analysis. Br J Dermatol 2011;164(4):776–84.

61. Bauer J, Curtin JA, Pinkel D, et al. Congenital melanocytic nevi frequently harbor NRAS mutations but no BRAF mutations. J Invest Dermatol 2007;127(1): 179–82.

62. Van Raamsdonk CD, Bezrookove V, Green G, et al. Frequent somatic mutations of GNAQ in uveal melanoma and blue naevi. Nature 2009;457(7229): 599–602.

63. Emley A, Nguyen LP, Yang S, et al. Somatic mutations in GNAQ in amelanotic/hypomelanotic blue nevi. Hum Pathol 2011;42(1):136–40.

64. Carvajal RD, Antonescu CR, Wolchok JD, et al. KIT as a therapeutic target in metastatic melanoma. JAMA 2011;305(22):2327–34.

65. Ross AL, Sanchez MI, Grichnik JM. Molecular nevogenesis. Dermatol Res Pract 2011;2011:463184.

66. Dessars B, De Raeve LE, Morandini R, et al. Genotypic and gene expression studies in congenital melanocytic nevi: insight into initial steps of melanotumorigenesis. J Invest Dermatol 2009; 129(1):139–47.

Update on Immunohistochemistry in Melanocytic Lesions

Tammie Ferringer, MD[a,b,*]

KEYWORDS

- Immunohistochemistry • Melanoma • Nevus

KEY POINTS

- Immunohistochemistry (IHC) should be used judiciously.
- In some circumstances, IHC is paramount to diagnosis.
- More often IHC simply provides additional information that must be weighed with the histomorphologic and clinical features to establish the most appropriate diagnosis or assist in planning patient management.
- Accurate interpretation relies on evaluation of appropriate staining pattern (cytoplasmic or nuclear), as well as independent and internal controls.
- Knowledge of the expected reactivity is required to correctly interpret immunohistochemical preparations.

Before the advent of immunohistochemistry (IHC), electron microscopy was required to identify tissue type in poorly differentiated neoplasms. Although electron microscopy still has its uses, IHC is now widely available and is less labor intensive and costly. Initially, a limited number of immunohistochemical markers were commercially available and use was limited mainly to fresh or frozen tissue. Today numerous commercially available antibodies applicable to formalin-fixed, paraffin-embedded tissue have greatly expanded the utility of IHC.

IHC is based on reagent antibody binding to a target epitope/antigen in tissue sections. Binding of the antibody to the antigen in tissue is visualized through use of a second immunohistochemical reaction, usually either an immunoperoxidase or alkaline phosphatase-based system, resulting in a stained reaction product. The 2 most common systems used include the diaminobenzidine (DAB) method, resulting in a brown product, and "Fast Red" or amino-9-ethylcarbozole (AEC), alternatively giving a red reaction.

Accurate interpretation of immunohistochemical preparations requires review of independent and internal controls to ensure appropriate staining. One must remember that immunoreactivity and true antigen expression are not necessarily synonymous, and several factors can account for immunostaining without true expression, including inappropriately high antibody concentration and/or excess antigen retrieval. By contrast, false negatives can occur because of too much or too little fixation time. The pattern of staining is also crucial. For example, faint staining of the cytoplasm with a nuclear marker should not be misinterpreted as a positive reaction. A thorough understanding of the expected reactivity for all

Disclosures and conflicts of interest: The author has no financial disclosures or conflicts of interest to express.
[a] Department of Dermatology, Geisinger Medical Center, Danville, PA, USA; [b] Department of Pathology, Geisinger Medical Center, Danville, PA, USA
* Department of Pathology, Geisinger Medical Center, 100 North Academy Avenue, MC 01-13, Danville, PA 17822.
E-mail address: tferringer@geisinger.edu

Dermatol Clin 30 (2012) 567–579
http://dx.doi.org/10.1016/j.det.2012.06.007
0733-8635/12/$ – see front matter © 2012 Elsevier Inc. All rights reserved.

entities in the differential diagnosis is required and, similar to most studies in medicine, IHC is not perfectly sensitive or specific, requiring correlation with the clinical scenario and histomorphology.

Despite numerous reports in the literature, reliable meta-analysis of immunohistochemical data in melanocytic lesions is limited by several variables, including differences in antibody source, antigen retrieval methods, and antibody concentrations. Other variables include differences in subtype of tumors included (eg, in melanoma: nodular, metastatic, desmoplastic, and so forth) and the criteria used to define positive and negative reactions.

Despite these limitations, IHC can, at times, be an adjunct to the hematoxylin and eosin (H&E) morphology when used appropriately. Some cases will still defy classification, even with extensive IHC. This article reviews the most recent advances of IHC in melanocytic lesions and provides guidance in a series of diagnostic dilemmas.

MELANOCYTIC MARKERS

In addition to morphologic clues, IHC can assist in distinguishing melanocytic from nonmelanocytic lesions when the tissue of origin is uncertain. Staining with S100 was one of the first and most enduring markers for melanocytic lesions. While S100 is considered the most sensitive marker and stains the great majority of melanocytic lesions, this marker lacks specificity and stains Langerhans cells, sweat glands, nerves, Schwann cells, myoepithelial cells, adipocytes, muscle cells, chondrocytes, and their tumors. Therefore other antibodies may be necessary to confirm the melanocytic nature of S100-positive neoplasms, particularly melanoma (**Table 1**). Although typically of high sensitivity, S100 is not always the preferred melanocytic marker in all settings. It should be used with caution for intraepithelial melanocytic proliferations of the nail matrix where sensitivity is low. Melan-A and HMB-45 (discussed below) are more sensitive in this small niche; however, S100 is still essential in identification of an invasive component, particularly when spindled.[1]

Melanoma antigen recognized by T cells (MART-1), also referred to as Melan-A, is expressed by normal melanocytes, nevi, and melanoma, but less frequently by desmoplastic malignant melanoma (DMM).[2,3] In addition, macrophages may aberrantly label with MART-1 using some antigen retrieval techniques; however, the staining is weak and granular, in contrast to the strong expression in melanocytic cells. Macrophage staining may be due to passive acquisition of antigens through phagocytosis.[4]

HMB-45 (anti-gp100), an organelle-specific, premelanosome marker, has been shown to mark only the intraepidermal and superficial dermal components of melanocytic nevi, with the exception of diffuse dermal staining in blue nevi and deep penetrating nevi.[5] When compared with MART-1, HMB-45 has been found to have weaker and more focal staining in both primary and metastatic melanomas, and rarely reacts in DMM. Therefore, HMB-45 is specific, only rarely staining other tumors (eg, perivascular epithelioid cell tumor [PEComa]) but does not stain all melanomas.[2,6] PEComas are tumors with immunophenotypic features of smooth muscle and melanocytic differentiation. While most are retroperitoneal or visceral, a subset arises in the skin. These lesions can mimic melanocytic neoplasms on routine sections and with IHC. HMB-45 is the most sensitive marker for PEComas, but Melan-A and microphthalmia transcription factor (MITF; discussed below) are also expressed in many cases. PEComas differ from melanocytic lesions by the absence of S100 expression.[7]

MITF is responsible for the normal embryonic development of melanocytes, mast cells, cells of the retinal pigment epithelium, and osteoclasts.[8] Immunohistochemical expression of MITF is nuclear. Reactivity is present in most melanomas, including some rare cases that do not express S100; however, a large proportion of desmoplastic and spindle-cell melanomas fail to react.[8,9] MITF positivity has been reported in 88% of conventional metastatic melanoma and although this is slightly less than the number of S100-positive metastases (90%), half of the S100-negative metastases were MITF positive, suggesting possible use in combination.[9] However, MITF is not specific, and staining has also been reported in

Table 1
Markers of primary cutaneous melanoma

Antibodies	Pattern	Positive (N)
S100	Nuclear/cytoplasmic staining	93.4% (91)
Sox-10	Nuclear staining	89.7% (68)
MART-1	Cytoplasmic staining	88.8% (89)
MITF	Nuclear staining	79.8% (89)
HMB-45	Cytoplasmic staining	75% (88)

Data based on review of primary melanomas at Geisinger Medical Laboratories. N is the number of cases studied. The percentage indicates cases with greater than 25% reactivity.

Data from Ferringer T. Skin. In: Lin F, Prichard J, editors. Handbook of practical immunohistochemistry. Springer; 2011. p. CH30.

PEComas, cellular neurothekeomas, neurofibromas, dermatofibromas, atypical fibroxanthomas (AFX), leiomyosarcomas, schwannomas, malignant peripheral nerve sheath tumors (MPNST), and dermal scars.[2,10,11]

Similarly, Sox-10 is an alternative nuclear melanocytic marker. It is a transcription factor found in neural crest–derived cells and is crucial for specification, maturation, and maintenance of Schwann cells and melanocytes. Although Sox-10 stains Schwann cells and myoepithelial cells in addition to melanocytes, it is much more specific than S100 for melanocytic lesions and has shown equal or better sensitivity.[12,13]

It is important to be aware that melanocytic lesions, particularly melanomas, can show aberrant expression of nonmelanocytic markers. Some melanomas exhibit aberrant expression with desmin, smooth muscle actin (SMA), CD138, MDM-2, synaptophysin, glial fibrillary acidic protein, CD30, CD68, carcinoembryonic antigen, and epithelial membrane antigen. Cytokeratin expression occurs in 4% to 6% of malignant melanomas; however, the staining tends to be focal and sparse.[14,15] There is increased aberrant expression of epithelial-associated markers in melanoma metastases. Use of a panel of immunostains, including the aforementioned melanocytic markers, should help to prevent misdiagnosis.

One of the problems with IHC in heavily pigmented melanocytic lesions is distinction of melanin in keratinocytes and melanophages from the brown (DAB) chromogen reaction. The color and texture of the melanin pigment are slightly different, but distinction can be cumbersome (**Fig. 1A**). One option is the use of AEC, resulting in a red product; however, this tends to smear and fade faster than DAB. Alternatively one can pretreat with melanin bleach, but this can be time consuming and may result in loss of immunohistochemical reactivity, incomplete melanin removal, or loss of cytologic detail. Kamino and colleagues[16–18] were the first to report replacement of the counterstain hematoxylin by azure B, which stains melanin green-blue and can be easily contrasted with DAB used in immunohistochemical staining. Thus, the melanocytes appear brown while the melanin granules are green-blue whether in melanocytes, melanophages, pigmented keratinocytes, or free in the dermis (**Fig. 1B**).

JUNCTIONAL MELANOCYTIC PROLIFERATIONS

While S100 is widely believed to be the most sensitive marker for melanocytic lesions, it is also expressed by the Langerhans cells in the epidermis. In addition, it may be easier to interpret nuclear immunohistochemical reactivity in junctional melanocytic proliferations on sun-damaged skin when compared with the often dendritic, cytoplasmic staining of other melanocytic markers that may simulate confluence, an important criterion for diagnosis of melanoma in situ.[19] Although S100 stains the nuclei of melanocytes, it is also a cytoplasmic stain. Therefore the purely nuclear stains, MITF and Sox-10, which do not highlight Langerhans cells, have shown superiority in this context. Sox-10 has the added advantage of also highlighting an occult spindle-cell or desmoplastic melanoma in the underlying dermis, whereas MITF can lack sensitivity in the spindled component.[20]

Caution is required because use of purely nuclear melanocytic markers can result in an initial tendency to undercall confluence, as adjacent nuclear staining will not appear to touch because of the intervening cytoplasm (**Fig. 2**).

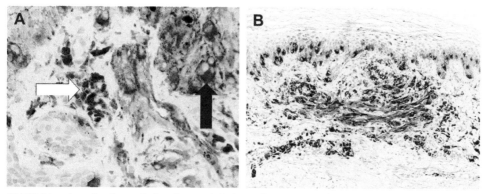

Fig. 1. MART-1 in a heavily pigmented melanocytic lesion using DAB, resulting in a brown product. (*A*) The color and texture of the MART-1 chromogen in the cytoplasm of the melanocytes (*black arrow*) differs subtly from the melanin in melanophages (*white arrow*). (*B*) Azure B counterstain converts the melanin to a green-blue color that contrasts nicely with the DAB brown product expressed in melanocytes (original magnification: *A* ×600; *B* ×200).

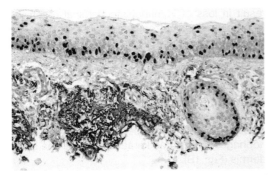

Fig. 2. MITF in melanoma in situ. Confluence of nuclear reactivity in the melanocytes at the dermal-epidermal junction can be less conspicuous owing to the intervening nonstaining cytoplasm (original magnification ×200).

Although uncommon, cells simulating junctional nests on routine sections can react with melanocytic markers and falsely suggest a melanocytic proliferation. These collections of cells have been referred to as pseudonests, and have been reported most commonly with MART-1/Melan-A in the setting of a lichenoid process (**Fig. 3**A).[21–24] However, a similar pitfall has been reported with MITF and Sox-10.[25,26] In reality these clusters of cells, when truly not incidental melanocytic nests, are likely an aggregate of cells including keratinocytes and macrophages, potentially in combination with rare melanocytes. The nonspecific staining may result from the lichenoid damage, allowing transfer of melanocyte antigens to adjacent nonmelanocytic cells. Clinical correlation and use of more than one melanocytic marker, including S100, should prevent a misdiagnosis of melanoma in situ (**Fig. 3**B).

MELANOMA VERSUS NEVUS

Of most interest are antibodies that may help in differentiating between benign and malignant melanocytic lesions. However, no single marker or panel of markers proves the diagnosis of melanoma unequivocally. Although trends have been identified, IHC alone cannot predict the biological behavior of a neoplasm.

The diminishing gradient of HMB-45 staining from the junction into the dermis suggests maturation in nevi (**Fig. 4**A). This finding is not surprising, considering there is a loss of premelanosomes with maturation. However, as already mentioned, blue and related nevi lack maturation and stain with HMB-45 throughout. Maturation and this orderly gradient is typically lacking in melanoma (**Fig. 4**B). Recently Leleux and colleagues[27] noted the additional caveat of HMB-45 labeling of nevus cells in scar or directly beneath it, creating the impression of loss of gradient, in healed traumatized benign nevi.

MIB-1, an antibody that detects Ki-67, is a marker of cell proliferation. Nuclear expression is identified in cells within the G1, M, G2, and S phases of the cell cycle but not in G0, the resting phase. Increasing expression and thus increasing proliferation is present in malignant melanocytic lesions and is highest in metastatic melanomas.[2] Nevi exhibit reactivity in very few to no dermal melanocytes. If there is reactivity, the proliferating cells tend to be near the dermal-epidermal junction.[3] MIB-1 is not melanocyte specific, and positive melanocytic nuclei must be distinguished from positive admixed, proliferating inflammatory cells. Dual labeling with a cytoplasmic melanocytic marker, such as MART-1, with a contrasting chromogen (AEC vs DAB) allows differentiation (**Fig. 5**).[28,29] Proliferating cell nuclear antigen (PCNA) and minichromosome maintenance protein (MCM) have been used similarly to MIB-1 as an indication of proliferation.[30–32]

Unlike MIB-1, which detects cells in any phase of the active cell cycle, the antibody against phosphohistone H3 (PHH3) only identifies cells in the

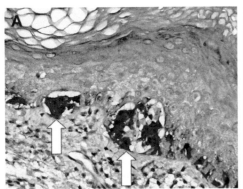

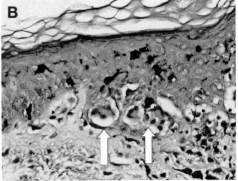

Fig. 3. Lichenoid dermatitis. The pseudonests, indicated by *white arrows*, were MART-1 positive (*A*) but S100 negative (*B*) (original magnification: *A, B* ×600).

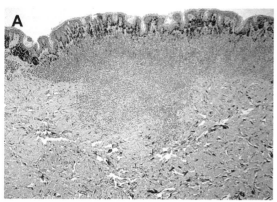
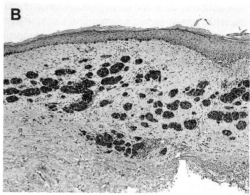

Fig. 4. HMB-45. (*A*) Maturing benign nevi reveal a diminishing gradient of HMB-45 with increasing depth into the dermis. (*B*) Melanomas can be positive, as in this case, or negative with HMB-45, but typically lack the orderly gradient seen in nevi (original magnification: *A* ×40; *B* ×100).

M phase. Phosphorylation of histone H3 is associated with decondensation of mitotic chromatin in the M phase. Use of this marker allows identification of mitoses at a lower power and improves interobserver and intraobserver agreement over routine microscopy of H&E-stained sections.[33,34] Negative-staining apoptotic and hyperchromatic nuclei can easily be distinguished from mitotic figures and identification of the mitotic "hot spot" is readily apparent using PHH3 (**Fig. 6**).[35] Similar to MIB-1, PHH3 is not cell specific, and dual staining with a cytoplasmic melanocytic marker improves reliable identification.[36]

The 2009 American Joint Committee on Cancer Staging and Classification (seventh edition) for melanoma introduced mitotic rate as a primary criterion for staging thin melanoma (≤1.0 mm).

Detection of a single mitotic figure will alter the staging and can alter management of these patients. PHH3 can clearly increase identification of mitoses; however, these staging guidelines were based on outcomes of patients in which mitoses were identified on routine microscopy. Use of this mitotic marker results in a higher mean mitotic rate when compared with H&E, therefore the impact on staging at this time is not fully established and requires further study.[35,37] Mitosis-specific phosphoprotein (MPM-2) is a mitotic marker similar to PHH3.

Kamino and colleagues[38] showed that immunohistochemical expression of elastin reveals elastic fibers between dermal nests and single cells of nevus, while melanoma showed a marked reduction of elastic fibers in the stroma and within the nests of melanocytes, often being compressed at the base of the invasive component. This finding seems to be of less utility in inflamed lesions.

Fig. 5. Dual labeling with MART-1 and MIB-1 in a melanoma. The cytoplasmic MART-1 staining is brown while the nuclear MIB-1 is red. Thus proliferating melanoma cells have brown cytoplasm and red nuclei (*black arrow*), and can be differentiated from nonmelanocytic proliferating lymphocytes, which only have red nuclei (*white arrow*) (original magnification ×600).

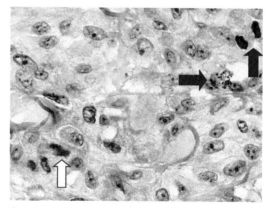

Fig. 6. PHH3 in a melanoma. Negative staining apoptotic or hyperchromatic nuclei (*white arrow*) are easily distinguished from mitotic figures (*black arrows*) (original magnification ×600).

The antibody D2-40 binds to podoplanin, a glycoprotein highly expressed in lymphatic endothelium. Because lymphovascular invasion in melanoma occurs predominantly via lymphatic vessels, this antibody facilitates accurate identification of lymphatic invasion in melanoma.[39] Identification can be further enhanced using dual staining for D2-40 and S100 or another melanocytic marker (**Fig. 7**).[40] However, the clinical implications of enhanced detection are debated. Some investigators have found no association between identification of lymphatic invasion with immunohistochemical markers and sentinel lymph node (SLN) positivity, relapse-free survival, or overall survival.[40,41] However, several other groups have found an association.[42–45] If the latter is true, use of these markers could potentially help identify patients who would benefit from observation over lymph node sampling.[44] The intratumoral lymphatic density, as determined by D2-40, has also been suggested to predict SLN metastasis.[46]

SPITZ NEVUS VERSUS SPITZOID MELANOMA

Differentiation of Spitz nevus from spitzoid melanoma can be problematic, as exemplified by the number of cases sent for consultation. In addition, lesions are often only partially sampled, further complicating diagnosis. Several immunohistochemical markers have been investigated to aid in characterization (**Table 2**). However, the search for a conclusive way to reliably distinguish these entities, with vastly different implications, continues.

HMB-45 can be used to indicate maturation, as already described. Although an increased proliferation rate of MIB-1 is concerning for melanoma,

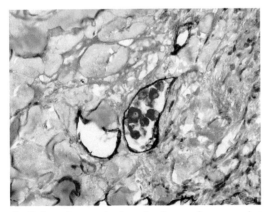

Fig. 7. Lymphovascular invasion in a melanoma using dual labeling with D2-40 and MART-1. The red MART-1–positive melanoma cells are easily identified within the lymphatic, highlighted brown with D2-40 (original magnification ×600).

Table 2		
Spitz nevus versus melanoma		
	Spitz	Melanoma
S100A6	+ Diffusely	Patchy or negative
HMB-45	Gradient from top to bottom	No gradient
MIB-1	<2%	>10%
P16	Prominent	Minimal

there is overlap between benign and malignant spitzoid lesions. Vollmer[47] found that a proliferation index greater than 10% as determined by MIB-1 favors melanoma, whereas a proliferation index below 2% favors Spitz nevus. Unfortunately, many lesions in question have an index between 2% and 10%. However, the pattern of MIB-1 expression may be useful. MIB-1 is similar to HMB-45, in that most reactivity is at the dermalepidermal junction or superficial dermis of nevi, in comparison with the more random expression in melanomas.[3]

The commercially available S100 antibody mainly stains cells containing the S100B polypeptide chains; however, it also reacts with many other protein subtypes of S100. Ribe and McNutt[48] found that the S100 subtype, S100A6 (calcyclin), strongly and diffusely stains Spitz nevi (**Fig. 8A**), whereas only one-third of melanomas expressed S100A6 and, when positive, revealed a weak and patchy pattern with minimal to no junctional expression (**Fig. 8B**). Although this may be helpful when comparing Spitz nevi and melanoma, other subtypes of nevi, including pigmented spindle-cell nevi, commonly are negative, weak, or patchy (**Fig. 8C**), similar to melanoma, and therefore S100A6 is of little use in differentiating nonspitzoid nevi from melanoma.[48,49] It is also important to recognize that S100A6 stains fibrohistiocytic lesions, including cellular neurothekeoma (**Fig. 9A–C**) and AFX, which can mimic melanocytic lesions.[50,51] Use of routine S100 in parallel can differentiate these S100-negative fibrohistiocytic lesions from S100-positive melanocytic proliferations.

The cell cycle inhibitor protein p16 is identified immunohistochemically in the majority of Spitz nevi (**Fig. 10A**); however, reactivity is not always homogeneous and can show a patchwork of immunostained and unstained nevus cells.[52] The p16 gene is deleted or mutated, resulting in loss of control of the cell cycle in a large percentage of melanomas.[53] Loss of both nuclear and cytoplasmic dermal reactivity is highly associated with melanoma (**Fig. 10B**).[54]

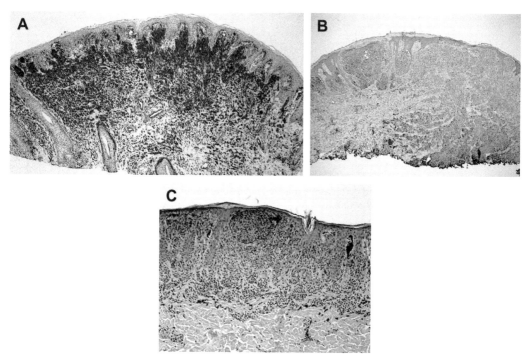

Fig. 8. S100A6. (*A*) Diffuse S100A6 reactivity in Spitz nevus. Weak and patchy S100A6 (*B*) in a spitzoid melanoma and (*C*) in a pigmented spindle-cell nevus (original magnification: *A, B* ×40; *C* ×100).

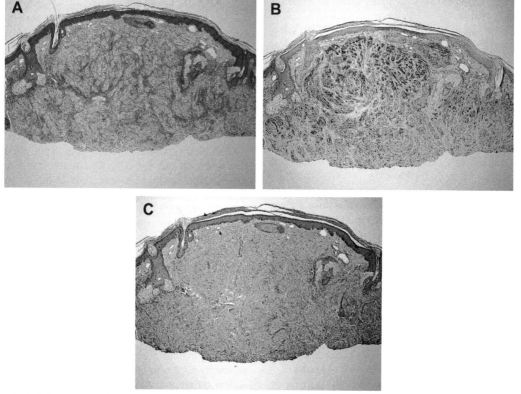

Fig. 9. Cellular neurothekeoma. (*A*) The nesting can mimic a melanocytic lesion (H&E). These lesions are positive with S100A6 (*B*) but negative with S100 (*C*) (original magnification: *A–C* ×40).

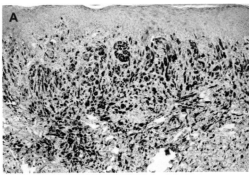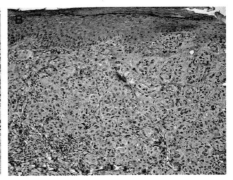

Fig. 10. p16. (*A*) Diffuse nuclear and cytoplasmic reactivity in a Spitz nevus. (*B*) Absence of p16 in a spitzoid melanoma (original magnification: *A, B* ×100).

DESMOPLASTIC MELANOMA VERSUS OTHER SPINDLE-CELL NEOPLASMS

The cells of DMM can appear remarkably bland, lack melanin, have sparse mitoses, and lack a junctional component. DMM can be confused with scar tissue, hypopigmented blue nevus, desmoplastic nevus, MPNST, AFX, leiomyosarcoma, and spindle-cell variant of squamous cell carcinoma (SSCC). The distinction becomes especially difficult in small biopsies. IHC can greatly facilitate diagnosis of DMM; however, expression of melanocytic markers in this melanoma subtype is unique (**Table 3**).

Nerve growth factor receptor (NGFR) (also known as p75) is normally expressed in neural crest cells and its tumor derivatives, such as neurofibromas, neurotized nevi, and neuroblastoma. It stains the majority of desmoplastic and neurotropic melanomas, often more intensely than S100.[55–58] Of interest, p75 stains predominantly type C, spindled melanocytes, therefore most nonneurotized nevi and nonspindled melanomas do not consistently stain with NGFR, and those that do stain only do so focally.[57]

S100 staining is nearly always present in DMM (**Fig. 11**A, B), and initial limited studies have shown similar reactivity with Sox-10 (**Fig. 11**C).[59] On the other hand, several other melanocytic antibodies are not reliable in this setting. MITF is poorly sensitive for spindle-cell and desmoplastic melanoma,

staining only 19% of 21 cases investigated in one study.[60] Kucher and colleagues[61] found that HMB-45 is usually negative in DMM, and Melan-A was positive in the spindle cells of DMM in only 7% of cases (**Fig. 11**D). In fact, expression of Melan-A in spindled melanocytic proliferations strongly supports desmoplastic nevus over DMM. When considering this differential, a low MIB-1 (Ki-67) proliferation index (<5%) alone is not sufficient to rule out DMM; however, a proliferative index above 10% suggests DMM.[61] Blue nevi lack NGFR expression. Consequently, NGFR has the potential to help distinguish cellular blue nevus from the positive-staining DMM.[62] By contrast, strong HMB-45 staining suggests blue nevus over DMM.

Usually the clinical scenario and deep soft-tissue predominance aid in distinguishing MPNSTs from DMM, but when these entities are considered in the histologic differential, MPNSTs typically stain in a patchy or weak pattern with S100, in contrast to the usual strong and diffuse staining in DMM.

Differentiation of DMM from scar tissue on routine sections can be difficult. Chorny and Barr[63] found S100-positive spindle cells in the majority of scars. The histogenesis of these S100-positive cells is uncertain, but they are typically sparse and arranged in a horizontal pattern (**Fig. 12**A). Nonetheless, this is a potential diagnostic pitfall in evaluating DMM, particularly in reexcision specimens.[63] Kanik and colleagues[57] considered NGFR a promising alternative in this setting; however, Otaibi and colleagues[64] found NGFR reactivity involving many cells in scar, including myofibroblasts, nerve twigs, and Schwann cells (**Fig. 12**B). To date there are no published reports of Sox-10 reactivity in scars[20]; however, the author has seen reactivity similar to S100 and NGFR (**Fig. 12**C).

The differential diagnosis of DMM, particularly those lacking pigment or junctional involvement, includes SSCC, AFX, and leiomyosarcoma. It

Table 3 Immunoreactivity in DMM	
Positive	**Negative**
S100	MITF
Sox-10	MART-1
NGFR	HMB-45

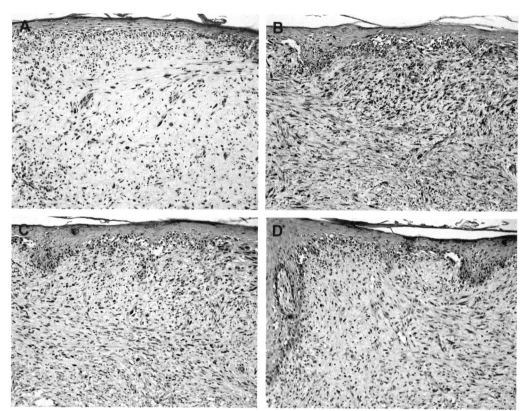

Fig. 11. Desmoplastic melanoma. (A) H&E. (B) S100 is nearly always positive in these lesions. (C) Sox-10 reacts in the nuclei but (D) MART-1 is negative (original magnification: A–D ×100).

must be remembered that CD68, cytokeratin, SMA, and desmin can be anomalously expressed in DMM.[65,66] Use of a panel of immunohistochemical markers including S100 will prevent misdiagnosis.

NODAL METASTATIC MELANOMA

Metastasis to SLN is undeniably a significant prognostic factor; however, the procedure otherwise is still of debatable use.[67] The 2009 American Joint Committee on Cancer Staging and Classification (seventh edition) considers identification of even one atypical melanocytic cell in the SLN to be stage N1. Identification of such small foci is a difficult problem. While adequate sampling and sectioning is required, IHC can further highlight small clusters or even single cells, and improve the sensitivity of detection by 10% to 45% over H&E alone.[4] The antigenicity of the primary tumor should be considered in selecting the markers used to evaluate the lymph node; however, the antigenic profile of metastatic lesions does not always reflect that of the primary tumor. Some pathologists recommend use of a cocktail of multiple melanocytic markers. However, as of

January 1, 2012, the Centers for Medicare and Medicaid Services' new National Correct Coding Initiatives policy does not allow billing of more than one unit of service per specimen per immunohistochemical procedure, even if it contains multiple separately interpretable antibodies.

S100 is highly sensitive for melanoma metastases; however, it is expressed in multiple cell types, including dendritic cells of the lymph node, and thus can make interpretation of melanoma troublesome. MART-1 does not exhibit the same background staining; however, weak granular cytoplasmic staining can occur in histiocytes, and Zubovits and colleagues[6] reported diffuse MART-1 staining in only 82% of metastases versus 98% of those stained with S100. Sox-10, on the other hand, has been found to be equivalent or better in identifying metastatic foci without the nonspecific cytoplasmic staining of MART-1 in nonmelanocytic cells or the distracting background dendritic cell staining of S100.[68]

Identification of S100, Sox-10, or MART-1 positive cells within a lymph node does not necessarily equate with metastatic melanoma. Benign nodal nevi have been detected in 0.33% to 7.3% of lymph nodes removed for nonmelanoma cases but in as

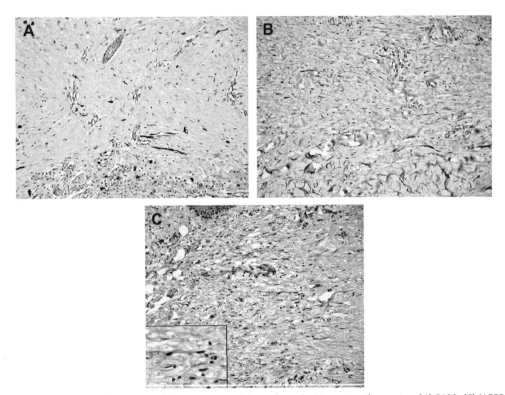

Fig. 12. Scattered nonmelanocytic cells in scar react with markers that target melanocytes. (*A*) S100, (*B*) NGFR, (*C*) Sox-10 (original magnification: *A–C* ×200; inset *C* ×600).

many as 22% of melanoma cases.[69] Nodal nevi are typically confined to the fibrous capsule or trabeculae of lymph nodes, but have been reported in the node parenchyma, whereas metastatic melanoma is typically present in a subcapsular location.[70] These nodal nevi can be a potential diagnostic pitfall in interpretation of immunohistochemically stained nodes. Identification of an immunopositive focus requires close examination of the corresponding H&E-stained sections for

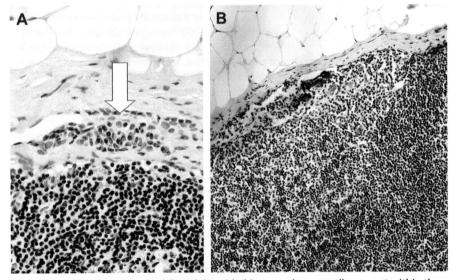

Fig. 13. HMB-45 in a sentinel lymph node. (*A*) Nodal nevi (*white arrow*) are usually present within the capsule and rarely express HMB-45. (*B*) Metastatic melanoma is often subcapsular and usually HMB-45 positive (original magnification: *A* ×600; *B* ×200).

cytologic atypia and comparison with the primary tumor cytology. Metastases usually reveal greater nuclear pleomorphism and tend to have nuclei that are more than 3 times the size of a lymphocyte.[71] According to Lohmann and colleagues,[72] MIB-1 may be helpful in distinction of nodal nevi and metastatic melanoma. All nodal nevi in their small study lacked immunoreactivity for this proliferative marker, but all metastases were MIB-1 positive, predominantly with more than 10% of the cells being MIB-1 positive. Because of the numerous MIB-1–positive lymphocytes in the node, dual staining with a melanocytic marker may be of assistance.[28] Similar to the dermal component of cutaneous nevi, nodal nevi are typically HMB-45 negative (**Fig. 13**A), with the exception of nodal blue nevi. Therefore, detection of an HMB-45–positive focus in a node, especially in a subcapsular location, supports a diagnosis of metastatic melanoma (**Fig. 13**B). While this might suggest that HMB-45 is the best marker for detection of melanoma in SLNs, HMB-45 does not detect all metastatic melanomas.[68,73] Jennings and Kim[68] found that 30 of 43 (69.8%) melanoma metastases to lymph nodes were highlighted by HMB-45.

SUMMARY

IHC will continue to be a rapidly evolving field with ever increasing new antibodies available in the armamentarium. Growth in this area parallels the advances in cytogenetics and molecular genetics. Immunohistochemical markers can increase the understanding of the pathogenesis of disease, serve as surrogate protein markers of underlying genetic events, and, by extrapolation, may suggest prognosis or be used to propose therapeutic alternatives and potentially to predict response.

ACKNOWLEDGMENTS

The author thanks Christine Cole, MD, Dirk Elston, MD, Jeffrey Graves, MD, Scott Dalton, DO, and William Tyler, MD for their kind review and comments.

REFERENCES

1. Theunis A, Richert B, Sass U, et al. Immunohistochemical study of 40 cases of longitudinal melanonychia. Am J Dermatopathol 2011;33:27–34.
2. Mangini J, Li N, Bhawan J. Immunohistochemical markers of melanocytic lesions: a review of their diagnostic usefulness. Am J Dermatopathol 2002; 24:270–81.
3. Prieto VG, Shea CR. Immunohistochemistry of melanocytic proliferations. Arch Pathol Lab Med 2011; 135:853–9.
4. Carlson JA, Ross JS, Slominski AJ. New techniques in dermatopathology that help to diagnose and prognosticate melanoma. Clin Dermatol 2009;27: 75–102.
5. Sun J, Morton TH Jr, Gown AM. Antibody HMB-45 identifies the cells of blue nevi. An immunohistochemical study on paraffin sections. Am J Surg Pathol 1990;14:748–51.
6. Zubovits J, Buzney E, Yu L, et al. HMB-45, S-100, NK1/C3, and MART-1 in metastatic melanoma. Hum Pathol 2004;35:217–23.
7. Liegl B, Hornick JL, Fletcher CD. Primary cutaneous PEComa: distinctive clear cell lesions of skin. Am J Surg Pathol 2008;32:608–14.
8. Vachtenheim J, Borovansky J. Microphthalmia transcription factor: a specific marker for malignant melanoma. Prague Med Rep 2004;105:318–24.
9. Miettinen M, Fernandez M, Franssila K, et al. Microphthalmia transcription factor in the immunohistochemical diagnosis of metastatic melanoma: comparison with four other melanoma markers. Am J Surg Pathol 2001;25:205–11.
10. Gleason BC, Nascimento AF. HMB-45 and Melan-A are useful in the differential diagnosis between granular cell tumor and malignant melanoma. Am J Dermatopathol 2007;29:22–7.
11. Page RN, King R, Mihm MC Jr, et al. Microphthalmia transcription factor and NKI/C3 expression in cellular neurothekeoma. Mod Pathol 2004;17:230–4.
12. Nonaka D, Chiriboga L, Rubin BP. Sox10: a panschwannian and melanocytic marker. Am J Surg Pathol 2008;32:1291–8.
13. Shin J, Vincent JG, Cuda JD, et al. Sox10 is expressed in primary melanocytic neoplasms of various histologies but not in fibrohistiocytic proliferations and histiocytoses. J Am Acad Dermatol 2012 Feb 9. [Epub ahead of print].
14. Korabiowska M, Fischer G, Steinacker A, et al. Cytokeratin positivity in paraffin-embedded malignant melanomas: comparative study of KL1, A4 and Lu5 antibodies. Anticancer Res 2004;24:3203–7.
15. Banerjee SS, Harris M. Morphological and immunophenotypic variations in malignant melanoma. Histopathology 2000;36:387–402.
16. Wiltz KL, Qureshi H, Patterson JW, et al. Immunostaining for MART-1 in the interpretation of problematic intra-epidermal pigmented lesions. J Cutan Pathol 2007;34:601–5.
17. Kamino H, Tam ST. Immunoperoxidase technique modified by counterstain with azure B as a diagnostic aid in evaluating heavily pigmented melanocytic neoplasms. J Cutan Pathol 1991;18: 436–9.
18. Kligora CJ, Fair KP, Clem MS, et al. A comparison of melanin bleaching and azure blue counterstaining in the immunohistochemical diagnosis of malignant melanoma. Mod Pathol 1999;12:1143–7.

19. Hillesheim PB, Slone S, Kelley D, et al. An immuno-histochemical comparison between MiTF and MART-1 with Azure blue counterstaining in the setting of solar lentigo and melanoma in situ. J Cutan Pathol 2011;38:565–9.

20. Ramos-Herberth FI, Karamchandani J, Kim J, et al. SOX10 immunostaining distinguishes desmoplastic melanoma from excision scar. J Cutan Pathol 2010; 37:944–52.

21. Demartini CS, Dalton MS, Ferringer T, et al. Melan-A/MART-1 positive "pseudonests" in lichenoid inflammatory lesions: an uncommon phenomenon. Am J Dermatopathol 2005;27:370–1.

22. Beltraminelli H, Shabrawi-Caelen LE, Kerl H, et al. Melan-A-positive "pseudomelanocytic nests": a pitfall in the histopathologic and immunohistochemical diagnosis of pigmented lesions on sun-damaged skin. Am J Dermatopathol 2009;31:305–8.

23. Nicholson KM, Gerami P. An immunohistochemical analysis of pseudomelanocytic nests mimicking melanoma in situ: report of 2 cases. Am J Dermatopathol 2010;32:633–7.

24. Maize JC Jr, Resneck JS Jr, Shapiro PE, et al. Ducking stray "magic bullets": a Melan-A alert. Am J Dermatopathol 2003;25:162–5.

25. Silva CY, Goldberg LJ, Mahalingam M, et al. Nests with numerous SOX10 and MiTF-positive cells in lichenoid inflammation: pseudomelanocytic nests or authentic melanocytic proliferation? J Cutan Pathol 2011;38:797–800.

26. Abuzeid M, Dalton SR, Ferringer T, et al. Microphthalmia-associated transcription factor-positive pseudonests in cutaneous lupus erythematosus. Am J Dermatopathol 2011;33:752–4.

27. Leleux TM, Prieto VG, Diwan AH. Aberrant expression of HMB-45 in traumatized melanocytic nevi. J Am Acad Dermatol 2012 Jan 27. [Epub ahead of print].

28. Nielsen PS, Riber-Hansen R, Steiniche T. Immunohistochemical double stains against Ki67/MART1 and HMB45/MITF: promising diagnostic tools in melanocytic lesions. Am J Dermatopathol 2011;33:361–70.

29. Puri PK, Valdes CL, Burchette JL, et al. Accurate identification of proliferative index in melanocytic neoplasms with Melan-A/Ki-67 double stain. J Cutan Pathol 2010;37:1010–2.

30. Gambichler T, Shtern M, Rotterdam S, et al. Minichromosome maintenance proteins are useful adjuncts to differentiate between benign and malignant melanocytic skin lesions. J Am Acad Dermatol 2009;60:808–13.

31. Boyd AS, Shakhtour B, Shyr Y. Minichromosome maintenance protein expression in benign nevi, dysplastic nevi, melanoma, and cutaneous melanoma metastases. J Am Acad Dermatol 2008;58:750–4.

32. Guerriere-Kovach PM, Hunt EL, Patterson JW, et al. Primary melanoma of the skin and cutaneous melanomatous metastases: comparative histologic features and immunophenotypes. Am J Clin Pathol 2004;122:70–7.

33. Casper DJ, Ross KI, Messina JL, et al. Use of anti-phosphohistone H3 immunohistochemistry to determine mitotic rate in thin melanoma. Am J Dermatopathol 2010;32:650–4.

34. Schimming TT, Grabellus F, Roner M, et al. pHH3 immunostaining improves interobserver agreement of mitotic index in thin melanomas. Am J Dermatopathol 2012;34:266–9.

35. Tapia C, Kutzner H, Mentzel T, et al. Two mitosis-specific antibodies, MPM-2 and phospho-histone H3 (Ser28), allow rapid and precise determination of mitotic activity. Am J Surg Pathol 2006;30:83–9.

36. Ikenberg K, Pfaltz M, Rakozy C, et al. Immunohistochemical dual staining as an adjunct in assessment of mitotic activity in melanoma. J Cutan Pathol 2012; 39:324–30.

37. Ladstein RG, Bachmann IM, Straume O, et al. Prognostic importance of the mitotic marker phosphohistone H3 in cutaneous nodular melanoma. J Invest Dermatol 2012;132:1247–52.

38. Kamino H, Tam S, Tapia B, et al. The use of elastin immunostain improves the evaluation of melanomas associated with nevi. J Cutan Pathol 2009;36:845–52.

39. Niakosari F, Kahn HJ, Marks A, et al. Detection of lymphatic invasion in primary melanoma with monoclonal antibody D2-40: a new selective immunohistochemical marker of lymphatic endothelium. Arch Dermatol 2005;141:440–4.

40. Petitt M, Allison A, Shimoni T, et al. Lymphatic invasion detected by D2-40/S-100 dual immunohistochemistry does not predict sentinel lymph node status in melanoma. J Am Acad Dermatol 2009;61:819–28.

41. Storr SJ, Safuan S, Mitra A, et al. Objective assessment of blood and lymphatic vessel invasion and association with macrophage infiltration in cutaneous melanoma. Mod Pathol 2012;25:493–504.

42. Rose AE, Christos PJ, Lackaye D, et al. Clinical relevance of detection of lymphovascular invasion in primary melanoma using endothelial markers D2-40 and CD34. Am J Surg Pathol 2011;35:1441–9.

43. Petersson F, Diwan AH, Ivan D, et al. Immunohistochemical detection of lymphovascular invasion with D2-40 in melanoma correlates with sentinel lymph node status, metastasis and survival. J Cutan Pathol 2009;36:1157–63.

44. Niakosari F, Kahn HJ, McCready D, et al. Lymphatic invasion identified by monoclonal antibody D2-40, younger age, and ulceration: predictors of sentinel lymph node involvement in primary cutaneous melanoma. Arch Dermatol 2008;144:462–7.

45. Fohn LE, Rodriguez A, Kelley MC, et al. D2-40 lymphatic marker for detecting lymphatic invasion in thin to intermediate thickness melanomas: association with sentinel lymph node status and prognostic

value-a retrospective case study. J Am Acad Dermatol 2011;64:336–45.

46. Massi D, Puig S, Franchi A, et al. Tumour lymphangiogenesis is a possible predictor of sentinel lymph node status in cutaneous melanoma: a case-control study. J Clin Pathol 2006;59:166–73.

47. Vollmer RT. Use of Bayes rule and MIB-1 proliferation index to discriminate Spitz nevus from malignant melanoma. Am J Clin Pathol 2004;122:499–505.

48. Puri PK, Elston CA, Tyler WB, et al. The staining pattern of pigmented spindle cell nevi with S100A6 protein. J Cutan Pathol 2011;38:14–7.

49. Ribe A, McNutt NS. S100A6 protein expression is different in Spitz nevi and melanomas. Modern Pathology 2003;16:505–11.

50. Fullen DR, Lowe L, Su LD. Antibody to S100a6 protein is a sensitive immunohistochemical marker for neurothekeoma. J Cutan Pathol 2003;30:118–22.

51. Fullen DR, Reed JA, Finnerty B, et al. S100A6 expression in fibrohistiocytic lesions. J Cutan Pathol 2001;28:229–34.

52. Scurr LL, McKenzie HA, Becker TM, et al. Selective loss of wild-type p16(INK4a) expression in human nevi. J Invest Dermatol 2011;131:2329–32.

53. Al Dhaybi R, Agoumi M, Gagne I, et al. p16 expression: a marker of differentiation between childhood malignant melanomas and Spitz nevi. J Am Acad Dermatol 2011;65:357–63.

54. George E, Polissar NL, Wick M. Immunohistochemical evaluation of p16INK4A, E-cadherin, and cyclin D1 expression in melanoma and Spitz tumors. Am J Clin Pathol 2010;133:370–9.

55. Sigal AC, Keenan M, Lazova R. P75 nerve growth factor receptor as a useful marker to distinguish spindle cell melanoma from other spindle cell neoplasms of sun-damaged skin. Am J Dermatopathol 2012;34:145–50.

56. Lazova R, Tantcheva-Poor I, Sigal AC. P75 nerve growth factor receptor staining is superior to S100 in identifying spindle cell and desmoplastic melanoma. J Am Acad Dermatol 2010;63:852–8.

57. Kanik AB, Yaar M, Bhawan J. p75 nerve growth factor receptor staining helps identify desmoplastic and neurotropic melanoma. J Cutan Pathol 1996;23:205–10.

58. Radfar A, Stefanato CM, Ghosn S, et al. NGFR-positive desmoplastic melanomas with focal or absent S-100 staining: Further evidence supporting the use of both NGFR and S-100 as a primary immunohistochemical panel for the diagnosis of desmoplastic melanomas. Am J Dermatopathol 2006;28:162–7.

59. Karamchandani JR, Nielsen TO, van de Rijn M, et al. Sox10 and S100 in the diagnosis of soft-tissue neoplasms. Appl Immunohistochem Mol Morphol 2012 Apr 10. [Epub ahead of print].

60. Granter SR, Weilbaecher KN, Quigley C, et al. Microphthalmia transcription factor: not a sensitive or specific marker for the diagnosis of desmoplastic melanoma and spindle cell (non-desmoplastic) melanoma. Am J Dermatopathol 2001;23:185–9.

61. Kucher C, Zhang PJ, Pasha T, et al. Expression of Melan-A and Ki-67 in desmoplastic melanoma and desmoplastic nevi. Am J Dermatopathol 2004;26:452–7.

62. Smith KS, Stahr BJ, White WL. Hypomelanotic blue nevus: an immunohistomorphologic and immunohistochemical comparison to desmoplastic malignant melanoma. J Cutan Pathol 1999;26:454.

63. Chorny JA, Barr RJ. S100-positive spindle cells in scars: a diagnostic pitfall in the re-excision of desmoplastic melanoma. Am J Dermatopathol 2002;24:309–12.

64. Otaibi S, Jukic DM, Drogowski L, et al. NGFR (p75) expression in cutaneous scars; further evidence for a potential pitfall in evaluation of reexcision scars of cutaneous neoplasms, in particular desmoplastic melanoma. Am J Dermatopathol 2011;33:65–71.

65. Zarbo RJ, Gown AM, Nagle RB, et al. Anomalous cytokeratin expression in malignant melanoma: one- and two-dimensional Western blot analysis and immunohistochemical survey of 100 melanomas. Modern Pathology 1990;3:494–501.

66. Folpe AL, Cooper K. Best practices in diagnostic immunohistochemistry: pleomorphic cutaneous spindle cell tumors. Arch Pathol Lab Med 2007;131:1517–24.

67. Satzger I, Volker B, Meier A, et al. Prognostic significance of isolated HMB45 or Melan A positive cells in melanoma sentinel lymph nodes. Am J Surg Pathol 2007;31:1175–80.

68. Jennings C, Kim J. Identification of nodal metastases in melanoma using sox-10. Am J Dermatopathol 2011;33:474–82.

69. Biddle DA, Evans HL, Kemp BL, et al. Intraparenchymal nevus cell aggregates in lymph nodes: a possible diagnostic pitfall with malignant melanoma and carcinoma. Am J Surg Pathol 2003;27:673–81.

70. Yan S, Brennick JB. False-positive rate of the immunoperoxidase stains for MART1/MelanA in lymph nodes. Am J Surg Pathol 2004;28:596–600.

71. Dalton SR, Gerami P, Kolaitis NA, et al. Use of fluorescence in situ hybridization (FISH) to distinguish intranodal nevus from metastatic melanoma. Am J Surg Pathol 2010;34:231–7.

72. Lohmann CM, Iversen K, Jungbluth AA, et al. Expression of melanocyte differentiation antigens and ki-67 in nodal nevi and comparison of ki-67 expression with metastatic melanoma. Am J Surg Pathol 2002;26:1351–7.

73. Busam KJ, Kucukgol D, Sato E, et al. Immunohistochemical analysis of novel monoclonal antibody PNL2 and comparison with other melanocyte differentiation markers. Am J Surg Pathol 2005;29:400–6.

Melanoma Staging
Where Are We Now?

Adriano Piris, MD[a], Alice Coelho Lobo, MD[b],
Lyn M. Duncan, MD[a],*

KEYWORDS

- American Joint Committee on Cancer • Melanoma staging • Melanoma classification

KEY POINTS

- Dermal primary melanoma mitogenicity is considered one of the 3 most powerful prognostic factors, along with ulceration and tumor thickness, in patients with localized melanoma.
- Tumor thickness remains the primary determinant of T staging and should be measured using the method described by Breslow.
- Dermal mitotic figures are counted using the hot spot method and are reported as the number of mitoses per squared millimeter.
- Ulceration is reported in the primary melanoma only if there is absence of epidermis with an underlying inflammatory infiltrate and traumatic ulceration has been ruled out.
- The presence of a single melanoma cell in a sentinel lymph node, visualized by hematoxylin-eosin stain or by one of the melanocytic markers, upstages the patient to IIIb.
- The most powerful predictors of survival in patients with regional disease are the number of lymph nodes affected, metastatic tumor burden, ulceration, and thickness of the primary tumor.

The seventh version of the American Joint Committee on Cancer (AJCC) Melanoma Staging guidelines, published in 2009, has significant revisions compared with the previous version. The current schema was developed based on the largest melanoma patient cohort analyzed to date and is the result of a multivariate analysis of 30,946 patients with stage I, II, and III melanoma and 7972 patients with stage IV melanoma.[1]

This article summarizes the findings and the new definitions included in the 2009 AJCC Melanoma Staging and Classification. The TNM categories for this seventh edition of the AJCC Staging Manual are defined in **Table 1**, and the stage groupings are defined in **Table 2**. Changes in the melanoma staging system are summarized in **Table 3**.

LOCALIZED MELANOMA: STAGES I AND II
Mechanics of Primary Melanoma Staging

For patients with T1 cutaneous melanoma (primary tumor thickness <1.0 mm), thickness, mitotic count, and ulceration of the primary tumor are the most powerful predictors of survival.

Primary tumor thickness

The staging thresholds of melanoma thickness are unchanged from the sixth edition of the AJCC.[2] A cutaneous melanoma staged as T1 is 1.0 mm thick or less. T2 includes tumors from 1.01 to 2.0 mm thick. T3 measures from 2.01 to 4.0 mm, and a T4 lesion is more than 4.0 mm thick. Because primary tumor thickness is the most powerful predictor of melanoma survival, it remains the cornerstone for patient management. It is therefore

[a] Dermatopathology Unit, Pathology Service, Massachusetts General Hospital, Harvard Medical School, 55 Fruit Street, WRN 820, Boston, MA 02114, USA; [b] Department of Dermatology, Hospital das Clinicas, University of Sao Paulo, Av Dr Eneas De Carvalho Aquiar, Sao Paulo, SP CEP 05403-900, Brazil
* Corresponding author. Dermatopathology Unit, Massachusetts General Hospital, 55 Fruit Street, WRN 827, Boston, MA 02114.
E-mail address: duncan@helix.mgh.harvard.edu

Dermatol Clin 30 (2012) 581–592
http://dx.doi.org/10.1016/j.det.2012.06.001
0733-8635/12/$ – see front matter © 2012 Elsevier Inc. All rights reserved.

Table 1
TNM staging categories for cutaneous melanoma

T	Thickness (mm)	Ulceration Status and Mitoses
T is	Not applicable	Not applicable
T1	≤1.00	T1a: without ulceration and mitoses <1/mm² T1b: with ulceration or mitoses ≥1/mm²
T2	1.01–2.00	T2a: without ulceration T2b: with ulceration
T3	2.01–4.00	T3a: without ulceration T3b: with ulceration
T4	≥4.01	T4a: without ulceration T4b: with ulceration
N	**No. of Metastatic Nodes**	**Nodal Metastatic Burden**
N0	0	Not applicable
N1	1	N1a: micrometastasis[a] N1b: macrometastasis[b]
N2	2–3	N2a: micrometastasis[a] N2b: macrometastasis[b] N2c: in transit metastases/satellites without metastatic nodes
N3	4+ metastatic nodes, or matted nodes, or in transit metastases/ satellites with metastatic nodes	
M	**Site**	**Serum Lactate Dehydrogenase**
M0	No distant metastases	Not applicable
M1a	Distant skin, subcutaneous, or nodal metastases	Normal
M1b	Lung metastases	Normal
M1c	All other visceral metastases	Normal
	Any distant metastasis	Increased

[a] Micrometastases are diagnosed after sentinel lymph node biopsy.
[b] Macrometastases are defined as clinically detectable nodal metastases confirmed pathologically.
　Data from Edge SB, Byrd DR, Compton CC, et al, editors. AJCC cancer staging manual. 7th edition. Chicago: Springer; 2009. p. 332.

a critical component of the pathology report and it must be determined with accuracy. The objective measurement of tumor thickness, as originally described by Breslow,[2] requires the use of an intraocular micrometer. A calibration table should be used to ensure accurate measurement across different brands and models of microscopes. The measurement is taken from the top of the granular cell layer to the deepest invasive melanoma cell. When ulceration is present, the measurement is taken from the base of the ulcer to the deepest point of tumor cell invasion. Deep tumoral cells along perineural and periadnexal (adventitial) dermis, as well as perivascular or intravascular extension, are not included in the primary tumor thickness measurement. When the primary tumor has a polypoidal architecture, the Breslow thickness is obtained by measuring across the largest diameter of the lesion perpendicular to the skin surface.[3]

Mitotic count

One of the most important changes in the revised staging system is the introduction of mitotic count as a criterion for category T1. The mitotic count, expressed as number of dermal mitoses/mm² (n/mm²), represents a strong and independent prognostic factor in this patient subset.[4–6] The conclusion of various statistical analyses was that the most significant correlation with survival was at a threshold of 1/mm² or more. A highly significant correlation between increasing mitotic count and declining survival rates has also been shown.[7] The identification of mitoses as an

Table 2
Anatomic stage groupings for cutaneous melanoma

	Clinical Staging[a]				Pathologic Staging[b]		
	T	N	M		T	N	M
0	Tis	N0	M0	0	Tis	N0	M0
IA	T1a	N0	M0	IA	T1a	N0	M0
IB	T1b	N0	M0	IB	T1b	N0	M0
	T2a	N0	M0		T2a	N0	M0
IIA	T2b	N0	M0	IIA	T2b	N0	M0
	T3a	N0	M0		T3a	N0	M0
IIB	T3b	N0	M0	IIB	T3b	N0	M0
	T4a	N0	M0		T4a	N0	M0
IIC	T4b	N0	M0	IIC	T4b	N0	M0
III	Any T	N >N0	M0	IIIA	T1-4a	N1a	M0
					T1-4a	N2a	M0
				IIIB	T1-4b	N1a	M0
					T1-4b	N2a	M0
					T1-4a	N1b	M0
					T1-4a	N2b	M0
					T1-4a	N2c	M0
				IIIC	T1-4b	N1b	M0
					T1-4b	N2b	M0
					T1-4b	N2c	M0
					Any T	N3	M0
IV	Any T	Any N	M1	IV	Any T	Any N	M1

[a] Clinical staging includes microstaging of the primary melanoma and clinical/radiologic evaluation for metastases. By convention, it should be used after complete excision of the primary melanoma with clinical assessment for regional and distant metastases.
[b] Pathologic staging includes microstaging of the primary melanoma and pathologic information about the regional lymph nodes after partial (ie, sentinel node biopsy) or complete lymphadenectomy. Pathologic stage 0 or stage IA patients are the exception; they do not require pathologic evaluation of their lymph nodes.

important independent predictor of survival in patients with thin primary tumors led to the inclusion of dermal mitotic activity of the primary tumor as a new component of the seventh edition of the melanoma staging system. For the staging system to be uniformly and universally applied, it is critical that the assessment and reporting of the pathologic variables are consistent. Because the studies that revealed mitoses as clinically significant were retrospective studies that used the hot spot technique of evaluating tumor mitogenicity, the AJCC Melanoma Staging Committee recommends that mitotic count be determined by this approach and reported as the number of mitoses per square millimeter of the primary tumor.[8] This measurement is accomplished by examination of routine hematoxylin-eosin–stained tissue sections of the most representative profile of the tumor. It is not necessary to perform exhaustive tissue sectioning. Once the area with the most mitotic figures (hot spot) has been identified, the count starts using a standard 10× ocular and a high power objective (40×). After determining the number of mitoses in the first high power field, the count is extended to adjacent fields until an area of 1 mm^2 is assessed. To ensure accuracy across observers, individual microscopes must be calibrated to determine the number of high power fields (400×) that correspond to 1 mm^2. The most common microscopes are sized such that 1 mm^2 equals approximately 4 high power fields. The final mitotic count must be reported as n/mm^2. If only 1 mitosis is found, this should be reported as 1/mm^2. If no dermal mitoses are identified, the count should be reported as 0/mm^2. In cases in which dermal mitotic figures are uniformly distributed or scarce, and do not aggregate in a hot spot, the count starts with a randomly selected mitotic figure and proceeds to adjacent fields, as outlined earlier. When the invasive component of the tumor measures less than 1 mm^2 the count should be performed on all of the dermal tumor and reported as n/mm^2. In small biopsies, one can also encounter partial sampling of the invasive component amounting to less than 1 mm^2; in these cases, the AJCC recommends that the count be recorded as at least n/mm^2. Alternatively, when the invasive tumoral compartment is extensive, encompassing several square millimeters, if only 1 mitotic figure is found, the count is reported as 1/mm^2. The AJCC Melanoma Staging Committee strongly discourages the use of <1/mm^2 in reporting melanoma. It is important to distinguish between the reporting function, which should always be in a whole number/mm^2, and the staging language, which is described as a range (eg, greater than or equal to 1/mm^2).

With regards to special stains, the detection of Ki-67 in more than 20% of dermal melanoma cells is associated with an increased risk of lymph node metastasis in patients with thin, less than 1 mm, primary melanoma. If this test is performed on primary cutaneous melanomas, it is recommended that it is reported as the percentage of dermal tumor cells staining, using a threshold of 20%.[9] Another immunohistochemical stain that holds promise is antiphosphohistone H3 (anti-PHH3). By highlighting mitotic figures at any stage of mitosis, this is a highly sensitive detection method. Additional studies that identify appropriate quantitative thresholds for reporting the results of anti-PHH3 are needed before its use in routine reporting of primary melanoma. The current

Table 3
Differences between the sixth edition (2002) and the seventh edition (2009) of the melanoma staging system

Factor	Sixth Edition Criteria	Seventh Edition Criteria	Comments
Thickness	Primary determinant of T staging	Same	Thresholds of 1.0, 2.0, and 4.0 mm
Level of invasion	Used only for defining T1 melanomas	Same	Used as a default criterion only if mitotic rate cannot be determined
Ulceration	Included as a secondary determinant of T and N staging	Same	Signifies a locally advanced lesion; dominant prognostic factor for grouping stages I, II, and III
Mitotic rate per mm²	Not used	Used for categorizing T1 melanoma	Mitosis $\geq$1/mm² used as a primary criterion for defining T1b melanoma
Satellite metastases	In N category	Same	Merged with in transit lesions
Immunohistochemical detection of nodal metastases	Not included	Included	Must include at least 1 melanoma-associated marker (eg, HMB-45, Melan-A, MART-1) unless diagnostic cellular morphology is present
0.2 mm threshold of defined N+	Implied	No lower threshold of staging N+ disease	Isolated tumor cells or tumor deposits <0.1 mm meeting the criteria for histologic or immunohistochemical detection of melanoma should be scored as N+
Number of nodal metastases	Primary determinant of N staging	Same	Thresholds of 1 vs 2–3 vs 4+ nodes
Metastatic volume	Included as a second determinant of N staging	Same	Clinically occult (microscopic) nodes are diagnosed at sentinel node biopsy vs clinically apparent (macroscopic) nodes diagnosed by palpation or imaging studies, or by the finding of gross (not microscopic) extracapsular extension in a clinically occult node
Lung metastases	Separate category as M1b	Same	Has a better prognosis than other visceral metastases
Increased serum LDH level	Included as a second determinant of M staging	Same	Recommend a second confirmatory LDH level if increased
Clinical vs pathologic staging	Sentinel node results incorporated into definition of pathologic staging	Same	Large variability in outcome between clinical and pathologic staging; sentinel node staging encouraged for standard patient care, should be required before entry into clinical trials

Abbreviation: LDH, lactate dehydrogenase.

recommendation is to examine a limited number of hematoxylin-eosin–stained tissue sections and to report the number of mitoses identified in 1 mm of tumor based on the hot spot technique.

Ulceration

The presence of ulceration in the primary tumor was described as a highly significant poor prognostic indicator as early as 1953.[10,11] However, it came to occupy its rightful place in the TNM classification and melanoma staging only after the thorough review that led to the sixth edition of the AJCC melanoma staging system.[12] Similar to tumor thickness, the current edition is unchanged with regards to ulceration. The presence of ulceration upgrades the corresponding T classification from Ta to Tb. For T1 melanomas, ulceration is used along with the presence or absence of dermal mitoses. A T1 melanoma without ulceration and with no dermal mitoses is designated as T1a. However, the presence of ulceration alone is enough to upgrade a thin melanoma from T1a to T1b, regardless of the mitogenicity of the tumor. Ulceration is defined as full-thickness interruption of the epidermis by tumor without previous history of mechanical trauma or surgery at the site. This finding must be accompanied by reactive changes (ie, fibrin deposition, granulation tissue, and mixed inflammatory infiltrate).

Other Important Factors not in the Schema

Clark level

In the sixth edition of the AJCC staging system, the anatomic level of invasion as described by Wallace Clark was discontinued as the primary determinant of T staging; nevertheless, this parameter was still used to stratify patients with a Breslow thickness of less than 1 mm.[13] However, the latest results showed that the level of invasion is no longer statistically significant when mitotic count and ulceration are included in the analysis.[1] Hence, the new recommendation is that the mitotic count be used as the primary criterion for considering a melanoma as T1b. The level of invasion is used only when the mitotic count cannot be reliably determined because of poor preparation of the histology slides. For example, on rare occasions, the histologic sections are too thick or overstained and mitotic figures cannot be distinguished in a dark cellular background. In such cases, the level of Clark can be used in place of the mitotic count, as described in the sixth edition.

Regression

The phenomenon of regression was described by Clark and colleagues as an important prognostic indicator and it has been associated with increased likelihood of metastasis, even in thin melanomas.[14,15] Regression is defined as the focal absence of tumor within or immediately adjacent to an otherwise viable melanoma. The regressed area is characterized by complete absence of melanoma cells in the epidermis and dermis, flanked on one or both sides by viable melanoma cells. Histologically this area can show a thin epidermis with underlying fibroplasia, increased vascularity, chronic inflammation, and melanophages (**Fig. 1**). When the criteria described earlier are strictly applied the presence of regression is indeed an important prognostic indicator. However, in many instances, there is an overcall of regression in primary melanomas and this is one of the main reasons why this phenomenon has not yet been validated in larger patient cohorts. Several secondary changes are commonly misinterpreted as regression, such as the presence of fibrosis, chronic inflammation, or melanophages in a background of viable melanoma cells, as well as the presence of focal reactive fibrosis as

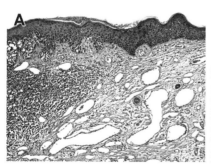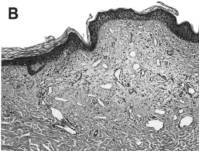

Fig. 1. Regression. (*A*) Focal complete absence of melanoma with replacement of the tumor by ectatic vessels and background fibroplastic stroma with scattered inflammatory cells (*right side of image*). Adjacent viable intraepidermal and dermal melanoma heavily infiltrated by lymphocytes (*left side of image*) (hematoxylin-eosin, ×200). (*B*) Different profile of the same tumor showing absence of epidermal rete ridges with dermal fibroplasia, ectatic vessels, and scattered melanophages. In this field, there is no residual melanoma (hematoxylin-eosin, ×200).

a result of trauma. As mentioned earlier, all these reactive changes are part of regression, but only when accompanied by a complete lack of viable tumor cells in the relevant area.

Host immune response (tumor-infiltrating lymphocytes)

The presence of cytotoxic T cells in the vertical growth phase of malignant melanoma has been associated with better prognosis.[14,16,17] The categories of the infiltrate have been described as brisk when the lymphocytes diffusely infiltrate throughout the tumor, nonbrisk when there is focal or multifocal infiltration, and absent when there are no lymphocytes infiltrating the tumoral compartment (**Fig. 2**). If a dense inflammatory infiltrate is present in the specimen adjacent to, but not infiltrating the melanoma, this is also termed absent. The prognosis was found to be better in patients with a brisk infiltrate, and worst in patients without tumor-infiltrating lymphocytes. However, despite the promising nature of these reports, many of the patients with a brisk host response still developed metastasis and disease progression. Several additional studies have further characterized these T cells, and besides cytotoxic T cells, there are also lymphocytes with regulatory functions.[18] Although present, these tumoral-infiltrating lymphocytes may not be immunologically active because of intrinsic regulatory influences. For staging purposes, this prognostic indicator has not been validated; however, it is important to consider this phenomenon when evaluating a primary melanoma, especially in light of the recent advances in immunotherapy.[19,20]

Lymphovascular invasion

The presence of lymphovascular invasion in a primary melanoma is considered to be an important predictor of metastasis in individual tumors.[21–24] This phenomenon is classically defined as the presence of viable tumor cells within the lumen of a vessel, preferably adhered to the vessel wall or admixed with fibrin. When the tumor cells are in the vessel wall, adjacent to the endothelium, but without luminal involvement, the finding has been described as uncertain vascular invasion. The tumoral cells can also surround the perivascular compartment, a phenomenon known as extravascular migratory metastasis or angiotropism.[25,26] This parameter is not part of the AJCC staging system. However, there are recent data that validate the identification of lymphatic invasion using a dual immunohistochemical stain (podoplanin/ D2-40 and S-100) as an independent prognostic indicator and predictor of metastasis, most specifically in clinical stages IB and IIA.[27] This powerful

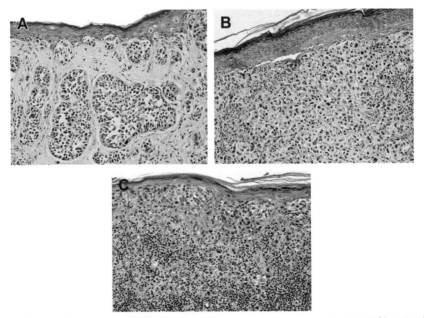

Fig. 2. Tumor-infiltrating lymphocytes. (*A*) Invasive malignant melanoma with no tumor-infiltrating lymphocytes (TILs), absent category (hematoxylin-eosin, ×200). (*B*) Invasive malignant melanoma with focally distributed TILs, nonbrisk. The lymphocytes can be observed to the right and left edges of the field, with no lymphocytes present in the center of the tumor (hematoxylin-eosin, ×200). (*C*) Invasive malignant melanoma with brisk TILs. The lymphocytes can be seen diffusely infiltrating across the entire base and percolating throughout the substance of the tumor (hematoxylin-eosin, ×200).

double-staining technique identifies S-100-positive melanoma cells within lymphatic vessels highlighted with D2-40 stain (**Fig. 3**).[28,29]

REGIONAL METASTASES: STAGE III
Microscopic Satellites, Clinical Satellites, and in Transit Metastases

Microscopic satellites (microsatellites) are identified in the tissue section of the primary tumor and are defined as a discontinuous group or nest of melanoma cells, greater than 0.05 mm in diameter, that are located at least 0.3 mm from the dermal invasive tumor mass and separated from it by normal dermis or panniculus not affected by fibrosis or inflammation.[30] This phenomenon was originally described as a primary tumor prognostic factor, which was found to be associated with poor prognosis.[31,32] In the sixth edition of the AJCC staging system, this feature was incorporated in the group of intralymphatic metastases, along with clinical satellites and in transit metastases.[13] Recent studies have revealed primary tumor microsatellites as an independent predictor of reduced disease-free survival in patients with positive sentinel lymph nodes.[33]

The term clinical satellite or satellite metastasis refers to tumor located no further than 5.0 cm from the primary lesion, although in transit metastases are foci located at a distance more than 5.0 cm from the primary tumor site, yet still proximal to the draining lymph node basin.

The terms intralymphatic regional metastases and in transit metastases/satellites are now used to describe these patterns of local spread.[1] Patients with intralymphatic metastases (microscopic satellites, satellite metastases or in transit metastases) without nodal metastases are classified as N2c (stage IIIB or IIIC), whereas those with combined intralymphatic metastases and nodal metastases are N3 (stage IIIC) and have a lower survival rate.

Sentinel Lymph Node Metastases

The identification of clinically occult nodal metastases is the most important independent predictor of prognosis in patients with stage I and II melanoma.[34] Sentinel lymph node mapping was described a quarter century ago as a minimally invasive tool for identifying patients with clinically localized melanoma who had microscopic metastases in regional lymph nodes.[35] Based on the patterns of lymphatic drainage from the skin, it has been shown that the sentinel node is the most likely lymph node to contain metastatic melanoma. Current techniques include the use of isosulfan blue dye and lymphoscintigraphy with technetium-99m (Tc99)–labeled sulfur colloid, followed by intraoperative identification of sentinel lymph nodes using a hand-held scanner with a γ-sensor probe to detect Tc99. After the hottest lymph node is identified and the Tc99 counts quantified, additional lymph nodes with more than 10% of the counts of this hottest lymph node may also be removed and considered sentinel.[36] Using this procedure, on average, 2 sentinel lymph nodes are removed.[37] If these sentinel lymph nodes do not contain metastatic melanoma, the remaining lymph nodes in the basin are unlikely to contain melanoma.[38] Patients who are diagnosed with sentinel lymph node metastases are usually offered completion lymphadenectomy and adjuvant therapy. Patients with negative lymph nodes are followed as melanoma patients and no additional regional surgery is recommended.

Pathology processing and analytical platforms
The histopathologic analysis of the sentinel lymph nodes includes the evaluation of hematoxylin-eosin–stained tissue sections and immunohistochemical-stained sections from multiple levels of each lymph node.[39,40] Although some elements are similar across institutions, there is marked overall variability in analytical platforms for the detection of melanoma in sentinel lymph nodes. The following represent practices used by most laboratories: (1) submit the lymph node tissue entirely; (2) perform level sections deep into the block (beyond the initial set of tissue sections); and (3) use immunohistochemical stains. Most institutions use S100 and either Melanoma Antigen Recognized by T-cells 1 (Mart-1) or Melanocyte antigen (Melan A); other less frequently used markers include Human

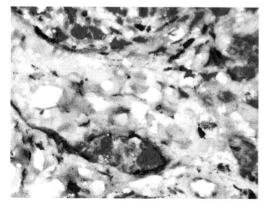

Fig. 3. Lymphovascular invasion in primary cutaneous melanoma. The endothelial cells mark positively for D240 (brown chromogen) and surround the intralymphatic S-100-positive melanoma cells (red chromogen) (×600).

Melanoma Black 45 (HMB-45) and Microphthalmia-associated transcription factor (MITF). In addition, some laboratories use a cocktail of reagents including MelanA/Mart1 and HMB-45/MelanA/tyrosinase. Protocols that do not include levels into the block or immunohistochemical stains are associated with a false-negative rate of approximately 15%.[39,41–43] Intraoperative frozen section analysis is less sensitive than the evaluation of formalin-fixed tissue and is not recommended.[44]

Histopathologic criteria

A major revision to the AJCC guidelines regarded the criteria for diagnosis of metastatic melanoma in a sentinel lymph node. In the past, the tumor was required to be identified on a hematoxylin-eosin–stained tissue section. In the current guidelines, the diagnosis of metastatic melanoma may be made if one melanoma cell is identified on any tissue section, whether stained with hematoxylin-eosin or with an immunohistochemical stain.[1] If melanoma is detected with immunohistochemical stains, efforts should be made to identify the tumor on an adjacent hematoxylin-eosin–stained tissue section. More specifically, the recommended criteria for the diagnosis of melanoma in sentinel lymph nodes include (1) the presence of individual cells or nests of epithelioid or spindle cells foreign to the lymph node, (2) cytologic atypia, defined as large cells with nuclear pleomorphism, prominent nucleoli, or dusty cytoplasmic melanin granules, and (3) positive staining for 1 or more melanocytic markers (eg, S-100, MART-1, Melan-A, HMB-45, MITF) (**Box 1, Fig. 4**). Sentinel lymph node metastases of melanoma are identified in 15% to 20% of patients who undergo this procedure.[45] The differential diagnosis of melanoma metastasis in this setting includes benign melanocytic rests (nodal nevus), usually observed in the lymph node capsule or

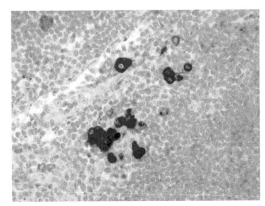

Fig. 4. Metastatic cells in the lymph node parenchyma. The tumor cells stain for Melan-A (red chromogen) and show irregular and pleomorphic nuclei. Some of the cells show multinucleation (×600).

fibrous trabeculae. The reported frequency of these benign melanocytic deposits ranges from a few percent to more than 20%; we found a rate of 9% in our series.[39] Diagnostic criteria for benign melanocytic nevi in lymph nodes include the following: (1) individual cells in a linear array or nests of epithelioid or spindle cells foreign to the lymph node, (2) no cytologic atypia, (3) positive staining for 1 or more melanocytic markers (S-100, MART-1, Melan-A, MITF; nodal nevi are usually negative for HMB-45), (4) identification of the cells on hematoxylin-eosin, and (5) cells are usually present in the fibrous capsule or trabeculae (**Box 2, Fig. 5**). In some cases, the presence of intranodal melanocytic rests may present a diagnostic challenge. Most reports indicate that HMB-45 does not stain nodal nevi, similar to the absence of staining for HMB-45 deep dermal nevomelanocytes of a cutaneous nevus. Others have reported an absence of Ki-67 staining in nodal nevi, leading to the

---

Box 1
Diagnostic criteria for the diagnosis of metastatic melanoma in sentinel lymph nodes

- Individual cells or nests of epithelioid or spindle cells foreign to the lymph node
- Cytologic atypia, defined as large cells with nuclear pleomorphism, prominent nucleoli, or dusty cytoplasmic melanin granules
- Positive staining for 1 or more melanocytic markers (S-100, MART-1, Melan-A, HMB-45, MITF)
- Identification of the cells on hematoxylin-eosin (not required)

Box 2
Diagnostic criteria for the diagnosis of nevic rests in sentinel lymph nodes

- Individual cells in a linear array or nests of epithelioid or spindle cells foreign to the lymph node
- No cytologic atypia
- Positive staining for 1 or more melanocytic marker (S-100, MART-1, Melan-A, MITF, usually negative for HMB-45)
- Identification of the cells on hematoxylin-eosin
- Cells are usually present in the fibrous capsule or trabeculae

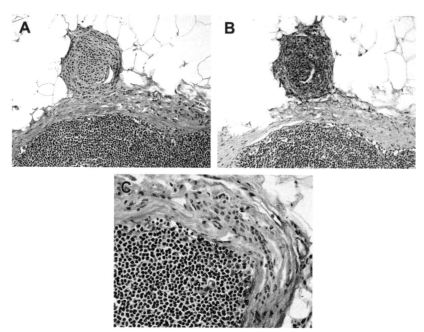

Fig. 5. Intracapsular rests of benign nevomelanocytes. (*A*) Periphery of a lymph node with pericapsular nevic nest composed of nevomelanocytes with bland cytologic features (hematoxylin-eosin, ×200). (*B*) The nevus cells display diffuse strong staining for S-100 (×200). (*C*) High power view of an adjacent focus of intracapsular nevus cells (hematoxylin-eosin, ×400).

adoption of a double MART-1/Ki-67 stain by some laboratories.[46]

Correlation of sentinel lymph node status with completion lymphadenectomy results and overall survival

The aims of sentinel lymph node biopsy include staging and regional disease control, with the overall hope of improving patient survival. As noted earlier, this technique is a relatively low-morbidity, accurate staging tool. Complications occur in 4% to 10% of patients who undergo sentinel lymph node mapping, usually infection, lymphedema, or seroma/hematoma. This is a low rate compared with the complication rate of 23% to 37% associated with complete lymph node dissection.[47] The false-negative rate is estimated to be less than 5%.[48] Regional disease control can be estimated by recurrence rates in the lymph node basin. The recurrence rate for patients with positive sentinel nodes and subsequent completion lymphadenectomy is less than 10%, in contrast to reported recurrence rates of 20% to 50% in patients with lymphadenectomy for clinically palpable tumor.[47,49] However, a clear survival benefit of sentinel lymph node mapping has not been shown in a statistically robust randomized trial. Some observers do not consider sentinel lymph node biopsy to be of therapeutic benefit.[50]

Others consider that micrometastases identified on histopathologic analysis of the sentinel lymph node will progress if left untreated. If this assumption is correct, then removal of sentinel lymph nodes containing microscopic tumor may be of therapeutic benefit.

On the other hand, the staging and prognostic value of sentinel lymph node status is not disputed. Tumor burden, regardless of the method of measurement, has been shown to correlate with risk of positive lymph nodes in the remainder of the basin, and also with overall survival.[51,52] Whereas 80% of patients with stage III disease have micrometastases, 20% of patients are diagnosed with clinically detectable macrometastases. The 5-year survival for these patients is 67% and 43%, respectively. Patients with microscopic metastases have widely varied prognosis; in these patients, multivariate analysis reveals that the number of tumor-containing lymph nodes, total metastasis size, primary tumor thickness, ulceration and tissue site, and patient age are independent predictors of survival. In addition, primary tumor mitotic count is the second most powerful predictor of survival after the number of involved lymph nodes.[53] On the other hand, for patients with nodal macrometastases, independent predictors of survival are number of tumor-containing nodes, primary tumor ulceration, and patient age.

Box 3
Quantitation and reporting of mitoses in primary cutaneous melanoma

- Routinely process primary cutaneous melanoma, do not perform excessive numbers of levels (3–5 tissue profiles is sufficient)
- Evaluate the dermal invasive melanoma with hematoxylin-eosin stain
- Use the hot spot technique
- Ki-67 is optional, report as less than 20% or more than 20% of the dermal melanoma cells
- If there is only 1 mitosis report as 1/mm^2 (not <1/mm^2)

Distant Metastases

Increase of serum lactate dehydrogenase (LDH) has been identified as an independent and highly significant predictor of survival in patients with stage IV melanoma.[12] This factor along with the sites of distant metastases are used to define the M categories. M1a includes patients with metastases to the skin, subcutaneous tissues, and nonregional lymph nodes and with a normal serum LDH. M1b includes patients with metastases to the lung and normal LDH levels. M1c is used for patients with increased serum LDH or visceral metastases (other than the lung). Although the number of metastases has been documented as an important prognostic factor, this was not included in the current schema because of significant variability in the use of tests to detect distant metastases.

SUMMARY

Changes to the AJCC staging schema for cutaneous melanoma resulted in several new definitions and changes in criteria. These new guidelines included: (1) for patients with stage I or II (eg, localized) melanoma, the most powerful prognostic indicators were found to be tumor thickness, mitotic count, and ulceration (all of these factors are now included in T staging), (2) mitotic count replaced Clark level of invasion in patients with thin primary tumors, (3) microscopic metastases of any size (including those with only 1 cell) are classified as stage III, and (4) in patients with regional lymph node metastases, the most powerful predictors of survival are the number of lymph nodes involved, metastatic tumor burden, and ulceration and thickness of the primary tumor.

The 2 factors likely to have the most impact on patient care are the inclusion of primary tumor mitotic count and the allowance of 1 cell micrometastases. If there is only 1 mitotic figure in the dermal component of the primary tumor, the mitotic count should be reported as 1/mm^2 rather than less than 1/mm^2 (even if the total tumor volume occupies several square millimeters) (**Box 3**). Thus, a patient with a primary tumor less than 1 mm thick and 1 dermal mitotic figure (stage IB) may be offered sentinel lymph node biopsy (**Table 4**). Similarly, cases with 1 metastatic melanoma cell identified in a sentinel lymph node are staged as IIIA, and are offered completion lymphadenectomy and most likely also adjuvant therapy.

Overall, the new staging guidelines enhance the capacity to identify patients at risk for metastatic melanomas.

Table 4
Decision tree for sentinel lymph node mapping in patients with clinically localized cutaneous melanoma

Thickness	Mitosis ≥1/mm^2		Ulceration		Clark Level IV or V, Lymphovascular Invasion, or Positive Deep Biopsy Margin	
	−	+	−	+	−	+
<0.5 mm	No	Consider	No	No	No	No
0.51–0.75	No	Offer	No	Offer	No	Consider
0.76–1.0	Consider	Offer	Consider	Offer	Consider	Offer
>1–4.0	Offer	Offer	Offer	Offer	Offer	Offer
>4.0	Offer	Offer	Offer	Offer	Offer	Offer

Data from National Comprehensive Cancer Network (NCCN). Clinical practice guidelines in oncology. Fort Washington (PA): NCCN; 2011. Available at: http://www.nccn.org/professionals/physician_gls/pdf/melanoma.pdf. Accessed July, 2012.

REFERENCES

1. Balch CM, Gershenwald JE, Soong SJ, et al. Final version of 2009 AJCC melanoma staging and classification. J Clin Oncol 2009;27:6199–206.
2. Breslow A. Thickness, cross-sectional area and depth of invasion in the prognosis of cutaneous melanoma. Ann Surg 1970;172:902–8.
3. Piris A, Mihm MC Jr, Duncan LM. AJCC melanoma staging update: impact on dermatopathology practice and patient management. J Cutan Pathol 2011;38:394–400.
4. Azzola MF, Shaw HM, Thompson JF, et al. Tumor mitotic rate is a more powerful prognostic indicator than ulceration in patients with primary cutaneous melanoma: an analysis of 3661 patients from a single center. Cancer 2003;97:1488–98.
5. Karakousis GC, Gimotty PA, Botbyl JD, et al. Predictors of regional nodal disease in patients with thin melanomas. Ann Surg Oncol 2006;13:533–41.
6. Kesmodel SB, Karakousis GC, Botbyl JD, et al. Mitotic rate as a predictor of sentinel lymph node positivity in patients with thin melanomas. Ann Surg Oncol 2005;12:449–58.
7. Thompson JF, Soong SJ, Balch CM, et al. Prognostic significance of mitotic rate in localized primary cutaneous melanoma: an analysis of patients in the multi-institutional American Joint Committee on Cancer melanoma staging database. J Clin Oncol 2011;29:2199–205.
8. Edge SB, Byrd DR, Compton CC, et al, editors. AJCC cancer staging manual. 7th edition. Chicago: Springer; 2009. p. 332.
9. Gimotty PA, Van Belle P, Elder DE, et al. Biologic and prognostic significance of dermal Ki67 expression, mitoses, and tumorigenicity in thin invasive cutaneous melanoma. J Clin Oncol 2005;23:8048–56.
10. Allen AC, Spitz S. Malignant melanoma a clinicopathological analysis of the criteria for diagnosis and prognosis. Cancer 1953;6:1–45.
11. Balch CM, Murad TM, Soong SJ, et al. A multifactorial analysis of melanoma: prognostic histopathological features comparing Clark's and Breslow's staging methods. Ann Surg 1978;188:732–42.
12. Balch CM, Buzaid AC, Atkins MB, et al. A new American Joint Committee on Cancer staging system for cutaneous melanoma. Cancer 2000;88:1484–91.
13. Balch CM, Buzaid AC, Soong SJ, et al. Final version of the American Joint Committee on Cancer staging system for cutaneous melanoma. J Clin Oncol 2001;19:3635–48.
14. Clark WH Jr, Elder DE, Guerry D, et al. Model predicting survival in stage I melanoma based on tumor progression. J Natl Cancer Inst 1989;81:1893–904.
15. Ronan SG, Eng AM, Briele HA, et al. Thin malignant melanomas with regression and metastases. Arch Dermatol 1987;123:1326–30.
16. Busam KJ, Antonescu CR, Marghoob AA, et al. Histologic classification of tumor-infiltrating lymphocytes in primary cutaneous malignant melanoma. A study of interobserver agreement. Am J Clin Pathol 2001;115:856–60.
17. Clemente CG, Mihm MC Jr, Bufalino R, et al. Prognostic value of tumor infiltrating lymphocytes in the vertical growth phase of primary cutaneous melanoma. Cancer 1996;77:1303–10.
18. Jacobs J, Nierkens S, Figdor C, et al. Regulatory T cells in melanoma: the final hurdle towards effective immunotherapy? Lancet Oncol 2012;13:e32–42.
19. Soiffer R, Hodi FS, Haluska F, et al. Vaccination with irradiated, autologous melanoma cells engineered to secrete granulocyte-macrophage colony-stimulating factor by adenoviral-mediated gene transfer augments antitumor immunity in patients with metastatic melanoma. J Clin Oncol 2003;21:3343–50.
20. Hodi FS, Oble DA, Drappatz J, et al. CTLA-4 blockade with ipilimumab induces significant clinical benefit in a female with melanoma metastases to the CNS. Nat Clin Pract Oncol 2008;5:557–61.
21. Petersson F, Diwan AH, Ivan D, et al. Immunohistochemical detection of lymphovascular invasion with D2-40 in melanoma correlates with sentinel lymph node status, metastasis and survival. J Cutan Pathol 2009;36:1157–63.
22. Schmidt CR, Panageas KS, Coit DG, et al. An increased number of sentinel lymph nodes is associated with advanced Breslow depth and lymphovascular invasion in patients with primary melanoma. Ann Surg Oncol 2009;16:948–52.
23. Barnhill RL, Fine JA, Roush GC, et al. Predicting five-year outcome for patients with cutaneous melanoma in a population-based study. Cancer 1996;78:427–32.
24. Doeden K, Ma Z, Narasimhan B, et al. Lymphatic invasion in cutaneous melanoma is associated with sentinel lymph node metastasis. J Cutan Pathol 2009;36:772–80.
25. Barnhill RL, Lugassy C. Angiotropic malignant melanoma and extravascular migratory metastasis: description of 36 cases with emphasis on a new mechanism of tumour spread. Pathology 2004;36:485–90.
26. Lugassy C, Barnhill RL. Angiotropic melanoma and extravascular migratory metastasis: a review. Adv Anat Pathol 2007;14:195–201.
27. Xu X, Chen L, Guerry D, et al. Lymphatic invasion is independently prognostic of metastasis in primary cutaneous melanoma. Clin Cancer Res 2012;18:229–37.
28. Yun SJ, Gimotty PA, Hwang WT, et al. High lymphatic vessel density and lymphatic invasion underlie the adverse prognostic effect of radial growth phase regression in melanoma. Am J Surg Pathol 2011;35:235–42.

29. Xu X, Gimotty PA, Guerry D, et al. Lymphatic invasion revealed by multispectral imaging is common in primary melanomas and associates with prognosis. Hum Pathol 2008;39:901–9.

30. Gershenwald JE, Soong SJ, Balch CM, American Joint Committee on Cancer Melanoma Staging Committee. 2010 TNM staging system for cutaneous melanoma... and beyond. Ann Surg Oncol 2010;17: 1475–7.

31. Day CL Jr, Harrist TJ, Gorstein F, et al. Malignant melanoma. Prognostic significance of "microscopic satellites" in the reticular dermis and subcutaneous fat. Ann Surg 1981;194:108–12.

32. Harrist TJ, Rigel DS, Day CL Jr, et al. "Microscopic satellites" are more highly associated with regional lymph node metastases than is primary melanoma thickness. Cancer 1984;53:2183–7.

33. Murali R, Desilva C, Thompson JF, et al. Factors predicting recurrence and survival in sentinel lymph node-positive melanoma patients. Ann Surg 2011; 253:1155–64.

34. Gershenwald J, Thompson W, Mansfield PF, et al. Multi-institutional melanoma lymphatic mapping experience: the prognostic value of sentinel lymph node status in 612 stage I or II melanoma patients. J Clin Oncol 1999;27:976–83.

35. Morton D, Wen DR, Wong J, et al. Technical details of intraoperative lymphatic mapping for early stage melanoma. Arch Surg 1992;127:392–9.

36. Liu LC, Lang JE, Jenkins T, et al. Is it necessary to harvest additional lymph nodes after resection of the most radioactive sentinel lymph node in breast cancer? J Am Coll Surg 2008;207:853–8.

37. Kroon HM, Lowe L, Wong S, et al. What is a sentinel node? Re-evaluating the 10% rule for sentinel lymph node biopsy in melanoma. J Surg Oncol 2007;95: 623–8.

38. Reintgen D, Cruse CW, Wells K, et al. The orderly progression of melanoma nodal metastases. Ann Surg 1994;220:759–67.

39. Yu LL, Flotte TJ, Tanabe KK, et al. Detection of microscopic melanoma metastases in sentinel lymph nodes. Cancer 1999;86:617–27.

40. Scolyer RA, Murali R, McCarthy SW, et al. Pathologic examination of sentinel lymph nodes from melanoma patients. Semin Diagn Pathol 2008;25:100–11.

41. Clary BM, Brady MS, Lewis JJ, et al. Sentinel lymph node biopsy in the management of patients with primary cutaneous melanoma: review of a large single-institutional experience with an emphasis on recurrence. Ann Surg 2001;233:250–8.

42. Shidham VB, Qi DY, Acker S, et al. Evaluation of micrometastases in sentinel lymph nodes of cutaneous melanoma: higher diagnostic accuracy with Melan-A and MART-1 compared with S-100 protein and HMB-45. Am J Surg Pathol 2001;25: 1039–46.

43. Abrahamsen HN, Hamilton-Dutoit SJ, Larsen J, et al. Sentinel lymph nodes in malignant melanoma: extended histopathologic evaluation improves diagnostic precision. Cancer 2004;100:1683–91.

44. Scolyer RA, Thompson JF, McCarthy SW, et al. Intraoperative frozen-section evaluation can reduce accuracy of pathologic assessment of sentinel nodes in melanoma patients. J Am Coll Surg 2005; 201:821–3.

45. Thompson JF. The value of sentinel node biopsy in patients with primary cutaneous melanoma. Dermatol Surg 2008;34:550–4 [discussion: 4–5].

46. Biddle DA, Evans HL, Kemp BL, et al. Intraparenchymal nevus cell aggregates in lymph nodes: a possible diagnostic pitfall with malignant melanoma and carcinoma. Am J Surg Pathol 2003;27: 673–81.

47. Gershenwald JE, Ross MI. Sentinel-lymph-node biopsy for cutaneous melanoma. N Engl J Med 2011;364:1738–45.

48. Veenstra HJ, Wouters MJ, Kroon BB, et al. Less false-negative sentinel node procedures in melanoma patients with experience and proper collaboration. J Surg Oncol 2011;104:454–7.

49. Gershenwald JE, Colome MI, Lee JE, et al. Patterns of recurrence following a negative sentinel lymph node biopsy in 243 patients with stage I or II melanoma. J Clin Oncol 1998;16:2253–60.

50. Kanzler MH. Sentinel node biopsy and standard of care for melanoma: a re-evaluation of the evidence. J Am Acad Dermatol 2010;62:880–4.

51. Gershenwald JE, Andtbacka RH, Prieto VG, et al. Microscopic tumor burden in sentinel lymph nodes predicts synchronous nonsentinel lymph node involvement in patients with melanoma. J Clin Oncol 2008;26:4296–303.

52. Cadili A, Scolyer RA, Brown PT, et al. Total sentinel lymph node tumor size predicts nonsentinel node metastasis and survival in patients with melanoma. Ann Surg Oncol 2010;17:3015–20.

53. Balch CM, Gershenwald JE, Soong SJ, et al. Multivariate analysis of prognostic factors among 2,313 patients with stage III melanoma: comparison of nodal micrometastases versus macrometastases. J Clin Oncol 2010;28:2452–9.

Medicolegal Issues with Regard to Melanoma and Pigmented Lesions in Dermatopathology

Amanda Marsch, MD[a], Whitney A. High, MD, JD, MEng[a,b,*]

KEYWORDS

- Medicolegal issues • Melanoma • Pigmented lesion • Dermatopathology

KEY POINTS

- The misdiagnosis of skin cancer is a substantial source of medical malpractice litigation.
- Multiple lines of evidence converge to suggest that melanoma represents a substantial source of risk within dermatology and dermatopathology.
- Before considering medicolegal issues involving the misdiagnosis of melanoma, it is both appropriate and necessary to outline important general tenets in malpractice law.

INTRODUCTION

The misdiagnosis of skin cancer is a substantial source of medical malpractice litigation. A recent analysis of claims submitted to a single large national malpractice insurance carrier revealed that 8.6% of all claims against pathologists and 14.2% of claims against dermatologists involved the terms skin cancer and/or melanoma.[1]

In a 2003 study, Troxel[1] reported on 362 pathology-related claims submitted to The Doctor's Company for the years 1995 to 2001; 46 (13%) involved the misdiagnosis of melanoma.[1] Melanoma ranked second only to breast cancer as the greatest source of pathology-related malpractice claims. In 2 later articles, using the same claims database but for the years 1998 to 2003, Troxel[2,3] identified 335 pathology-based malpractice claims. The missed diagnosis of melanoma was the single most common occurrence for litigation, accounting for 42 (13%) of 335 cases. Furthermore, a recent examination of data from the Physician's Insurance Association of America found melanoma to be the most common cause of medical misadventure among dermatologists, many of whom interpret histologic specimens themselves.[4]

Multiple lines of evidence converge to suggest that melanoma represents a substantial source of risk within dermatology and dermatopathology.[1–5] The risk associated with melanoma is understandable because (1) melanocytic lesions are perhaps the most common neoplasm in humans; (2) melanoma is arguably one of the most lethal of all malignancies; (3) the distinction between benign and malignant melanocytic lesions is often vexing, even for the most skilled of dermatopathologists; and (4) melanoma is a disease that affects both the young and old, causing more years of lost life than any other malignancy except leukemia.[6,7]

With the incidence of melanoma in the United States increasing annually at 4% to 6%,[8] and the inherent medicolegal risks involved in the histologic interpretation of pigmented lesions, a review

[a] Department of Dermatology, University of Illinois at Chicago, Chicago, IL, USA; [b] Department of Pathology, University of Colorado School of Medicine, Anschutz Medical Campus, Denver, CO, USA
* Corresponding author. University of Colorado Dermatopathology Consultants, 1999 N. Fitzsimons Parkway, Bioscience East, Suite 120, Aurora, CO 80045.
E-mail address: whitney.high@ucdenver.edu

Dermatol Clin 30 (2012) 593–615
http://dx.doi.org/10.1016/j.det.2012.06.011
0733-8635/12/$ – see front matter © 2012 Elsevier Inc. All rights reserved.

of relevant medicolegal principles, suggestions to optimize care, and strategies to mitigate risk is very useful.

BASIC TENETS AND PRINCIPLES OF MALPRACTICE LITIGATION

Before considering medicolegal issues involving the misdiagnosis of melanoma, it is both appropriate and necessary to outline important tenets in malpractice law in a general sense. Malpractice is adjudicated using state law. Even for cases filed in a federal court, most substantive decisions are based on the law of the state in which the events transpired.[9] Substantial overlap exists among the states, so only a generalized overview can be provided here. Important variations may be encountered. Should readers become involved in an issue with medicolegal implications, they should consult their malpractice insurance carrier and/or a licensed attorney in the state in which they practice and/or where the event transpired. This article is not intended to provide legal advice.

COMPONENTS OF MEDICAL MALPRACTICE

The underlying principle of medical malpractice is to identify a party (the plaintiff) who has received care beneath an established standard, and also to identify a party responsible for the substandard care (the Defendant), and to compensate the injured, or the kin of the expired, to the extent that money can, for an injury or death. Malpractice therefore is a matter of civil law, and, more specifically, it is a form of tort law, or law that deals with situations in which the actions of a liable party have unfairly harmed another individual. However, few of the malpractice cases that arise in medicine are that definite or straightforward.

In the United States, which follows a common law system of justice, there are 6 requisite elements that must be established in an case of malpractice: (1) duty, (2) standard of care, (3) breach of duty, (4) cause-in-fact, (5) proximate cause, and (6) damages. These elements must be established individually for each case, and failure to prove any element (typically to a standard of more likely than not, or greater than a 50% likelihood), results in victory for the defense. To provide a better understanding of the legal process, each of these elements is discussed in greater detail later.

Duty

Duty arises through the establishment of a patient-physician relationship. In a clinical setting, duty typically is realized through taking a history and performing a physical examination. In the realm of pathology, it occurs when tissue is accessioned and examined, and a report issued.

Duty arising from so-called curbside consultations (occurrences that occur sometimes in dermatopathology) may result in a great deal of uncertainty.[10] Differing court decisions on the matter exist.[11,12] For this reason, avoidance of curbside consultation is often advocated.[13] When curbside consultation does transpire, some record of the event, even if only handwritten notes, is recommended to prevent the consulting physician's use of the advice from becoming the only documentation of the event.[13,14]

In dermatopathology, another less formal means of consultation often used is an intradepartmental second opinion. Experts suggest that intradepartmental second opinions are of great usefulness in providing optimal care in difficult cases,[15,16] but the rendering of an intradepartmental consultation should be well documented, including the names and qualifications of those involved, the date consensus was achieved, and the title of any conference at which the material was reviewed. Failure to do so renders the reasonable and prudent approach of multiple physicians undocumented.[14]

In addition, pathologists and dermatopathologists, like clinical brethren, may be vicariously liable for the actions of laboratory employees under their control/supervision, so long as the employees are acting within the scope of their duties.[17] Physicians working in education are similarly responsible for the dutiful but negligent actions of students, residents, and fellows following the legal theory of respondeat superior.

Standard of Care

The term standard of care refers to a minimum level of care owed to a patient by a physician who has incurred a duty to a patient. The term reasonable and prudent physician may appear in reference to the standard of care, but standard of care often is a matter assessed by custom. Physicians must act with the minimum knowledge and skill common to members of their profession in good standing. Although it might seem that the standard of care is simply the manner of practice for most physicians in a particular community,[18] in the legal setting the standard of care is not simply what most providers do, because courts routinely recognize the concept of a respectable minority.[19] Therefore a jury is not bound to accept only the majority approach, but may opt instead to apply a different standard, promulgated by a reasonable and respectable minority.

Furthermore, an incident occurring 5 years earlier involves the standard of care, and the state of medical knowledge, widely held at the time the care was rendered. A situation cannot be fairly judged by medical knowledge or additional testing options accrued and/or disseminated since the incident transpired. The standard of care historically was subject to geographic variation, and legal situations are still encountered that are decided on this basis; however, with improved communications, overnight couriers, and standardized national medical education, the modern trend is increasingly toward a uniform national standard.[20,21] The standard of care also may vary with respect to the level of training for a provider.

For example, a general pathologist might be held to different standard than a board-certified dermatopathologist, but, because the standard of care is established independently in each case, through expert witnesses and evidence, it is not presumed and is open to argument. Although there is little research into the matter, Trotter and Bruecks[22] showed only a 1.4% incidence of major discrepancies between general pathologists and dermatopathologists, and such evidence may be used by a plaintiff to suggest that the standard of care for a general pathologist who voluntarily interprets skin samples and a dermatopathologist is much the same. The defense may counter that the existence of a separate training process and board examination, administered jointly by the specialties of dermatology and pathology, and recognized by the American Board of Medical Specialties, suggests a more limited standard of care for general pathologists.

Furthermore, when physicians voluntarily represent themselves as experts (eg, an internist acting as medical director at a laser center, or a general pathologist electing to interpret skin specimens at an institution or in a geographic area where dermatopathology expertise is available), the plaintiff will likely contended that the physician has committed to a standard of care commensurate with this expert representation.[23] Also, a general pathologist attempting to diagnose a specialized problem that normally would call for a referral to a specialist may be held to the standard of such a specialist.[24] This detail must also be remembered when a dermatopathologist elects to interpret specimens on the cusp of dermatopathology, such as ocular or oral lesions.

In the end, with the exception of licensing requirements and/or restrictions on a scope of practice (more common for nonphysician providers than for allopathic or osteopathic physicians), the standard of care is not legislated; it is established through the testimony of 'expert witnesses. It is

the trial judge who determines whether an expert is qualified to testify about the standard of care.[25] To be qualified, an expert witness must, in general, either possess expertise equivalent to that of the accused provider, the subject matter must be of substantial overlap between disciplines of the defendant provider and the witness, or the expert must have reasonable knowledge of the scope of training of the defendant provider.

Illustrative Example 1

A plaintiff files a complaint against a podiatrist regarding an ankle injury and wishes to call an orthopedic surgeon to testify against the podiatrist. An orthopedic surgeon may not be allowed to testify as to the standard of care for a podiatrist, unless the judge finds that the orthopedic surgeon has either a detailed knowledge regarding the training and practices afforded within podiatric medicine, or the subject matter has substantial overlap between the disciplines.

Published practice guidelines, consensus conferences, or peer-reviewed articles of particular impact or merit may also be used to establish the standard of care. Regulations or societal recommendations pertaining to the operation of a pathology laboratory might be germane to the standard of care for lawsuits based on procedural or processing errors.

A suit may, rarely, be brought for which expert testimony regarding a standard of care is unnecessary, and such cases are proffered based on a legal theory of res ipsa loquitor (the thing speaks for itself).[26] For example, if a pathologist allowed a dog into the grossing room, and the dog ate a large tissue sample, res ipsa loquitor may apply to such a case, because there is no reasonable way this error could occur without negligence; experts are not required.

Breach

Breach occurs when the care rendered is less than an established standard, and it leads to a physician's liability in a malpractice action.[18] To discourage baseless suits, many states require an affidavit from a licensed physician, filed at the outset of a legal action, that states that a review of the facts justifies a reasonable likelihood of negligence existing.

Cause-in-Fact

Justice requires that an injury claimed must be the result of the alleged malpractice. Cause-in-fact causation is also referred to as but-for causation, meaning that, but for the provider's action (or inaction), the injury would not have transpired.

Proximate Cause

Proximate cause is a different legal principle, distinct from cause-in-fact, and it can be a difficult principle for laypersons to appreciate. In simple terms, proximate cause is akin to the ability to foresee a consequence of a negligent act.[27] Attacks on proximate cause are made by asserting that, considering the quality of a negligent act, any outcome was so unforeseen that it would be unjust to assign liability.

Illustrative Example 2

- A 53-year-old man was diagnosed (mistakenly) with metastatic melanoma and was informed of a poor prognosis. Based on this erroneous diagnosis, and assuming that he had no time left, the patient abandoned his family, traveled to Thailand, and spent all his money on alcohol, gambling, and brothels. He contracted human immunodeficiency virus (HIV). The error was discovered a week later, the medical record corrected, and all reasonable attempts to contact him were made, but he had left the country. The patient sues the pathologist for his financial losses and for acquisition of HIV.
- In this situation, purposefully preposterous, although the misdiagnosis might be the cause-in-fact, some of the ramifications encountered were so unforeseen that proximate cause should be contested. It would be unjust to assign liability for all the consequences (many of which might also be contested for being illegal in the United States). In contrast, if the patient sued for unnecessary diagnostic procedures and/or additional therapy or surgery, performed after the errant diagnosis was issued, both cause-in-fact and proximate cause would likely be met.

Damages

For a malpractice action to foment, harm must transpire. Compensatory damages awarded to an injured party may include special damages (tangible items) or general damages (intangible items). Special damages include medical costs (past, current, or future) and/or lost wages (past, current, or future) caused by the injury. General damages include pain, suffering, and loss of enjoyment or consortium. Punitive damages, designed to punish an offender for egregious and willful acts and to deter similar actions in the future, are not covered by insurance policies; hence, they are both infrequently sought and infrequently awarded in malpractice actions.

The severity of an injury, and the age/occupation of a patient, may affect total damages. Calculation methods may be contested fiercely, even when fault is agreed on. For example, speculation regarding potential career advancement by a plaintiff will be opposed vigorously by a defendant because of the effect it might have on damages. In general, plaintiffs often request general damages be calculated on a per diem basis (eg, $1000/d for pain and suffering for the period in question), whereas defendants often seek a lump-sum payment. Without quantifiable damages, there is no viable malpractice case, particularly to an attorney paying the bills.

Illustrative Example 3

- A melanoma is missed during initial examination of histology slides and a misdiagnosis of a benign nevus is issued instead. The dermatopathologist, later suspicious of the result, realizes his mistake a week later. An amended report is issued, and care resumes at the correct anatomic location.
- Note the difficulty in assessing damages in this case. Has the effectiveness of any potential treatment diminished over such a short time span? Emotional stress (special damages), in the absence of firm general damages, is a difficult (ie, risky) claim for a plaintiff's attorney, who will be accepting the case on a contingency basis (meaning that the attorney will only be paid if the case is settled or won). Damages in this scenario are so difficult to ascertain that it is probably unlikely that a lawsuit will result, even though the error was serious, and could have been grave had it not be detected in a timely fashion.
- As a mental exercise, keep adding 1 week to the delay in diagnosis until you think that real (ie, easily proven) damages ensue. There is no correct answer. Instead, it is a matter of opinion, and it is something that a plaintiff's attorney must evaluate carefully (with the assistance of expert medical consultants) when considering a potential suit.

OTHER AFFIRMATIVE DEFENSES

A provider may contest, legitimately, any of the 6 requisite elements of a prima facie malpractice case. To this end, defendants may use their own experts to contest a duty, to provide an alternative standard of care, or even to contest causation or damages. However, other affirmative defenses may exist, the most common of which is a case that is outside of the statute of limitations for that particular jurisdiction and circumstances.

Statute of Limitations

Malpractice suits must be filed in a timely manner; it would not be practical or just for a physician to be sued for an incident occurring 30 years previously because records may be destroyed, witnesses may have died, memories of the events may be unreliable. Therefore, each state has a statute of limitation applicable to medical malpractice. These statutes bar prosecution of a case that was not commenced within a prescribed period of time. In most states, the allocated time period ranges from 1 to 5 years, but exceptions exist. For example, the time period may not commence at the moment of the negligence but instead may begin when a reasonable person would have been made aware of the injury.

Illustrative Example 4

A patient sought care for a mole from a dermatologist who then performed a biopsy, and interpreted the lesion himself as a benign nevus. Two years later, the patient sought care for the same lesion from a plastic surgeon, who called for the earlier tissue to be reexamined by another facility. The original dermatologist reexamined the tissue before release and realized it was a melanoma. The dermatologist amended his report more than 2 years after the original date of service, and the state had a 2-year statute of limitations. The patient sued, and the dermatologist claimed the statute of limitations had expired before assertion of her claim.

The court had several ways to dispose of this case. It could have ruled the statute of limitations had commenced (1) at the time of the initial biopsy (as the defendant contended), (2) when the patient sought additional care for the recurrent neoplasm, or (3) when the report was amended (as contended by the plaintiff).

The court ruled that the statute of limitation began to toll when the injury occurred, and that injury occurred at the point when the patient's melanoma moved from the epidermis to the dermis.[28] The court concluded that, absent evidence to the

contrary, this event had occurred within the last 2 years; hence, the case was timely. The matter was settled.

The decision in illustrative example 4 highlights several important points:

1. The timing as it relates to the statute of limitations may be contested and does not simply begin to toll from a date of service or from when a histology report is issued.
2. Any affirmative defense pertaining to a statute of limitation must be raised by the defendant, and evidence must be supplied.
3. The court may decide medical matters in a way that is counterintuitive to physicians, but is designed to achieve an equitable end.

In addition, for minors, the statute of limitations may be suspended until a patient reaches a specified age of majority (often 18 years of age, but varying from state to state). This exception substantially prolongs the susceptibility of providers to suits arising from the care of children.[29] In dermatopathology, this issue may be of particular relevance to experts who render diagnoses of Spitz nevi or atypical spitzoid proliferations in children.

BUSINESS ASPECTS OF MEDICAL MALPRACTICE

In general, a private law firm is a business. Expenses are incurred for front office staff, paralegals, society memberships, licensing fees, and continuing legal education, just as is the case for most private medical practices. Most malpractice cases are accepted on a contingency basis; the attorney accepts a percentage of ultimate collections, but in turn provides all the money for expenses. If no verdict or settlement is reached, these expenses become losses to the firm. The economic realities of this system affect the cases that a law firm will accept. From the perspective of a plaintiff's attorney, an ideal case consists of easily proven substandard care that resulted in readily quantifiable damages. Two separate studies showed that 67% to 82% of medical malpractice cases were disposed of without any type of indemnity payment[30,31]; however, there is an escalating trend in the amount of indemnity payments,[32] perhaps changing the aggregate dynamics over time.

As such, it seems that a plaintiff's attorney is not interested in close calls, or cases exemplified by subtle differences of opinion that may be difficult for a jury to comprehend. It is estimated that only about 1 in every 30 calls to law offices results in a medical malpractice case that the firm is willing to pursue.[24] Although persuasive articles have been written about the detrimental consequences of a judicial system based on contingency fees, the resultant economic incentives and disincentives act as a screen against cases of lesser merit.[33]

DAMAGE CAPS

Damages caps are statutory limits placed on damages. Such caps may apply only to general damages, for noneconomic harms such as pain or emotional distress, or, more rarely, state legislatures may impose total damage cap, particularly with regard to public entities. For example, physicians employed by the University of Colorado and caring for patients under those auspices have a total damage cap of $150,000 per person per incident.[34] Other states, most notably Oregon, have had a varied experience with damage caps, having experienced periods with low damage caps ($200,000) for public entities, as well as periods without a damage cap at all, even for public entities. During the period with an absence of damage caps, Oregon Health Sciences University, the public medical entity for the state of Oregon, estimated that an additional $20 million per year was spent on additional insurance costs because of the uncontained risk. Damage caps may also affect decisions attorneys make about accepting cases.

INCLUSION OF PHOTOMICROGRAPHS

There has recently been debate regarding the inclusion of photomicrographs in pathology reports. With the constant advancements in color digital photography and photomicrography, more and more facilities are opting to include these images as part of the final pathology report. However, opponents to the inclusion of images in pathology reports suggest that this act may distribute liability, making the clinician obligated to also correctly interpret the image.[35]

Although to the best of our knowledge this remains a theoretic debate, without any substantive case law on the matter, the situation may be of greater peril to dermatologists, because their training includes substantial training in dermatopathology, and this expertise is publicly acknowledged by the American Board of Dermatology. In response to this situation, some laboratories have added legal disclaimers to reports containing images that state that any inclusion is for illustrative purposes only. In addition, because digital photography permits manipulation of an image, it

may also pose a potential risk for unintentional misrepresentation or even fraudulent activity.[36]

INTERPRETATION OF HISTOLOGY SPECIMENS ACROSS STATE LINES

The American Medical Association and the College of American Pathologists (CAP) define telemedicine as "the delivery of health care services via electronic or digital means from a health care provider in one location to a patient in another."[37,38] Although telepathology is often considered to be only the correlate of other forms of traditional telemedicine, such as teledermatology, and assume that this means that the image must be viewed electronically, this is not the case, and the sending of pathology reports to another state suffices to bring the practice under the auspices of telemedicine legislation in states that have such regulations.[38]

Therefore, simply having a medical license in the state in which you reside/practice does not permit you to participate in medicine that affects citizens of other states. State law may differ, but it may be necessary for those practicing medicine on citizens of one state to have either a telemedicine license from that state, or even a full license, depending on circumstances.[39] However, some state laws do not address the issue of interstate practice of medicine.[37,39]

CAP defines the sending of wet-tissue specimens (specimens in formalin) from one state to another state for processing and interpretation as the "interstate practice of pathology." According to CAP, pathologists interpreting specimens, slides, or images sent through interstate commerce should be fully licensed in the state where the patient presents for diagnosis, with the exception being occasional cases sent in consultation.[38] Most states allow for consultations sent to out-of-state consultants so long as participation in care is infrequent, and such out-of-state experts do not consult directly with, or provide medical services directly to, patients in the state from which the consultation originated.

Table 1 shows the penalties potentially incurred for practicing medicine across a state lines without appropriate licensure, as they currently exist or can be deciphered from legislation and case law. Should a dermatopathologist be anticipating regular and routine business from an out-of-state provider, in the form of wet tissue and first opinions, as opposed to infrequent consultation, it would be prudent to either ascertain the specific licensing requirements in the state from which the tissue is to originate (full license vs special-purpose/telemedicine license, and so forth), or

Table 1
Potential penalties for the practice of medicine across state lines without appropriate licensure

Violation is a Misdemeanor	Violation is Felony	Exempt from Licensure Requirement Violations if Holding an Active License in Home State	Penalty for Violation Determined on an Individual Basis/Current Statutes are Unclear
Alaska	Arizona	Minnesota	Connecticut
Alabama	Delaware	South Carolina	Nebraska
Arkansas	Florida	Utah	New Jersey
California	Georgia	—	—
Colorado[a]	Guam	—	—
District of Columbia	Idaho	—	—
New Hampshire	Illinois	—	—
Hawaii	Indiana	—	—
Iowa	Kentucky	—	—
Kansas	Michigan	—	—
Louisiana	Missouri	—	—
Maine	New Mexico	—	—
Maryland	New York	—	—
Massachusetts	Nevada	—	—
Mississippi	North Carolina		
Montana	Ohio	—	—
New Hampshire	Oklahoma	—	—
North Dakota	Oregon	—	—
Pennsylvania	Puerto Rico	—	—
Rhode Island	Vermont	—	—
South Dakota	Virgin Islands	—	—
Tennessee	—	—	—
Texas	—	—	—
Virginia[a]	—	—	—
West Virginia[b]	—	—	—
Wisconsin	—	—	—
Wyoming	—	—	—

[a] First violation is a misdemeanor, second or third violations are felonies.
[b] Violations that occur for more than 90 days may be felonies.

simply to follow the CAP recommendation of seeking full licensure in the state of interest.

SELF-INTERPRETATION OF DERMATOPATHOLOGY CASES AND CONSULTATION

Some dermatologists prefer to interpret histologic specimens generated by their dermatology practice. A recent study identified male dermatologists and dermatologists practicing in the western United States to be more likely to interpret their own specimens.[40] In defense of this practice, it has been reported that dermatology trainees receive more dermatopathology training than do general pathology trainees, and board certification in dermatology includes testing on the correct interpretation of dermatopathology material.[41] It is estimated that dermatology residency training programs devote twice as many training hours to dermatopathology compared with general pathology residency programs.[42]

However, cases are often of sufficient difficulty to justify consultation with an expert. In dermatopathology, this may be a dermatologist consulting a dermatopathologist, but it may also be a general pathologist, or even a dermatopathologist, consulting another dermatopathologist with unique and recognized expertise in some domain. In general terms, dermatologists and general pathologists tend to consult most often on benign melanocytic lesions, benign nonmelanocytic lesions, and inflammatory conditions, whereas dermatopathologists tend to consult other dermatopathologists most often on benign and malignant melanocytic lesions.[43]

Dermatopathology is a subspecialty recognized by the American Board of Medical Specialties. Therefore, in a medicolegal situation, it will be asserted that dermatopathologists are most qualified to interpret difficult pigmented lesions.[44,45] Jean Bolognia, Professor of Dermatology at Yale, has likened the relationship between dermatologists, general pathologists, and dermatopathologists to overlapping bell curves.[44] Summarizing Dr Bolognia's argument, although it is possible that a non-dermatopathologist (dermatologist or general pathologist) might be far enough to the right of a bell curve measuring diagnostic prowess in dermatopathology to surpasse an individual of lesser prowess who is to the left of a separate bell curve measuring the prowess of dermatopathologists, in most circumstances, at least in theory (and perhaps in the opinion of a jury), the average dermatopathologist would be superior in assessing disease of the skin under the microscope.

Therefore, it is likely prudent that consultative expertise be sought, particularly in regard to problematic melanocytic neoplasms and other lesions that are not routinely encountered by the general pathologist, or by the dermatologist interpreting his/her own specimens. In a 2003 examination of melanoma litigation, Troxel[1] noted that a significant number of lawsuits against pathologists involved melanoma mistaken for a Spitz nevus. Troxel[1] advised that, if a general pathologist is not routinely involved in the interpretation of Spitz nevi (ie, has sufficient experience and regular exposure), and the patient is more than 20 years of age, the case should be sent to an expert.[2] He advised that, even if Spitz nevi are being seen on a regular basis in a general pathology practice and the patient is more than 20 years of age, unless all of the diagnostic criteria are present for a Spitz nevi (ie, the case is textbook in its features), the case should still be sent to an expert.[1]

One recent study involving 1887 lesions submitted for consultation to an expert panel found that a second opinion from an expert pathologist on melanocytic neoplasms prevented significant misdiagnosis (defined by changes in patient management) in 27% of cases.[46] The most frequently submitted differential diagnosis for consultation was Spitz nevus versus melanoma.[46] Furthermore, a recent study by Shoo and colleagues[47] observed a discordance rate for melanoma of 15% during a 2-year period when comparing the diagnoses of referring centers with 1 large expert dermatopathology center in California, suggesting that consultation affected the results and, therefore, patient care. In sum, there should likely be a low threshold for seeking consultative opinion on difficult melanocytic neoplasms among prudent dermatologists, general pathologists, and dermatopathologists.[48]

OPPORTUNITIES TO IMPROVE CARE FOR MELANOMA AND PIGMENTED LESIONS

In 1990, a review of 30,000 hospital records in New York reported that a medical error was discovered in the care of 1 of every 25 patients, but a lawsuit was filed in less than 4% of cases in which error transpired.[49,50] Nevertheless, even if malpractice lawsuits are rarer than news headlines suggest, the process of being sued, whether merited or unwarranted, is traumatic for the physician involved. Prevention is the best strategy.

To this end, this article presents a dozen suggestions to improve the quality of care of pigmented lesions. These suggestions are culled from multiple sources, the authors' experiences, and the shared experiences of colleagues and mentors.

Suggestion 1: Beware of Low-Power Imitators of Benignity (Nevoid Melanoma)

Examination of pigmented lesions at low magnification is often an excellent indicator of benignity, but it is not an infallible tool. Use of productivity standards in dermatopathology, with an emphasis on high slide throughput and rapid turnaround time, may lead to medical error.[1] Under these pressures, melanoma with the low-power architecture of a benign nevus, but the biologic (and lethal) behavior of melanoma, may be missed under such a system. Although the nosology of nevoid melanoma may be debated, the existence of melanoma with features that, on low magnification, resemble a benign nevus is an undeniable occurrence[51–57]; thus, the concept should not be discounted because of semantics alone.

Nevoid melanoma presents clinically as a dome-shaped or verrucous lesion with little, if any, junctional activity or pagetoid extent in the epidermis.[51] Lateral symmetry may be deceiving for benignity, but nevoid melanoma typically is not symmetric at the base.[52] On histology, there may be an appearance of maturation (pseudomaturation) in nevoid melanoma, but examination at higher magnification often refutes this perception, because nuclei are roughly the same size at all levels of the dermis, although cells may seem smaller in the deeper dermis because nests are smaller.[53] The most helpful histologic features for recognizing nevoid melanoma are hypercellularity, cytologic atypia, and the presence of dermal mitoses (**Fig. 1**A and B), but such features are difficult to detect without a careful examination at higher magnification.[1,52]

Immunohistochemical analysis using HMB-45 and Ki67 may be of some use in showing lack of maturation or an increased proliferative index, respectively. Lack of maturation may be evidenced either by abnormal preservation of HMB-45 expression in the deep dermis in the bulk of the lesion (a lack of zonation), or by an irregular patchy staining that does not conform to any orderly pattern.[53] Use of HMB-45 is not an infallible means of detection for nevoid melanoma, because HMB-45 negative cases have been reported.[54] In addition, fluorescence in situ hybridization (FISH) analysis has been used to distinguish nevoid melanoma from benign nevi with mitotic figures, but the data supporting this practice, at present, are limited.[55] Key features of nevoid melanoma are summarized in **Box 1**.

Suggestion 2: Beware of a Partial Biopsy

Partial biopsy, as a concept, assumes that a clinician can reasonably predict, by inspection with the naked eye alone, the portion of a larger and suspicious lesion that, when sampled, will provide the relevant histologic findings to diagnose the whole of the lesion. In dermatopathology, as in all of pathology, in which diagnoses are based on subjective morphologic assessment, it is intuitive that errors in diagnosis and staging will be more frequent with partial sampling.[58–62]

Partial biopsy was responsible for more than 50% of false-negative melanoma misdiagnoses among surgical pathology claims to a US medical indemnity provider.[1,63] Biopsies of all suspicious melanocytic processes likely to be melanoma would ideally be a complete excision, with a margin

> **Box 1**
> Key features of nevoid melanoma
>
> 1. Predominance of nevoid-appearing cells[53]
> 2. General overall lateral symmetry at low magnification
> 3. Subtle lack of maturation among melanocytes at high magnification[53]
> 4. Slight pleomorphism and nuclear atypia at high magnification[53]
> 5. Prominent nucleoli[56]
> 6. Possible features of melanoma in situ in the overlying junctional component[53]
> 7. Mitotic figures in the deeper portions of the lesion[53,56]
> 8. Lack of zonation or patchy immunostaining with HMB-45, or possibly overexpression of leptin by immunostaining[53,57]
> 9. An increased proliferative index by Ki67 immunostaining[53]
> 10. Copy number abnormalities in chromosome 6 or 11 as assessed by FISH-based testing[55]

of adjacent normal skin. However, this is rarely the case, and many experts think that increased use of shave biopsies is driven by cost considerations.[64] It is therefore ironic that any cost savings realized by partial sampling may be trivial compared with the cost and emotional turmoil associated with a malpractice claim.[1]

In addition to misdiagnosis, partial sampling may also lead to inaccurate assessments of tumor thickness, affecting prognosis in melanoma (**Fig. 2**). Significant microstaging inaccuracy has been reported in 16% to 43% of partial biopsies.[63] Therefore, we contend that at a minimum, it is imperative that the care provider inform the dermatopathologist when a partial sampling is being submitted, and, furthermore, it is equally important that the dermatopathologist inform the referring

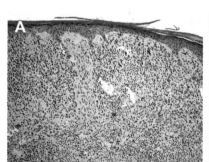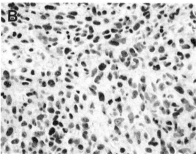

Fig. 1. Nevoid melanoma may at first mimic a simple dermal or compound nevus, particularly on low power (*A*; hematoxylin and eosin [H&E], 50×) but one of the most reliable histologic findings on close inspection is that of increased dermal mitotic figures (*B*; H&E, 200×).

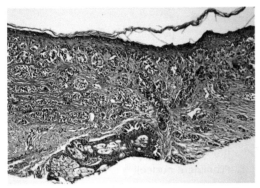

Fig. 2. Partial sampling of a lesion may complicate analysis. In this case, involving a 79-year-old man, a diagnosis of melanoma was rendered at 2 different academic centers, with genetic abnormalities detected by FISH-based analysis. However, the first shave sampling revealed a depth of at least 0.5 mm to the deep surgical margin, but subsequent reexcision revealed a melanoma of 1.5 mm in greatest depth (H&E, 50x).

practitioner when a sample is inadequate for analysis, in particular for exclusion of a particular diagnosis of interest.

Nevertheless, it is important to understand that, on occasion, circumstances may render it detrimental, or even impossible, to obtain an excisional specimen. For example, there may be cosmetic or functional considerations associated with use of a partial biopsy. Lentigo maligna, a form of melanoma in situ most commonly seen on faces of elderly patients, can reach a diameter of several centimeters or more, making an excisional biopsy difficult and excessively morbid, particularly if the lesion is ultimately deemed benign. In such situations, a broad shave or multiple punches or multiple incisional ellipses may be useful, with emphasis on the thickest and/or darkest areas of the lesion.[65] Furthermore, when a partial sampling is used, it is incumbent on the practitioner to communicate the degree of clinical suspicion and the size of the overall lesion (as discussed later). In addition, the practitioner may guide the pathologist further by providing a clinical and/or dermoscopic image to ensure that clinical features are understood and histologic sampling is optimal.[58]

Other than excisional technique, there are 4 additional methods of cutaneous biopsy that may acceptably be used under certain conditions: superficial shave biopsy, saucerization (deep shave or scoop shave), punch biopsy, and incisional biopsy (with a scalpel). Punch biopsies are typically most appropriate when the melanocytic lesion is suspected to be deep, and especially if the entirety of the lesion can be captured within

the trephine.[66] Care must be taken not to crush the specimen with forceps when using a punch technique. Incisional biopsy uses a scalpel and surgical technique similar to excision except that the entirety of the lesion is not sampled. This technique is most appropriate when lesions are too large to be completely excised, or when time does not permit a full excision.[66] Incisional biopsies should generally attempt to include the most heavily pigmented or thickest parts of a pigmented lesion.

Superficial shave biopsies are a topic of recent debate. One study assessed this technique by retrospectively analyzing melanomas initially diagnosed by shave biopsy with a Breslow depth less than 2 mm.[67] The deep margin on the shave biopsy was positive in 224 (37%) of the 600 patients. After definitive wide excision, residual tumor was found in 133 patients (22%), and a potential change in staging, with a new recommendation for sentinel lymph node biopsy, occurred in 8 patients (1.3% of the cohort). The investigators reported an insignificant impact on recurrence, disease-specific survival rates, and overall survival rates, although the median follow-up was only 12 months.[67] Although this is an intriguing study, with such a short median follow-up, superficial shave specimens are still generally considered to be inappropriate for the sampling of pigmented lesions that are reasonably suspected to be melanoma, with the exception of lentigo maligna, a clinically distinct and histologically junctional process.

Another point of controversy in dermatology involves the saucerization of lesions. Unlike a superficial shave biopsy, saucerization is a deep shave, going beneath the lesion, to accomplish a sampling similar to an excision but with greater expediency for the physician and patient alike. Experts in skin cancer have expressed favorable opinions regarding saucerization.[68] Evidence suggests that, when saucerization is performed by a skilled and experienced physician, the results are comparable with those rendered by excision.[69]

Suggestion 3: Beware of Inflamed Lesions

A vigorous inflammatory host response can be an important sign of a malignant process that is being rejected by the body, and urges careful and close examination of all lichenoid processes occurring on sun-damaged skin for evidence of a malignant condition (**Fig. 3**A–C). Nevertheless, there are also cases of a lichenoid inflammatory reaction leading to inflammatory pseudomelanocytic nests along the dermoepidermal junction that mimic melanoma in situ.[70,71]

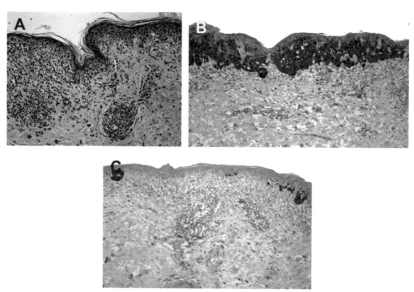

Fig. 3. Highlighting the difficulty in analyzing densely inflamed lesions, this lesion manifested a lichenoid infiltrate complicating identification of a melanocytic proliferation (*A*; H&E, 100×), but an immunohistochemical stain with Melan-A on a subsequent excisional sampling revealed a contiguous atypical melanocytic neoplasm (*B*, Melan-A with counterstain 100×), and areas of marked regression of the junctional component (*C*, Melan-A with counterstain, 100×).

To this end, the identification of a melanocytic neoplasm at the dermoepidermal junctional may be facilitated by use of monoclonal antibody stains like S100, HMB-45, Melan-A, Microphthalmia-associated transcription factor (MITF), and tyrosinase, but recent studies have highlighted cases in which the use of these immunohistochemical stains gives rise to false-positive immunoreactivity among inflammatory pseudomelanocytic nests. In particular, Melan-A has been implicated in these cases of immunopositive pseudonesting. One study described several diagnoses of melanoma in situ on sun-damaged skin that were based on strong Melan-A positivity; however, clinicopathologic correlation revealed the presence of lichenoid dermatitis in all 3 cases.[70]

A subsequent report described a series of 2 similar cases that were initially misdiagnosed as melanoma in situ, likely as a result of Mart-1 positivity of the pseudomelanocytic nests that were then distinguished by MITF.[72] These investigators concluded that MITF is a more useful marker for evaluating lentiginous proliferations along the dermoepidermal junction, particularly when dealing with the differential diagnosis of lichenoid reaction with pseudomelanocytic nests versus melanoma in situ.[72] However, complicating this assertion is the report of MART-1/Melan-A–positive staining in pseudomelanocytic nests as well as focal S100 protein, MITF, and SOX10 positivity.[73] The mixed experience of multiple immunostains in falsely

marking inflammatory pseudonesting confounds any single approach to distinguishing inflammatory pseudonesting from true melanocytic nesting, and, taken in aggregate, it suggests a need for clear communication of the clinical situation and emphasizes the importance of clinicopathologic correlation in evaluating difficult cases.

Suggestion 4: Beware of Spitz Nevi and Other Spindled Melanocytic Neoplasms

Spitz nevi were first described by Sophie Spitz[74] in 1948 and were referred to as juvenile melanoma. Spitz nevi are difficult melanocytic lesions that possess melanoma-like features, but typically, at least in classic form, are distinguishable from melanoma.[75] In contrast, spitzlike melanoma shares some microscopic features with Spitz nevi, but is expected to have a preponderance of malignant features. In addition, borderline or atypical spitzoid neoplasms seemingly have features that overlap significantly with both Spitz nevi and melanoma. It seems that these borderline spitzoid neoplasms are likely the most controversial entities with regard to diagnosis and treatment because of the uncertain biologic potential (**Fig.** 4A–C) and sentinel node involvement in a large number of cases, without any observed detriment in survival.[76]

One of the best initial clinical discriminators is the age of the patient: Spitz nevi are common in children, accounting for approximately 1% of

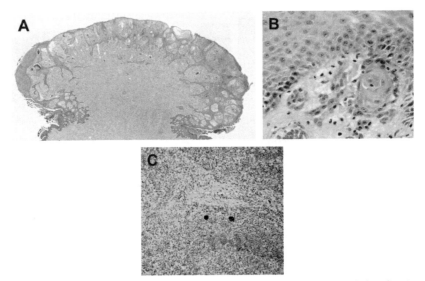

Fig. 4. Spitzoid neoplasms in young adults can be problematic and defy conventional classification, such as this exophytic atypical spitzoid neoplasm arising over a reported period of 3 weeks on the leg of a 19-year-old woman (*A*; H&E, 12.5×). The lesion manifested some nesting, poor maturation but also Kamino bodies, and other spitzoid features (*B*; H&E 200×). Although signed out as an atypical Spitz tumor with uncertain biologic potential, sentinel lymph node sampling revealed just 2 Melan-A–positive cells in the lymph node (*C*, Melan-A with counterstain, 100×), the significance of which remains unclear because the patient is without disease after 4 years of follow-up.

excised nevi,[75] whereas melanoma is not common in this same population. Nearly half to two-thirds of all Spitz nevi occur in individuals younger than 20 years.[75] In adults, melanoma is more prominent, and Spitz nevi, particularly newly arising Spitz nevi, occur more rarely.

Most Spitz nevi are characterized by spindled and epithelioid cells, with superior clefting at the dermoepidermal junction, fascicular recapitulation in the dermis, and Kamino bodies at the interface between the nests and the epidermis. Overlapping features with melanoma may include limited pagetoid extension and a few superficial mitotic figures. Criteria for classifying atypical Spitz lesions have been proposed but are inconsistently practiced and are without firm consensus.[77] These criteria are based on the size of the lesion, the presence of pathologic features (ulceration and mitotic activity), and the age of the patient. Scores reflect the potential for malignancy. Such criteria attempt to remove subjective, nonvalidated criteria for these atypical lesions.[75] These criteria also emphasize that distinguishing Spitz nevi from melanoma is best achieved by assessing evidence taken in the context of the clinical presentation.

Potential histologic clues that favor Spitz nevus include symmetry of the lesion and the absence of significant pleomorphism, deep mitoses, pagetoid spread, and extension into surrounding structures.[75] In contrast, melanoma is typically a larger,

asymmetric, poorly demarcated lesion in which nests are variable in size, shape, and orientation; Kamino bodies are typically absent but can be present in early melanoma.[75,78] Immunohistochemistry can help support a diagnosis of a Spitz lesion rather than melanoma; however, there is often overlap. Ki67/MIB-1 is a particularly helpful marker for distinguishing Spitz nevi from melanoma.[75,79–81] In this regard, at least some experts have postulated the general rule that, for difficult spitzoid neoplasms, benignity is favored by a Ki67/MIB-1 proliferative index of less than 2%, whereas malignancy is favored by a Ki67/MIB-1 proliferative index of greater than 10%, with indeterminate lesions suggested by 2% to 10%.[82,83]

Emerging studies reporting use of comparative genomic hybridization (CGH) and array CGH as ancillary evidence for distinguishing Spitz nevi from melanoma seem promising.[84,85] These studies have shown significant genetic differences between histologically benign nevi, including Spitz nevi, and melanoma. Although preliminary, studies using FISH-based genotypic assays may also facilitate the evaluation of atypical spitzoid proliferations.[86] The issue of sentinel lymph node sampling for atypical spitzoid proliferations is still a matter of debate. However, it is uniformly recommended that a Spitz nevus with atypical features should always be sent for expert review by a dermatopathologist.[87,88] Furthermore, it is the recommendation of many experts that all spitzoid neoplasms be completely excised, irrespective of a patient's age.[89]

Pigmented spindled cell nevus (of Reed) was once thought to be a variant of Spitz nevus, but it is now considered by many experts to be a distinct entity that, like Spitz nevi, may be confused and misdiagnosed as melanoma.[90] Because of the pigmentary incontinence associated, a spindled cell nevus (of Reed) may mimic a regressing melanoma with nodular melanosis.[91] Features suspicious for melanoma include larger lesions, more hyperchromatic nuclei, and a paucity of epidermal rete. The presence of solar elastosis in the background also seemingly favors melanoma. Other factors favoring a spindled cell nevus include younger age, monomorphic and banal-appearing melanocytes, even distribution of pigment, and a superficial quality, with restriction to the epidermis and papillary dermis. Because of diagnostic difficulties in distinguishing a spindled cell nevus (of Reed), from a Spitz nevus or a melanoma, consultation in these cases is also likely to be appropriate.

Suggestion 5: Beware of Regressed Lesions

The prognostic implication of regression in a primary melanoma is a controversial issue, and it cannot be handled in full in this article, but it is estimated that partial regression occurs in 10% to 35% of cases of melanoma.[92] Partial regression may consist only of dermal fibrosis and a chronic inflammatory infiltrate. Complete regression, albeit more rare, is also well recognized, with many well-documented cases reported in the literature.[93,94] Of the documented cases of complete regression in malignant melanoma, survival has been variable, ranging from 6 weeks to 11 years after diagnosis.[94] It is likely that this variation is even more substantial when considering all the untoward and unreported cases that occur.

On histopathology, complete regression may show attenuation of the epidermis, decreased epidermal melanocytes, papillary dermal fibrosis, a chronic inflammatory infiltrate, and telangiectasias. Nodular melanosis or tumoral melanosis are terms describing extensive deposition of dermal melanophages, but this appearance is not invariably caused by regressed melanoma alone.[95]

The importance of identifying regression in a biopsy or excision is 2-fold. First, partial regression may alter a therapeutic approach to an otherwise thin melanoma. Some investigators have found partial regression to be an adverse prognostic indicator,[96–101] probably because of preexisting deeper extent of the melanoma, whereas others failed to show this relationship.[102–111] Although immediate consensus is unlikely, the prudent pathologist/dermatopathologist may decrease medicolegal risk by noting the presence of regression and informing the clinician and/or patient of the observation so that additional investigation can commence. Counseling with regard to management or prognosis may be broadened or adjusted. Although some institutions have proposed sentinel lymph node examinations on what normally would be considered thin melanomas when extensive regression is noted,[97,112,113] other investigations have identified no association between regression and lymph node status.[114,115]

Second, when evidence of complete regression of a pigmented lesion is observed, a prudent pathologist/dermatopathologist should clearly communicate the finding of tumoral melanosis or nodular melanosis to the clinician, so that additional clinical and historical correlation may transpire.[93] Perhaps the clinician will be privy to data that would readily explain, in some manner, the observation of such histologic findings, or perhaps a more vigorous search for malignancy will be commissioned, such as a full skin examination, ocular examination, chest radiograph, imaging of the body or central nervous system, or even lymph node sampling; in each case, the manner of investigation is guided by unique clinical and historical circumstances, including the age of the patient, the size of the lesion, relevant past medical history, and other clinical and historical factors.

Suggestion 6: Beware of Desmoplastic Melanoma

Desmoplastic melanoma (DM) is a rare spindle cell malignancy that usually develops on the sun-damaged skin of elderly patients. However, these elderly patients are also predisposed to other spindle cell neoplasms, such as spindle cell squamous carcinoma and atypical fibroxanthoma. Characteristic histopathologic features of DM include spindle-shaped melanocytes, prominent desmoplasia, and frequent neurotropism. Pure DM and combined melanomas (with both desmoplastic and epithelioid components) have been described (**Fig. 5**A–C). Although a better prognosis has been postulated for DM, at least when matched for depth with conventional melanoma, in most cases a DM is more often diagnosed in longer-standing, and thereby thicker, melanomas and this may complicate the prognostic situation.

In a recent study of 113 cases of DM, it was discovered that the dermal process was associated with overlying melanoma in situ in 81% of

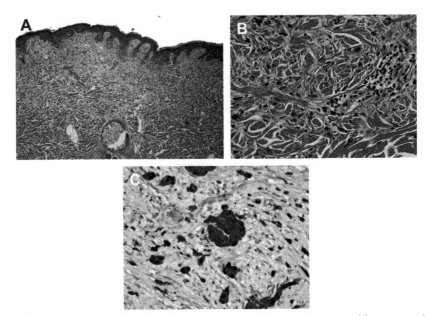

Fig. 5. Desmoplastic melanoma can be difficult to recognize. In this case, interpreted by a general pathologist, the melanoma in situ was recognized (A; H&E, 12.5×), but the subtle atypical spindled melanocytic process in the dermis, intercalated between and among the collagen bundles, was not initially recognized as a dermal, invasive, desmoplastic component (B; H&E, 200×) until later review by a dermatopathologist, and confirmation with an immunostain (C; S100 with counterstain, 200×).

cases, usually of the lentigo maligna subtype.[116] Solar elastosis was seen in 82% of the cases and the mean Breslow thickness at diagnosis was 4.1 mm.[113–116] The mitotic rate among the malignant melanocytes was low, being less than 1 mitosis/mm^2 in 72% of cases. With regard to pigmentation, 71% of the cases of DM were amelanotic.[116] Although a significant portion of DM is amelanotic, when DM does arise with melanoma in situ, the pigmented junctional component often provides an important clue to the melanocytic lineage of the process.[56] Therefore, a major diagnostic dilemma occurs when DM arises without an associated junctional melanocytic proliferation. In cases such as this, lesions may mimic a cicatrix, dermatofibroma, nevus, basal cell carcinoma, neuroma, or cyst.[56] DM is often bottom heavy, with cellular atypia being more pronounced in the deeper extents of the process.[52] If the possibility of desmoplastic melanoma is being entertained for a lesion that is only superficially sampled, it is wise to recommend consideration of a second, and more generous, biopsy.

In addition, immunohistochemical studies may be necessary to confirm the diagnosis, but it is important to recall that DM may often be HMB-45 negative. In the present literature, the 2 most useful immunohistochemical markers are S100 protein and p75 nerve growth factor receptor (Fig. 6A–C).[116] However, caution must be exercised when interpreting S100 stains in regard to reexcision specimens because nonneoplastic, S100-reactive cells are common in scars associated with prior biopsies or excisions.[56,117] These markers, in combination with careful histopathologic analysis, facilitate early diagnosis and thus improve prognosis (**Box 2**).

Suggestion 7: Beware of Confusion with Atypical/Dysplastic Nevi and Atypical Lentiginous Melanocytic Lesions

In many areas of the United States, the degree of atypia within dysplastic nevi is graded, although the practice is controversial.[118,119] In some areas, grading of dysplastic nevi is an expectation of patients and clinicians alike.[120] However, there remains little agreement about which criteria are most significant within grading schemes. Despite the controversy, the degree of atypia has been shown to correlate with risk of melanoma.[119] Even for those who do not formally grade lesions, reexcision of Clark nevi that have troubling features, or indeterminate biologic potential, or features of incipient melanoma, is often recommended. Regardless of the terminology or philosophy used, it seems to be understood that certain abnormal nevi (atypical/dysplastic nevi or Clark

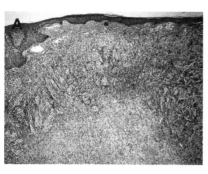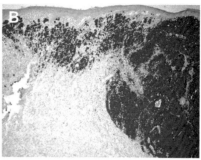

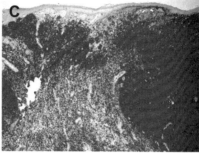

Fig. 6. In a melanoma with multiple morphologic clones, both epithelioid and spindled in appearance (*A*; H&E, 50×), Melan-A fails to mark affirmatively the spindle cell population (*B*; Melan-A with counterstain, 50×), whereas S100, widely regarded as among the most sensitive of immunohistochemical stains for melanocytes, marks affirmatively both the epithelioid and spindled populations (*C*; S100 with counterstain, 50×). This case shows the limitations of some immunostains in detecting spindled melanocytic neoplasms.

nevi) show histopathologic features that overlap with melanoma, often to such a degree that distinction is difficult.

In this situation, several additional pieces of information must be considered in making the diagnosis. For example, the nature of the biopsy

---

Box 2
Key features of DM

1. Mitotic figures may be present, but generally there is a low mitotic rate among the spindled cells[116]

2. Cytologic atypia is often more pronounced in deeper regions of the desmoplastic process

3. Lymphoid aggregates may be present[56]

4. There may be an overlying intraepidermal melanocytic proliferation (often lentigo maligna)[116]

5. Mucinous stroma is possible[56]

6. Perineural invasion may be present and is thought to explain the observation of greater local recurrence than was expected

7. S100 and p75 are reportedly of greatest sensitivity in detecting the proliferation[116]

(partial vs complete), and/or the status of surgical margins may prompt further advice to the referring clinician. In addition, the clinical history of a new-onset lesion or changing lesion may provoke additional concern, especially in an older patient. Dysplastic nevi are uncommon on the face compared with other sites, and therefore a diagnosis of lentigo maligna, or another form of melanoma, must be firmly and carefully excluded on this anatomic site.[119]

Astute or informative clinicians may describe specific portions of the lesions that are suspicious, such as nevus with peripherally-located black spot or central nodule. In this case, the dermatopathologist should ensure that these areas are well shown in histologic sections.[119] In addition, a prior history of sampling or other trauma is essential, because recurrent nevi (those continuing to persist in the cytokine and growth factor milieu of healing) often exhibit increased atypia and may even mimic malignant melanoma (pseudomelanoma). Studies evaluating the use of FISH-based genotypic studies to classify ambiguous melanocytic lesions are promising, although the results are preliminary.[121,122]

Atypical lentiginous melanocytic lesions continue to pose diagnostic challenges, especially when partially sampled. Such lesions often show histologic features that overlap with both simple lentiginous nevus and melanoma in situ. One group recently defined the term lentiginous melanoma as a "slowly progressing variant of melanoma typically found on the trunk and proximal extremities of middle-aged and older individuals."[123] Dermatopathologist Dr David Weedon[124] acknowledged use of this term, but he considered lentiginous melanoma as synonymous with atypical lentiginous junctional dysplastic nevus (of the elderly).

Key characteristics in distinguishing lentiginous melanomas from lentiginous nevi and dysplastic lentiginous nevi are (1) large size (rarely provided by the clinician), (2) confluent growth of atypical melanocytes (spanning the entirety of the sampling), and (3) pagetoid spread.[123] In contrast with most other forms of dysplastic nevi, lentiginous melanoma is not reported to be associated with other architectural alterations of the dermoepidermal junction, such as lamellar fibroplasia.[123] In addition, in contrast with melanoma in situ (lentigo maligna subtype), lentiginous melanoma lacks prominent solar elastosis and is characterized by preservation of the retiform epidermis.[123]

Suggestion 8: Beware of Miscommunication with the Clinician and Neglect of Clinicopathologic Correlation

A referring clinician is still sometimes encountered who declines to share any clinical impression because of a concern that this information will prejudice the dermatopathologist. It is our opinion that this practice and philosophy is both dangerous and misguided. Even the simple indication that a pigmented lesion was encountered would be preferable to sending in all specimens with a generic clinical impression, such as rule out cancer, rule out malignancy, neoplasm of uncertain behavior, or even simply 238.2 (the International Classification of Diseases-9 code for neoplasm of uncertain behavior).

For example, noting that the lesion was pigmented may prevent a melanoma with intense lichenoid inflammation from being mistaken for benign lichenoid keratosis, which is often perceived clinically to mimic a nonmelanoma skin cancer. Furthermore, clinicians must reasonably conclude that any financial savings realized by not taking time to record a meaningful clinical impression (literally seconds) are profoundly outstripped by the injurious and emotional impact of a malpractice claim.

Even the mismarking of check boxes regarding the nature of the specimen (shave, punch, excision), although seemingly trivial to the clinician, may lead to concerns of specimen misidentification, either in the physician's office or in the pathology laboratory, and this concern is amplified when the clinical suspicion is inaccurate or omitted.

A recent study reported that indication of the type of specimen submitted (punch, shave, ellipse) influences the process of margin evaluation (gross dissection, inking, ordering of additional levels), and, ultimately, the terminology in the final report.[125] A different study, reviewing the clinical information on dermatopathology requisition forms, found significant shortcomings and miscommunication between the dermatologist and the dermatopathologist.[126] These latter investigators echoed our opinion that, "the most useful clinical information to be communicated to dermatopathologists regarding melanocytic lesions includes lesion size, whether the lesion has previously been biopsied or traumatized, and whether the biopsy specimen represents only a partial sample."[126]

In sum, reliable communication between the clinician and the dermatopathologist enhances the accuracy of the end result, thereby improving the quality of care. Neglect of this communication can result in unnecessary medical error and heightened risk.

Suggestion 9: Beware of Overcall

In response to medicolegal pressures, it is understandable that pathologists and dermatopathologists adopt an attitude of hypervigilance, often manifesting as a lower threshold of suspicion toward malignancy. However, repeated studies have shown that the overcall of malignancy, when the lesion is benign, may result in damages to the patient and resultant malpractice litigation.[1-3]

A recent review of medicolegal issues in neoplastic dermatology noted that melanocyte activation in the setting of psoralen and ultraviolet light therapy, nevi occurring on special sites (the breasts, flexural areas, ears, genitalia, and acral skin), spindle cell nevus (of Reed), combined nevus (a lesion consisting of more than 1 distinct morphologic component), and deep penetrating nevi all have the potential for overcall among dermatopathologists.[48]

Hence, simply becoming more likely to suspect malignancy does not render clinicians impervious to claims of malpractice. Despite documenting the largest single series of deep penetrating nevi and clonal nevi in the literature,[127] all of which showed benign behavior, one author (W.A.H.)

often recommends complete excision when margins are involved (so long as it is not excessively morbid), chiefly out of recognition that a recurrent lesion of this type, when admixed with reactive atypia from the healing process, will lead to further diagnostic confusion and consternation, possibly with patient detriment and injury, particularly if the recurrence is sent to a laboratory that does not have knowledge of, or access to, the original material.

Suggestion 10: Beware of Being Blue

Blue nevi (BN) are dendritic or spindled melanocytic neoplasms, located in the dermis, that, because of the Tyndall effect, take on a blue hue.[78] Variants of BN include common (dendritic) BN, cellular BN (CBN), and epithelioid BN (EBN). In particular, CBN may be confused with malignancy because of their larger size, dense cellularity, infiltrative growth (often with extension into the subcutaneous fat), and even the presence of occasional mitotic figures.[128,129]

The controversial term malignant blue nevus has been used to denote melanomas arising in association with, or exhibiting some morphologic similarities to a blue nevus.[129,130] Some investigators prefer other terminology, such as blue nevus–like melanoma (BNLM) or atypical blue nevus–like lesion of uncertain malignant potential. BNLM are most common on the scalp and face, and occur most often in older persons (**Fig. 7A–C**). The clinical course and prognosis are generally poor, with many investigators reporting local invasion or widespread metastasis.[129] This phenomenon might also be caused by reporting bias, or by a delay in diagnosis and treatment, because it is known that BNLM tend to present at a more advanced stage and with a thicker primary tumor than do other melanomas.[131] In a recent study from Australia, involving 23 patients with BNLM,

researchers found that clinical outcome was similar to that of conventional melanoma compared with matched controls.

BNLM is distinguished from cellular blue nevus by the presence of variable necrosis, a high mitotic rate, abnormal mitotic figures, vascular invasion, expansive or destructive growth, marked cytologic atypia, and infiltrative margins.[131] BNLM are often associated with CBN, whereas melanoma arising in association with a common BN is extremely rare.[129] Distinguishing BNLM from metastatic or nodular melanoma can be difficult because both types of processes typically lack a junctional component.[132] The presence of a background benign blue nevus of some sort, typically a CBN, might favor the diagnosis of BNLM. Clinicopathological correlation is also helpful, because a history of melanoma and/or other evidence of metastatic disease might militate against a second primary process. As with studies involving other diagnostic mimics of melanoma, FISH-based genotypic analysis has been reported to be useful in distinguishing BNLM as well. A recent study showed that FISH-based assays targeting 4 areas of chromosomes 6 and 11 could distinguish EBN from BNLM.[133]

Atypical CBN (ACBN) is a term used to describe rare variants of CBN that also have some overlapping features of melanoma. They are mostly characterized by solitary, predominately dermal nodules occurring on the buttock or sacral region of younger adults.[129] There is controversy among pathologists about the definitions and biologic nature of such tumors, but distinguishing ACBN from melanoma presents additional diagnostic challenges. Factors that favor melanoma include high mitotic activity, atypical mitotic figures, marked cytologic atypia, cell crowding, and variable necrosis.[129] The finding of atypical mitotic figures may be the most helpful distinguishing feature.[129,134] Until additional data emerge, the

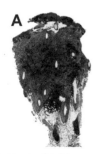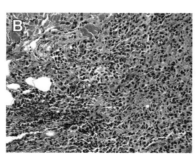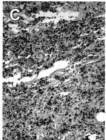

Fig. 7. At low power, this blue nevuslike melanoma (malignant blue nevus) occurring on the scalp of an 84-year-old woman could be confused with a cellular blue nevus (A; H&E, 50×), but, in addition to concerning atypia and mitotic figures at higher power (B; H&E, 100×), a Ki67 immunostain showed a markedly increased proliferative index confirming the diagnosis (C; Ki67 with counterstain, 100×).

consensus remains to treat them as being of indeterminate malignant potential and to proceed with complete resection, followed by close clinical follow-up for local recurrence or regional/distant spread.[129]

Suggestion 11: Beware of Recurrent Nevi

Recurrent/residual nevi represent melanocytic proliferations that regrow and/or persist after some type of sampling or subtotal removal. Various theories have been proposed regarding the origin of recurrent nevi, including repopulation of melanocytes from the adjacent epidermis,[135,136] repopulation of melanocytes from adnexal structures,[137,138] or, more simply, regrowth of a nevomelanocytic processes that was left behind after subtotal removal.

Recurrent nevi present clinically as flat lesions with irregular areas of pigmentation, admixed scarring, and a size generally less than 1.5 cm.[139] These characteristics promote concern regarding the possibility of malignancy. It may be impossible to distinguish recurrent nevi from melanoma, even with dermoscopy,[140] and, appropriately, this may culminate in biopsy of the lesion. However, even on histologic examination, recurrent nevi are problematic, and it has long been recognized that such lesions may manifest features that overlap significantly with melanoma (pseudomelanoma),[141] including cytologic atypia, confluent growth of melanocytes along the dermoepidermal junction, pagetoid extent, unusual horizontal growth, and associated dermal fibrosis and inflammation, perhaps even with pigmentary incontinence and associated pigmented melanophages. In turn, this may lead to unique diagnostic challenges, particularly in distinguishing a recurrent nevomelanocytic proliferation from either frank recurrent melanoma (possibly missed on a prior sampling) or melanoma with regression.[142]

In general, recurrent nevi show pagetoid spread and variable cytologic atypia, but any pagetoid component is typically confined to the area overlying the scar.[78] Nests of normally maturing residual nevomelanocytes, with less cytologic atypia, may be found either deep to or at the edge of the scarring process.[141] Although immunohistochemistry studies may manifest increased HMB-45 expression in the junctional aspects of the recurrent process, at least compared with the original sampling,[143] the dermal aspects of the recurrent lesion typically still manifest normal diminished HMB-45 staining with descent and the proliferative index is still generally low.[144]

It is often appropriate to call for, examine, and reassess the original sampling to ensure that a melanoma has not been missed. Furthermore, many dermatopathologists assert that, in the case of an incompletely excised dysplastic nevus, reexcision of the entire process is often the best management approach, particularly because further recurrence may be associated with an increasing degree of reactive atypia, and, when examined by dermatopathologists in the future who are not privy to the entirety of the clinical situation, may lead to diagnostic confusion and consternation.

Suggestion 12: Beware of Hubris

It was pride that changed angels into devils; it is humility that makes men as angels.
    —d'Saint Augustine (354–430 AD)

Humility is not only good for the soul: it is also a useful strategy for minimizing unnecessary or unintended medicolegal actions. For example, when a lesion is difficult, and reasonable physicians could come to differing conclusions, all parties should acknowledge this fact, both openly and honestly. Although there are many verbose ways to do this, at the University of Colorado, we often use a simple and direct statement in the Comment section of a report, such as, "This is a difficult case, and reasonable opinions, even among experts, may vary."

The purpose of such a statement is multifaceted: (1) it informs the clinician that differing opinions regarding this lesion may exist; (2) it alerts patients to any legitimate uncertainty with regard to the ultimate biologic behavior of a lesion, so the patient may consider this uncertainty when soliciting further opinions or consenting to treatment; (3) it signals to other dermatopathologists that conflicting signs were observed, and that differences of opinion may exist, and should be expected and respected. Even considering the myriad of morphologic, immunohistochemical, and even genotypic studies (FISH-based studies or CGH) that are available, it is truthful to state that there are some melanocytic processes that are not classifiable with complete certainty; we question the objectivity of any dermatopathologist unwilling to acknowledge diagnostic limitations with regard to some melanocytic neoplasms.

SUMMARY

Understanding malpractice risk and practicing risk management strategies results in better care and a less stressful environment of practice; it is therefore good for both the patient and the dermatopathologist. Although the numbers of closed claims against dermatologists are few, and the annual number has remained constant for the past 21 years, errors in diagnosis are most commonly related to melanoma and neoplasms of the skin.[32] To offset this constant, but subtle, threat of malpractice litigation, malpractice data can be used to focus safety efforts on common diagnostic errors.

Major patient safety issues identified by the American Academy of Dermatology Ad Hoc Task Force included misdiagnosis and delayed diagnosis, errors in pathology specimen processing, and errors in the timely and accurate communication of biopsy results as points of concern.[32] With these points in mind, some researchers have suggested novel techniques for histopathologic analysis and the issuance of results, such as the use of dermoscopic images of a lesion, to guide sampling of suspicious areas during histopathologic analysis.[58]

In addition, many laboratories have moved toward electronic specimen tracking systems that allow for affirmative identification of a specimen, via a barcode, at each step of laboratory processing, from initial accession, through grossing, embedding, cutting, staining, and case assembly. Techniques such as this also allow the efficient capture of quality assurance data to analyze trends and prevent future errors within the laboratory. By analogy, recognition of sources of error in the analysis of pigmented lesions by dermatopathologists, and the development of new immunohistochemical or genotypic techniques for the recognition and distinction of malignant disease from benign pigmented lesions, will also provide important improvements in care and diagnosis in the future.

REFERENCES

1. Troxel DB. Pitfalls in the diagnosis of malignant melanoma: findings of a risk management panel study. Am J Surg Pathol 2003;27(9):1278–83.
2. Troxel DB. An insurer's perspective on error and loss in pathology. Arch Pathol Lab Med 2005; 129(10):1234–6.
3. Troxel DB. Medicolegal aspects of error in pathology. Arch Pathol Lab Med 2006;130(5): 617–9.
4. Read S, Hill HF 3rd. Dermatology's malpractice experience: clinical settings for risk management. J Am Acad Dermatol 2005;53(1):134–7.
5. Lydiatt DD. Medical malpractice and cancer of the skin. Am J Surg 2004;187(6):688–94.
6. Glusac EJ. Under the microscope: doctors, lawyers, and melanocytic neoplasms. J Cutan Pathol 2003;30(5):287–93.
7. Albert VA, Koh HK, Geller AC, et al. Years of potential life lost: another indicator of the impact of cutaneous malignant melanoma on society. J Am Acad Dermatol 1990;23(2 Pt 1):308–10.
8. Baade PD, Green AC, Smithers BM, et al. Trends in melanoma incidence among children: possible influence of sun-protection programs. Expert Rev Anticancer Ther 2011;11(5):661–4.
9. Erie Railroad v. Tompkins, 304 U.S. 64 (1938).
10. Fox BC, Siegel ML, Weinstein RA. "Curbside" consultation and informal communication in medical practice: a medicolegal perspective. Clin Infect Dis 1996;23(3):616–22.
11. Kelley v. Middle Tennessee Emergency Physicians, P.C., 133 S.W.3d 587 (Tenn. 2004).
12. Scafide v. Bazzone, 962 So.2d 585 (Miss. Ct. App. 2006).
13. Epstein JI. Pathologists and the judicial process: how to avoid it. Am J Surg Pathol 2001;25(4): 527–37.
14. Troxel DB, Sabella JD. Problem areas in pathology practice. Uncovered by a review of malpractice claims. Am J Surg Pathol 1994;18(8):821–31.
15. Tomaszewski JE, LiVolsi VA. Mandatory second opinion of pathologic slides: is it necessary? Cancer 1999;86(11):2198–200.
16. Dahl J. Quality, assurance, diagnosis, treatment, and patient care. Pathology review - patient safety and quality healthcare. 2006. Available at: http://www.psqh.com/marapr06/pathologist. html. Accessed November 5, 2011.
17. Martello J. Basic medical legal principles. Clin Plast Surg 1999;26(1):9–14, v.
18. Goldberg DJ. Legal issues in dermatology: informed consent, complications and medical malpractice. Semin Cutan Med Surg 2007;26(1):2–5.
19. Furrow BR. Health law. 2nd edition. St. Paul (MN): West Publishing; 2000. xxxviii, 1121 p.
20. Kinney ED, Wilder MM. Medical standard setting in the current malpractice environment: problems and possibilities. Spec Law Dig Health Care (Mon) 1990;(135):7–36.
21. Vergara v. Doan, 593 N.E.2d 185 (Ind. 1992).
22. Trotter MJ, Bruecks AK. Interpretation of skin biopsies by general pathologists: diagnostic discrepancy rate measured by blinded review. Arch Pathol Lab Med 2003;127(11):1489–92.
23. Goldberg DJ. Legal issues in laser operation. Clin Dermatol 2006;24(1):56–9.
24. Gittler GJ, Goldstein EJ. The elements of medical malpractice: an overview. Clin Infect Dis 1996; 23(5):1152–5.
25. Hirsch P. The medical expert witness: legal and ethical issues. Clin Dermatol 2010;28(2):240–2.
26. Marshall JC. Credibility: the key to the successful physician witness. Surv Ophthalmol 1995;40(1): 69–72.

27. Palsgraf v. Long Island Railway Co, 284 N.Y. 339 (N.Y. 1928).

28. St. George v. Pariser, 484 S.E.2d 888 (Va. 1997).

29. American Academy of Pediatrics. Committee on Medical Liability. Professional liability coverage for residents and fellows. Pediatrics 2000;106(3):605–9.

30. Ellington DP, Rosenthal RS. Medical malpractice. The defense perspective. Mo Med 1997;94(7):323–7.

31. Moran T. So you've been sued. Tips for enduring and avoiding the malpractice roller coaster ride. Texas Med 1995;91(3):24–31.

32. Elston DM, Taylor JS, Coldiron B, et al. Patient safety: part I. Patient safety and the dermatologist. J Am Acad Dermatol 2009;61(2):179–90 [quiz: 191].

33. Kessler DP, Summerton N, Graham JR. Effects of the medical liability system in Australia, the UK, and the USA. Lancet 2006;368(9531):240–6.

34. Colorado Governmental Immunity Act. Colorado revised statutes, Section 24-10-101 (2006).

35. White WL, Stavola JM. The dark side of photomicrographs in pathology reports: liability and practical concerns hidden from view. J Am Acad Dermatol 2006;54(2):353–6.

36. Pritt BS, Gibson PC, Cooper K. Digital imaging guidelines for pathology: a proposal for general and academic use. Adv Anat Pathol 2003;10(2):96–100.

37. American Medical Association. Regulations on the practice of telemedicine and out-of-state consulting physicians. State medical licensure requirements and statistics. Chicago, IL: American Medical Association; 2012.

38. College of American Pathologists. Licensure requirements for interstate diagnosis, including interstate telemedicine practice. Available at: http://www.cap.org/apps/cap.portal?_nfpb=true&cntvwrPtlt_actionOverride=%2Fportlets%2Fcontent Viewer%2Fshow&_windowLabel=cntvwrPtlt&cntvwr Ptlt{actionForm.contentReference}=policies%2F policy_appZZ.html&_state=maximized&_page Label=cntvwr. Accessed December 6, 2011.

39. Olsen TG, Feeser TA, Jenkins PL. Interstate dermatopathology interpretations–50 separate licenses? J Am Acad Dermatol 2004;51(3):454–7.

40. Brauer JA, Shin DB, Troxel AB, et al. Characteristics of dermatologists who read dermatopathology slides. J Cutan Pathol 2007;34(9):687–92.

41. Hancox JG, Neville JA, Chen J, et al. Interpretation of dermatopathology specimens is within the standard of care of dermatology practice. Dermatol Surg 2005;31(3):306–9.

42. Singh S, Grummer SE, Hancox JG, et al. The extent of dermatopathology education: a comparison of pathology and dermatology. J Am Acad Dermatol 2005;53(4):694–7.

43. Goldenberg G, Camacho F, Gildea J, et al. Who sends what: a comparison of dermatopathology referrals from dermatologists, pathologists and dermatopathologists. J Cutan Pathol 2008;35(7):658–61.

44. Grant-Kels JM. The whys and wherefores of who reads dermatopathology slides. J Am Acad Dermatol 2005;53(4):703–4.

45. Ackerman AB. Dermatologist not equal to dermatopathologist: no place in a profession for pretenders. J Am Acad Dermatol 2005;53(4):698–9.

46. van Dijk MC, Aben KK, Van Hees F, et al. Expert review remains important in the histopathological diagnosis of cutaneous melanocytic lesions. Histopathology 2008;52(2):139–46.

47. Shoo BA, Sagebiel RW, Kashani-Sabet M. Discordance in the histopathologic diagnosis of melanoma at a melanoma referral center. J Am Acad Dermatol 2010;62(5):751–6.

48. Crowson AN. Medicolegal aspects of neoplastic dermatology. Mod Pathol 2006;19(Suppl 2):S148–54.

49. Brennan TA, Leape LL, Laird NM, et al. Incidence of adverse events and negligence in hospitalized patients: results of the Harvard Medical Practice Study I. 1991. Qual Saf Health Care 2004;13(2):145–51 [discussion: 151–2].

50. Localio AR, Lawthers AG, Brennan TA, et al. Relation between malpractice claims and adverse events due to negligence. Results of the Harvard Medical Practice Study III. N Engl J Med 1991;325(4):245–51.

51. Schmoeckel C, Castro CE, Braun-Falco O. Nevoid malignant melanoma. Arch Dermatol Res 1985;277(5):362–9.

52. Magro CM, Crowson AN, Mihm MC. Unusual variants of malignant melanoma. Mod Pathol 2006;19(Suppl 2):S41–70.

53. Diwan AH, Lazar AJ. Nevoid melanoma. Clin Lab Med 2011;31(2):243–53.

54. McNutt NS, Urmacher C, Hakimian J, et al. Nevoid malignant melanoma: morphologic patterns and immunohistochemical reactivity. J Cutan Pathol 1995;22(6):502–17.

55. Gerami P, Wass A, Mafee M, et al. Fluorescence in situ hybridization for distinguishing nevoid melanomas from mitotically active nevi. Am J Surg Pathol 2009;33(12):1783–8.

56. DiCaudo DJ, McCalmont TH, Wick MR. Selected diagnostic problems in neoplastic dermatopathology. Arch Pathol Lab Med 2007;131(3):434–9.

57. Diwan AH, Dang SM, Prieto VG, et al. Lack of maturation with anti-leptin receptor antibody in melanoma but not in nevi. Mod Pathol 2009;22(1):103–6.

58. Marghoob AA, Terushkin V, Dusza SW, et al. Dermatologists, general practitioners, and the best method to biopsy suspect melanocytic neoplasms. Arch Dermatol 2010;146(3):325–8.

59. Molenkamp BG, Sluijter BJ, Oosterhof B, et al. Non-radical diagnostic biopsies do not negatively influence melanoma patient survival. Ann Surg Oncol 2007;14(4):1424–30.

60. Bong JL, Herd RM, Hunter JA. Incisional biopsy and melanoma prognosis. J Am Acad Dermatol 2002;46(5):690–4.

61. Karimipour DJ, Schwartz JL, Wang TS, et al. Microstaging accuracy after subtotal incisional biopsy of cutaneous melanoma. J Am Acad Dermatol 2005; 52(5):798–802.

62. Ng PC, Barzilai DA, Ismail SA, et al. Evaluating invasive cutaneous melanoma: is the initial biopsy representative of the final depth? J Am Acad Dermatol 2003;48(3):420–4.

63. Ng JC, Swain S, Dowling JP, et al. The impact of partial biopsy on histopathologic diagnosis of cutaneous melanoma: experience of an Australian tertiary referral service. Arch Dermatol 2010;146(3):234–9.

64. Fernandez EM, Helm T, Ioffreda M, et al. The vanishing biopsy: the trend toward smaller specimens. Cutis 2005;76(5):335–9.

65. Pardasani AG, Leshin B, Hallman JR, et al. Fusiform incisional biopsy for pigmented skin lesions. Dermatol Surg 2000;26(7):622–4.

66. Tran KT, Wright NA, Cockerell CJ. Biopsy of the pigmented lesion–when and how. J Am Acad Dermatol 2008;59(5):852–71.

67. Zager JS, Hochwald SN, Marzban SS, et al. Shave biopsy is a safe and accurate method for the initial evaluation of melanoma. J Am Coll Surg 2011; 212(4):454–60 [discussion: 460–2].

68. Ho J, Brodell RT, Helms SE. Saucerization biopsy of pigmented lesions. Clin Dermatol 2005;23(6):631–5.

69. Pariser RJ, Divers A, Nassar A. The relationship between biopsy technique and uncertainty in the histopathologic diagnosis of melanoma. Dermatol Online J 1999;5(2):4.

70. Demartini CS, Dalton MS, Ferringer T, et al. Melan-A/MART-1 positive "pseudonests" in lichenoid inflammatory lesions: an uncommon phenomenon. Am J Dermatopathol 2005;27(4):370–1.

71. Maize JC Jr, Resneck JS Jr, Shapiro PE, et al. Ducking stray "magic bullets": a Melan-A alert. Am J Dermatopathol 2003;25(2):162–5.

72. Nicholson KM, Gerami P. An immunohistochemical analysis of pseudomelanocytic nests mimicking melanoma in situ: report of 2 cases. Am J Dermatopathol 2010;32(6):633–7.

73. Silva CY, Goldberg LJ, Mahalingam M, et al. Nests with numerous SOX10 and MiTF-positive cells in lichenoid inflammation: pseudomelanocytic nests or authentic melanocytic proliferation? J Cutan Pathol 2011;38(10):797–800.

74. Spitz S. Cutaneous tumors of childhood. Disparity between clinical behavior and histologic appearance. J Am Med Womens Assoc 1951;6(6):209–19.

75. Lyon VB. The Spitz nevus: review and update. Clin Plast Surg 2010;37(1):21–33.

76. Ludgate MW, Fullen DR, Lee J, et al. The atypical Spitz tumor of uncertain biologic potential: a series of 67 patients from a single institution. Cancer 2009;115(3):631–41.

77. Spatz A, Calonje E, Handfield-Jones S, et al. Spitz tumors in children: a grading system for risk stratification. Arch Dermatol 1999;135(3):282–5.

78. de Giorgi V, Sestini S, Massi D, et al. Melanocytic aggregation in the skin: diagnostic clues from lentigines to melanoma. Dermatol Clin 2007;25(3): 303–20, vii–viii.

79. Kamino H. Spitzoid melanoma. Clin Dermatol 2009; 27(6):545–55.

80. Bergman R, Malkin L, Sabo E, et al. MIB-1 monoclonal antibody to determine proliferative activity of Ki-67 antigen as an adjunct to the histopathologic differential diagnosis of Spitz nevi. J Am Acad Dermatol 2001;44(3):500–4.

81. Li LX, Crotty KA, McCarthy SW, et al. A zonal comparison of MIB1-Ki67 immunoreactivity in benign and malignant melanocytic lesions. Am J Dermatopathol 2000;22(6):489–95.

82. Vollmer RT. Use of Bayes rule and MIB-1 proliferation index to discriminate Spitz nevus from malignant melanoma. Am J Clin Pathol 2004;122(4): 499–505.

83. Barnhill RL. The Spitzoid lesion: rethinking Spitz tumors, atypical variants, 'Spitzoid melanoma' and risk assessment. Mod Pathol 2006;19(Suppl 2):S21–33.

84. Bastian BC, LeBoit PE, Pinkel D. Mutations and copy number increase of HRAS in Spitz nevi with distinctive histopathological features. Am J Pathol 2000;157(3):967–72.

85. Ali L, Helm T, Cheney R, et al. Correlating array comparative genomic hybridization findings with histology and outcome in spitzoid melanocytic neoplasms. Int J Clin Exp Pathol 2010;3(6):593–9.

86. Massi D, Cesinaro AM, Tomasini C, et al. Atypical Spitzoid melanocytic tumors: a morphological, mutational, and FISH analysis. J Am Acad Dermatol 2011;64(5):919–35.

87. Urso C, Borgognoni L, Saieva C, et al. Sentinel lymph node biopsy in patients with "atypical Spitz tumors." A report on 12 cases. Hum Pathol 2006; 37(7):816–23.

88. Roaten JB, Partrick DA, Bensard D, et al. Survival in sentinel lymph node-positive pediatric melanoma. J Pediatr Surg 2005;40(6):988–92 [discussion: 992].

89. Gelbard SN, Tripp JM, Marghoob AA, et al. Management of Spitz nevi: a survey of dermatologists in the United States. J Am Acad Dermatol 2002;47(2):224–30.

90. Webber SA, Siller G, Soyer HP. Pigmented spindle cell naevus of Reed: a controversial diagnostic

entity in Australia. Australas J Dermatol 2011;52(2): 104–8.

91. Massi G. Melanocytic nevi simulant of melanoma with medicolegal relevance. Virchows Arch 2007; 451(3):623–47.

92. Blessing K, McLaren KM. Histological regression in primary cutaneous melanoma: recognition, prevalence and significance. Histopathology 1992; 20(4):315–22.

93. High WA, Stewart D, Wilbers CR, et al. Completely regressed primary cutaneous malignant melanoma with nodal and/or visceral metastases: a report of 5 cases and assessment of the literature and diagnostic criteria. J Am Acad Dermatol 2005;53(1): 89–100.

94. Emanuel PO, Mannion M, Phelps RG. Complete regression of primary malignant melanoma. Am J Dermatopathol 2008;30(2):178–81.

95. Flax SH, Skelton HG, Smith KJ, et al. Nodular melanosis due to epithelial neoplasms: a finding not restricted to regressed melanomas. Am J Dermatopathol 1998;20(2):118–22.

96. Clark WH Jr, Elder DE, Guerry D 4th, et al. Model predicting survival in stage I melanoma based on tumor progression. J Natl Cancer Inst 1989; 81(24):1893–904.

97. Slingluff CL Jr, Vollmer RT, Reintgen DS, et al. Lethal "thin" malignant melanoma. Identifying patients at risk. Ann Surg 1988;208(2):150–61.

98. Ronan SG, Eng AM, Briele HA, et al. Thin malignant melanomas with regression and metastases. Arch Dermatol 1987;123(10):1326–30.

99. Naruns PL, Nizze JA, Cochran AJ, et al. Recurrence potential of thin primary melanomas. Cancer 1986;57(3):545–8.

100. Sondergaard K, Hou-Jensen K. Partial regression in thin primary cutaneous malignant melanomas clinical stage I. A study of 486 cases. Virchows Arch 1985;408(2–3):241–7.

101. Gromet MA, Epstein WL, Blois MS. The regressing thin malignant melanoma: a distinctive lesion with metastatic potential. Cancer 1978;42(5):2282–92.

102. Fontaine D, Parkhill W, Greer W, et al. Partial regression of primary cutaneous melanoma: is there an association with sub-clinical sentinel lymph node metastasis? Am J Dermatopathol 2003;25(5):371–6.

103. Skov L, Clemmensen O, Baadsgaard O. Thin cutaneous malignant melanoma and the MIN terminology. Lancet 1997;350(9087):1264–5.

104. Cooper PH, Wanebo HJ, Hagar RW. Regression in thin malignant melanoma. Microscopic diagnosis and prognostic importance. Arch Dermatol 1985; 121(9):1127–31.

105. Kelly JW, Sagebiel RW, Blois MS. Regression in malignant melanoma. A histologic feature without independent prognostic significance. Cancer 1985; 56(9):2287–91.

106. Briggs JC, Ibrahim NB, Hastings AG, et al. Experience of thin cutaneous melanomas (less than 0.76 mm and less than 0.85 mm thick) in a large plastic surgery unit: a 5 to 17 year follow-up. Br J Plast Surg 1984;37(4):501–6.

107. Trau H, Rigel DS, Harris MN, et al. Metastases of thin melanomas. Cancer 1983;51(3):553–6.

108. McGovern VJ, Shaw HM, Milton GW. Prognosis in patients with thin malignant melanoma: influence of regression. Histopathology 1983;7(5):673–80.

109. Sartore L, Papanikolaou GE, Biancari F, et al. Prognostic factors of cutaneous melanoma in relation to metastasis at the sentinel lymph node: a case-controlled study. Int J Surg 2008;6(3):205–9.

110. Kaur C, Thomas RJ, Desai N, et al. The correlation of regression in primary melanoma with sentinel lymph node status. J Clin Pathol 2008;61(3):297–300.

111. Socrier Y, Lauwers-Cances V, Lamant L, et al. Histological regression in primary melanoma: not a predictor of sentinel lymph node metastasis in a cohort of 397 patients. Br J Dermatol 2010; 162(4):830–4.

112. Slingluff CL Jr, Seigler HF. "Thin" malignant melanoma: risk factors and clinical management. Ann Plast Surg 1992;28(1):89–94.

113. Nahabedian MY, Tufaro AP, Manson PN. Sentinel lymph node biopsy for the T1 (thin) melanoma: is it necessary? Ann Plast Surg 2003;50(6):601–6.

114. Wong SL, Brady MS, Busam KJ, et al. Results of sentinel lymph node biopsy in patients with thin melanoma. Ann Surg Oncol 2006;13(3):302–9.

115. Liszkay G, Orosz Z, Péley G, et al. Relationship between sentinel lymph node status and regression of primary malignant melanoma. Melanoma Res 2005;15(6):509–13.

116. de Almeida LS, Requena L, Rütten A, et al. Desmoplastic malignant melanoma: a clinicopathologic analysis of 113 cases. Am J Dermatopathol 2008; 30(3):207–15.

117. Chorny JA, Barr RJ. S100-positive spindle cells in scars: a diagnostic pitfall in the re-excision of desmoplastic melanoma. Am J Dermatopathol 2002; 24(4):309–12.

118. Tripp JM, Kopf AW, Marghoob AA, et al. Management of dysplastic nevi: a survey of fellows of the American Academy of Dermatology. J Am Acad Dermatol 2002;46(5):674–82.

119. Clarke LE. Dysplastic nevi. Clin Lab Med 2011; 31(2):255–65.

120. Smoller BR, Egbert BM. Dysplastic nevi can be diagnosed and graded reproducibly: a longitudinal study. J Am Acad Dermatol 1992;27(3): 399–402.

121. Gerami P, Jewell SS, Morrison LE, et al. Fluorescence in situ hybridization as an ancillary method for the distinction of desmoplastic melanomas

from sclerosing melanocytic nevi. J Cutan Pathol 2011;38(4):329–34.

122. Gaiser T, Kutzner H, Palmedo G, et al. Classifying ambiguous melanocytic lesions with FISH and correlation with clinical long-term follow up. Mod Pathol 2010;23(3):413–9.

123. King R. Lentiginous melanoma. Arch Pathol Lab Med 2011;135(3):337–41.

124. Weedon D. Lentiginous melanoma. J Cutan Pathol 2009;36(11):1232.

125. Kolman O, Hoang MP, Piris A, et al. Histologic processing and reporting of cutaneous pigmented lesions: recommendations based on a survey of 94 dermatopathologists. J Am Acad Dermatol 2010;63(4):661–7.

126. Waller JM, Zedek DC. How informative are dermatopathology requisition forms completed by dermatologists? A review of the clinical information provided for 100 consecutive melanocytic lesions. J Am Acad Dermatol 2010;62(2):257–61.

127. High WA, Alanen KW, Golitz LE. Is melanocytic nevus with focal atypical epithelioid components (clonal nevus) a superficial variant of deep penetrating nevus? J Am Acad Dermatol 2006;55(3): 460–6.

128. Rook A, Burns T. Rook's textbook of dermatology. 8th edition. Chichester (United Kingdom); Hoboken (NJ): Wiley-Blackwell; 2010.

129. Murali R, McCarthy SW, Scolyer RA. Blue nevi and related lesions: a review highlighting atypical and newly described variants, distinguishing features and diagnostic pitfalls. Adv Anat Pathol 2009; 16(6):365–82.

130. Allen AC, Spitz S. Malignant melanoma; a clinico-pathological analysis of the criteria for diagnosis and prognosis. Cancer 1953;6(1):1–45.

131. Martin RC, Murali R, Scolyer RA, et al. So-called "malignant blue nevus": a clinicopathologic study of 23 patients. Cancer 2009;115(13):2949–55.

132. Connelly J, Smith JL Jr. Malignant blue nevus. Cancer 1991;67(10):2653–7.

133. Gammon B, Beilfuss B, Guitart J, et al. Fluorescence in situ hybridization for distinguishing

cellular blue nevi from blue nevus-like melanoma. J Cutan Pathol 2011;38(4):335–41.

134. Rodriguez HA, Ackerman LV. Cellular blue nevus. Clinicopathologic study of forty-five cases. Cancer 1968;21(3):393–405.

135. Cox AJ, Walton RG. The induction of junctional changes in pigmented nevi. Arch Pathol 1965;79: 428–34.

136. Cox AJ, Walton RG. Pigmented nevi. Induced changes in the junctional component. Calif Med 1966;104(1):32–4.

137. Park HK, Leonard DD, Arrington JH 3rd, et al. Recurrent melanocytic nevi: clinical and histologic review of 175 cases. J Am Acad Dermatol 1987; 17(2 Pt 1):285–92.

138. Imagawa I, Endo M, Morishima T. Mechanism of recurrence of pigmented nevi following dermabrasion. Acta Derm Venereol 1976;56(5):353–9.

139. Marghoob AA, Changchien L, DeFazio J, et al. The most common challenges in melanoma diagnosis and how to avoid them. Australas J Dermatol 2009;50(1):1–13 [quiz: 14–5].

140. Botella-Estrada R, Nagore E, Sopena J, et al. Clinical, dermoscopy and histological correlation study of melanotic pigmentations in excision scars of melanocytic tumours. Br J Dermatol 2006; 154(3):478–84.

141. Kornberg R, Ackerman AB. Pseudomelanoma: recurrent melanocytic nevus following partial surgical removal. Arch Dermatol 1975;111(12):1588–90.

142. King R, Hayzen BA, Page RN, et al. Recurrent nevus phenomenon: a clinicopathologic study of 357 cases and histologic comparison with melanoma with regression. Mod Pathol 2009;22(5): 611–7.

143. Sexton M, Sexton CW. Recurrent pigmented melanocytic nevus. A benign lesion, not to be mistaken for malignant melanoma. Arch Pathol Lab Med 1991;115(2):122–6.

144. Hoang MP, Prieto VG, Burchette JL, et al. Recurrent melanocytic nevus: a histologic and immunohistochemical evaluation. J Cutan Pathol 2001;28(8): 400–6.

Dermatopathology Updates on Melanocytic Lesions

Wang L. Cheung, MD, PhD[a],*, Bruce R. Smoller, MD[b]

KEYWORDS

• Melanocytes • Nevi • Melanoma • Special site

KEY POINTS

- Special site nevi such as those on the breast and genitalia tend to have more cytologic and architectural atypia but can be considered benign changes.
- The histopathology of melanocytic proliferations during pregnancy does not appear to differ significantly.
- Atypical dermal melanocytic proliferations are difficult to diagnose and tend to have a better outcome after adequate treatment.
- Additional histopathologic studies along with longer clinical follow-up are required to determine if atypical dermal melanocytic proliferations and special site nevi will behave as low grade malignant neoplasms or benign neoplasms.

This article examines some of the recent studies on interesting melanocytic lesions, such as site-specific nevi, "Spark's" nevi, nevi during pregnancy, and atypical dermal melanocytic proliferation, including pigmented epithelioid melanocytoma, proliferating nodules, and atypical Spitzoid tumor. In general, the studies with both histopathologic findings and clinical outcome are most informative, allowing dermatopathologists and dermatologists to identify the histologic features that are most helpful. Although newer immunohistochemical and molecular tests are available, they currently confirm the hematoxylin and eosin (H&E) findings and remain ancillary studies. More histopathologic studies with clinical follow-up are still needed to help understand the behavior of some melanocytic lesions.

SITE-SPECIFIC NEVI (DYSPLASTIC NEVI OR NOT?)

Normal skin biopsies from different anatomic locations from 97 patients in Australia were examined for the distribution of melanocytes using an immunohistochemical stain for tyrosinase-related protein 1.[1] This study showed that overall melanocyte density decreases with age, and the density is highest on the back, shoulder, and limbs. In addition, patients with more nevi had a higher density of melanocytes. Hair color, eye color, and freckling did not have an impact on the density of melanocytes. Another study of 506 Australian children showed that the highest number of nevi were on the arms, neck, and face. Girls had more nevi on the lower leg and thigh than boys.[2] These simple and eloquent studies show that the density of melanocytes and nevi differ, suggesting that the biology of melanocytes from different locations and genders may vary. Reasoning would follow that melanocytic proliferations from different locations and genders also will probably be different.

Hosler and colleagues[3] recently wrote an excellent review on nevi with site-related atypia., categorizing them into 4 groups: acral, genital, special-site, and conjunctival. And they review on nevi with site-related atypia, the special-site category included breast, flexural, scalp, and auricular

The authors have nothing to disclose.
[a] Department of Pathology, Orlando Health, 1414 Kuhl Avenue, Orlando, FL 32806, USA; [b] United States and Canadian Academy of Pathologist, 3643 Walton Way Extension, Augusta, GA 30909, USA
* Corresponding author.
E-mail address: wang.cheung@orlandohealth.com

sites.[4] These special-site nevi can have more cyto-logic atypia and architectural disorder than other sites (**Fig. 1**). For example, 101 breast nevi showed more dermal fibroplasia, cytologic atypia, and in-traepidermal melanocytes compared with 97 other nevi.[5] Similar studies from other special sites have also been reported. However, these studies do not address whether these atypical nevi really repre-sent completely benign nevi or whether dysplastic nevi occur more frequently at these sites. Recogni-tion is important to ensure that melanoma is not overdiagnosed. However, in some instances, whether atypia is attributed to site-specific changes is not straightforward, and some derma-topathologists might still recommended complete conservative removal.[6]

Atypical genital nevi, regarded as nevi of a special site, have unique histopathologic findings. These nevi, especially in premenopausal women, consist of large and irregular junctional nests with focal single cells in a lentiginous growth pattern and in the spinous layer of the epidermis and adnexal structures.[7] The melanocytes can also have mild to severe cytologic atypia but are uniform. Usually superficial dermal fibrosis is present, likely from prior trauma. The dermal component can be very dense, containing nests and many single melano-cytes, again with cytologic atypia. Focally, an increase in mitoses can be seen, but maturation is present and no deep dermal or atypical mitoses are identified (**Fig. 2**). Although limited data are available, atypical genital nevi may recur when incompletely excised.[7] The most important distinc-tion is vulvar melanoma, but usually these are larger clinically and present in older women with histo-pathologic features of frank melanoma.

Recently, the histopathologic features of dysplastic nevi on the lower leg were further exam-ined.[8] The authors examined 62 dysplastic nevi of the lower leg from women and men and compared them with 20 dysplastic nevi from the back and 20 superficial spreading melanoma of the lower leg. The women showed more pagetoid spread, more cytologic atypia, and larger melanocytes in dysplastic nevi. The authors also noted that lesions larger than 4 mm are more likely to be diagnosed as melanoma.[8] These types of studies are informative but again do not address whether these changes are really benign or precursors to a malignant process, and do not address whe-ther these lesions from the lower leg represent distinct site-specific change of benign nevi or are dysplastic nevi.

Whether dysplastic nevi are a precursor to mela-noma is not certain, but presence of multiple nevi (especially dysplastic) definitely is a risk factor for melanoma. Many studies have found that mela-noma is strongly associated with total number of nevi, such that the relative risk is 6.89 for patients with more than 100 nevi versus those with fewer than 15 nevi.[9] The relative risk is even higher for atypical nevi. One study from Queensland, Australia showed that people with low numbers of nevi who are exposed to frequent sunlight tend to develop head and neck melanomas, whereas people with many nevi who are exposed to rare sunlight tend to develop truncal melanomas.[10] A more recent study showed a site-specific correla-tion of number of nevi to risk of melanoma on the back, but not on other locations.[11] In other words, increasing numbers of nevi in a particular location might not increase the risk of developing melanoma in that same location, rather the general increase in risk is seen throughout the body. These clinical studies might support that the special-site nevi as described earlier are benign nevi with distinct atyp-ical features. By themselves, these special-site nevi probably do not increase the risk of melanoma in

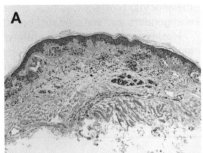
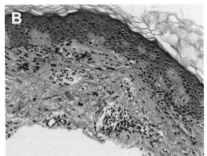

Fig. 1. A melanocytic lesion from the breast of a 25-year-old woman. The low-power histopathologic examina-tion shows architectural disorder (ie, lamellar fibroplasia, bridging of the rete ridges, irregular and enlarged nests, and scattered single melanocytes in the epidermis). The dermal component contains smaller melanocytes (*A*). The higher-power view shows more architectural disorder and moderate cytologic atypia (*B*). Even though cytologically atypical cells are present, many of the junctional melanocytes appear similar.

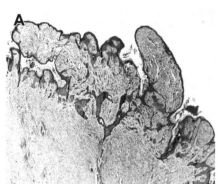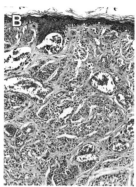

Fig. 2. A melanocytic lesion from the vulva of a 14-year-old girl. The low-power view shows a large melanocytic lesion with pedunculation. Enlarged nests of melanocytes are present in the epidermis and superficial dermis. However, the cells in the dermis seem to mature even in this low-power view (*A*). With higher magnification, irregular-shaped nests are seen, predominately at the dermoepidermal junction. In the dermis, many melanocytes appear as single cells and in nests. Although cytologic atypia is present, it is uniform (*B*). Of course, more importantly, the dermal melanocytes do mature and the proliferation index remains low.

that location. The only exception might be the back.[11] This finding also might mean that the atypia seen in nevi from the back probably should not be considered as changes attributed to a special site.

"SPARK'S" NEVI

Recently, the name *Spark's nevi* was proposed for nevi with features of Spitz and Clark's dysplastic nevi.[12] Histologically, the authors reported 27 cases having epithelioid and spindle cells at the dermoepidermal junction and in the papillary dermis. These lesions were well circumscribed, symmetric, and had melanocytes of similar size, shape, and small diameter. Furthermore, most (23/27) of these lesions had Kamino bodies. Clinically, these patients were predominately young (mean age, 33 years) with a female predominance (63%). These nevi were most common on the trunk or lower extremity (20/27). Toussaint and Kamino[13] also reported lesions similar to these, which they called "dysplastic Spitz's nevus." They described 67 of these cases. Similarly, these lesions were usually seen in younger patients (mean age, 34.7 years) and located on the lower extremity (44%). The recent study by Ko and colleagues[12] included an average of 10 years' follow-up in 12 patients, showing no recurrences or metastasis in any of these patients.

PREGNANCY EFFECT ON MELANOCYTIC PROLIFERATION

During pregnancy, hyperpigmentation of the areola, axilla, and other locations is noted. In addition, darker melanocytic nevi have also been documented during pregnancy. One objective

study that followed melanocytic nevi in 22 patients using photographs and, in some cases, biopsy showed no significant difference during the pregnancy.[14] Two earlier studies also found little or no histologic differences in nevi of pregnant women versus control women.[15,16]

A recent study examining in more detail the histologic features of melanocytic nevi in pregnancy compared 16 melanocytic nevi from pregnant women with 15 melanocytic nevi from nonpregnant women matched for location and age.[17] The investigators found an increased number of epithelioid melanocytes in the superficial dermis (**Fig. 3**A), termed *superficial micronodules of pregnancy.* The pregnancy nevi were also more likely to have dermal mitotic figures (62.5% vs 13.3%) and higher mitotic rate (1.44 vs 0.2 mitoses per mm^2) than non–pregnancy-related nevi (see **Fig. 3**B). However, despite a trend, the difference in Ki-67 staining was not statistically significant, suggesting that the overall proliferation rate may not differ between the groups (see **Fig. 3**C, D). Although Ki-67 levels might become statistically significant with more cases, the mitotic rate determined by mitoses counted and Ki-67 index may be slightly different. After all, Ki-67 immunostain will highlight cells that are entering mitoses before any evidence is detectable on H&E-stained sections. Another unexpected finding was that the multinucleated melanocytes common in benign nevi were not noted in pregnancy nevi. The relationship of these findings to the hormonal state of pregnant women is not clear, but at least some histologic difference seems to be present between nevi from pregnant women and those in controls.[17]

Spectrophotometric intracutaneous analyses (SIAscopy) were performed in vivo on 381

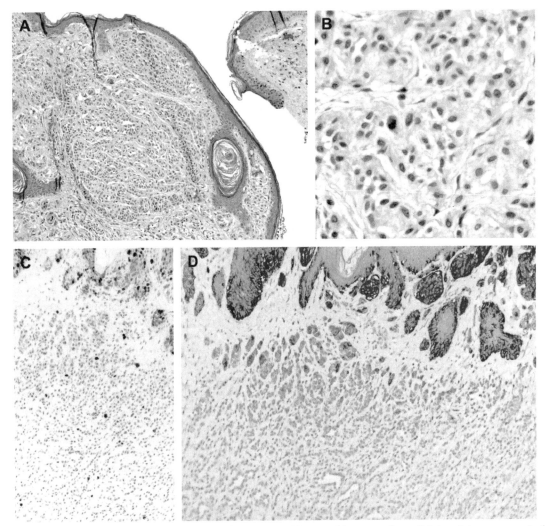

Fig. 3. A melanocytic lesion from mons pubis of a pregnant 28-year-old woman. Superficial nodules composed of slightly enlarged melanocytes are seen (*A*). Scattered mitoses are noted in the mid dermis (*B*). However, the Ki-67 still shows a low proliferation index with epidermis as control (*C*). An HMB-45 immunostain shows loss of staining in the deeper dermal cells as an indicator of maturation, supporting that this is a benign lesion (*D*).

melanocytic nevi of pregnant women during early pregnancy and before birth, and compared with 163 melanocytic nevi of nonpregnant women.[18] SIA-scopy uses different light sources to build a model of where melanin pigment is located in the skin, and supplements information that can be obtained with only a dermatoscope. In the pregnant group, only 2.1% of nevi increased in size and 1.8% decreased in size. Only one nevus increased in pigmentation, whereas 3.7% of nevi decreased in pigmentation. When compared with the nonpregnant group, no statistical differences were found. These data suggest that no significant changes are found in nevi from women during pregnancy. Whether any changes in nevi occur postdelivery would be interesting to determine. Nonetheless, all of these studies

do not support the notion that melanocytic lesions change during pregnancy. Therefore, a changing melanocytic lesion in a pregnant woman should be treated as though it is an atypical finding and warrants biopsy.

ATYPICAL DERMAL MELANOCYTIC PROLIFERATIONS

Atypical dermal melanocytic proliferations pose a unique problem for dermatopathologists. When marked cytologic atypia is seen along with higher proliferation index, a dermal melanoma can be diagnosed. However, in some dermal melanocytic lesions, all of the criteria for dermal melanoma are not met. These lesions create problems for the pathologist because an accurate prognosis cannot be given to the clinician. Furthermore, the threshold and description of atypia can be subjective among different observers.

Proliferative Nodules in Congenital Nevi

One type of atypical dermal melanocytic proliferation is the proliferative nodule that can arise in a congenital nevus. These nodules are clinically soft and may regress, but some proliferative nodules can have atypia. Differentiating them from melanoma arising in a congenital nevus can be challenging. According to the literature, the giant congenital nevus can have a 6% to 14% lifetime risk of developing melanoma.[19] Therefore, atypical proliferative nodules are important to distinguish from melanoma and benign proliferative nodules. Phadke and colleagues[20] studied 18 benign and 25 atypical proliferative nodules using various immunohistochemical proliferation markers and molecular analyses. Atypical proliferative nodules differed from the benign counterpart in that they displayed sharp demarcation, expansile growth, epidermal effacement, nuclear pleomorphism, and increased mitoses. Molecular analysis showed that more NRAS mutations are found in giant congenital nevi and their proliferative nodules, whereas medium or small congenital nevi and their proliferative nodules have more BRAF mutations. These mutational studies are interesting, but they do not discriminate different types of proliferative nodules. Both proliferation markers, Ki-67 and pHH3, were noted to be higher in atypical versus benign proliferative nodules. When comparing atypical proliferative nodules with dermal melanoma, the proliferation index is very similar, suggesting that these atypical lesions are borderline and perhaps have a potential to become malignant.[20]

Pigmented Epithelioid Melanocytoma

Another example of an atypical dermal melanocytic proliferation is pigmented epithelioid melanocytoma (PEM). PEM was initially described in 2004 as a low-grade melanoma that metastasized to lymph nodes but with better prognosis than conventional melanoma.[21] PEM includes epithelioid blue nevus of Carney complex, which has been found to have loss of cyclic adenosine 3′,5′ monophosphate (AMP)–dependent protein kinase A regulatory subunit 1α (R1α).[22] Histologically, PEMs have distinct cytology, with epithelioid and spindle cells that are heavily pigmented with a very infiltrative pattern. To further understand the malignant potential of these lesions, a more recent study examined 26 cases of PEM with median follow-up of 67 months (range, 39–216 months).[23] The study showed that PEM behaves much better than conventional melanoma. Even though 8 of 18 patients who underwent sentinel lymph node biopsy had positive results, all 26 patients (including those who were positive for lymph node metastasis) are alive. Therefore, these limited data support that PEM is a low-grade tumor that can metastasize but does not cause significant mortality.[23]

Other atypical dermal melanocytic proliferations include nevoid borderline tumor, atypical Spitzoid tumor, and atypical lesions arising from a deep penetrating nevus. Magro and colleagues[24] examined cases of each of these lesions and PEMs, with an average follow-up of 4.2 years. They found a total of 32 cases, and all but one patient was alive and well. Many of these cases underwent treatment similar to melanoma, with wide excision and sentinel lymph node biopsy. The lymph node positivity ranged from 14% to 57%, depending on the category of atypical dermal melanocytic proliferation (25% [1/4] nevoid borderline tumors, 35% [5/14] atypical Spitzoid tumors, 14% [1/7] pigmented epithelioid melanocytomas, and 57% [4/7] borderline tumors in deep penetrating nevi). At first, this finding would support that, even though these lesions have positive sentinel lymph nodes, their biologic behavior is benign. However, the only patient (a 36-year-old man) who died had an atypical proliferation arising from a deep penetrating nevus. This lesion was diagnosed as a benign lesion 2 years before metastasis. Although it would be difficult to prove, the question remains whether adequate treatment of these lesions might explain the more benign behavior of these lesions. In other words, the current treatment for these atypical dermal melanocytic proliferations is the same as for melanoma.

SUMMARY

In summary, special-site nevi, such as those on the breast and genitalia, tend to have more cytologic and architectural atypia, but these differences can be considered benign. The histopathology of melanocytic proliferations during pregnancy does not seem to differ significantly. Atypical dermal melanocytic proliferations are difficult to diagnose and tend to have a better outcome after adequate treatment. Additional histopathologic studies along with longer clinical follow-up are required to determine if atypical dermal melanocytic proliferation will behave as a low-grade malignant neoplasm or a benign neoplasm. These types of studies are also needed for nevi of special (or different) sites and other difficult melanocytic lesions.

REFERENCES

1. Whiteman DC, Parsons PG, Green AC. Determinants of melanocyte density in adult human skin. Arch Dermatol Res 1999;291:511–6.

2. Harrison SL, Buettner PG, MacLennan R. Body-site distribution of melanocytic nevi in young Australian Children. Arch Dermatol 1999;135:47–52.

3. Hosler GA, Moresi JM, Barrett TL. Nevi with site-related atypia: a review of melanocytic nevi with atypical features based on anatomic site. J Cutan Pathol 2008;35:889–98.

4. Saad AG, Patel S, Mutasim DF. Melanocytic nevi of the auricular region: histologic characteristics and diagnostic difficulties. Arch Dermatol Res 2005;27:111–5.

5. Ronglioletti F, Urso C, Batolo D, et al. Melanocytic nevi of the breast: a histologic case-control study. J Cutan Pathol 2004;31:137–40.

6. Elder D. Precursors to melanoma and their mimics: nevi of special sites. Mod Pathol 2006;19:S4–20.

7. Gleason BC, Hirsh MS, Nucci MR, et al. Atypical genital nevi: a clinicopathologic analysis of 56 cases. Am J Surg Pathol 2008;32:51–7.

8. Coras B, Landthaler M, Stolz W, et al. Dysplastic melanocytic nevi of the lower leg: sex- and site-specific histopathology. Am J Dermatopathol 2010;32:599–602.

9. Gandini S, Sera F, Cattaruzza MS, et al. Meta-analysis of risk factors for cutaneous melanoma: I. common and atypical naevi. Eur J Cancer 2005;41:28–44.

10. Whiteman DC, Watt P, Purdine DM, et al. Melanocytic nevi, solar keratoses, and divergent pathways to cutaneous melanoma. J Natl Cancer Inst 2003;95:806–11.

11. Randi G, Naldi L, Gallus AD, et al. Number of nevi at a specific anatomical site and its relation to cutaneous malignant melanoma. J Invest Dermatol 2006;126:2106–10.

12. Ko CJ, McNiff JM, Glusac EJ. Melanocytic nevi with features of Spitz nevi and Clark's/dysplastic nevi ("Spark's" nevi). J Cutan Pathol 2009;36:1063–8.

13. Toussaint S, Kamino H. Dysplastic changes in different types of melanocytic nevi. A unifying concept. J Cutan Pathol 1999;26:84–90.

14. Grin CM, Rojas AI, Grants-Kels JM. Does pregnancy alter melanocytic nevi? J Cutan Pathol 2001;28:389–92.

15. Foucar E, Bentley TJ, Laube DW, et al. A histopathologic evaluation of nevocellular nevi in pregnancy. Arch Dermatol 1985;121:350–4.

16. Sanchez JL, Figueroa LD, Rodriguez E. Behavior of melanocytic nevi during pregnancy. Am J Dermatopathol 1984;6(Suppl):89–91.

17. Chan MP, Chan MM, Tahan SR. Melanocytic nevi in pregnancy: histologic features and Ki-67 proliferation index. J Cutan Pathol 2010;37:843–51.

18. Wyo Y, Synnerstad I, Fredrikson M, et al. Spectrophotometric analysis of melanocytic naevi during pregnancy. Acta Derm Venereol 2007;87:231–7.

19. Bittencourt FV, Marghoob AA, Kopf AW, et al. Large congenital melanocytic nevi and the risk for development of malignant melanoma and neurocutaneous melanocytosis. Pediatrics 2000;106:736–41.

20. Phadke PA, Rakheja D, Le LP, et al. Proliferative nodules arising within congenital melanocytic nevi: a histologic, immunohistochemical, and molecular analyses of 43 cases. Am J Surg Pathol 2001;35:656–69.

21. Zembowicz A, Carney JA, Mihm MC. Pigmented epithelioid melanocytoma. Am J Surg Pathol 2004;28:31–40.

22. Zembowicz A, Knoeepp SM, Bei T, et al. Loss of expression of protein kinase a regulatory subunit 1alpha in pigmented epithelioid melanocytoma but not in melanoma or other melanocytic lesions. Am J Surg Pathol 2007;31:1764–75.

23. Mandal RV, Murali R, Lundquist KF, et al. Pigmented epithelioid melanocytoma: favorable outcome after 5 year follow-up. Am J Surg Pathol 2009;33:1778–82.

24. Magro CM, Crowson AN, Mihm MC, et al. The dermal-based borderline melanocytic tumor: a categorical approach. J Am Acad Dermatol 2010;62:469–79.

Dermatology Clinics
What's New in Dermatopathology: News in Nonmelanocytic Neoplasia

Harleen K. Sidhu, MD[a], Rita V. Patel, MD[b],
Gary Goldenberg, MD[a,b],*

KEYWORDS

- Nonmelanocytic neoplasia • Dermatopathology • Merkel cell carcinoma
- Squamous cell carcinoma • Muir-Torre syndrome • Sebaceous

KEY POINTS

- The proposed oncogenic role of Merkel cell polyomavirus in Merkel cell carcinoma has prompted researchers to explore its role in several human cancers, including non-Merkel skin cancers, neuroblastoma, and lung cancer.
- In the seventh edition of the American Joint Committee of Cancer's recommended staging criteria manual, new staging systems for Merkel cell carcinoma and squamous cell carcinoma (with the exception of those affecting the eyelid, vulva, or penis) were introduced, which separated these entities from the existing nonmelanoma skin cancer staging system because of their increased metastatic potential.
- The entity known as reticulated acanthoma/epithelioma with sebaceous differentiation is controversial and there is a need to develop clear-cut diagnostic criteria. A possibility of association of this entity with Muir-Torre syndrome (MTS) has been raised.
- Sebaceous neoplasms, including sebaceous adenomas, sebaceomas and sebaceous carcinomas, and multiple keratoacanthomas, may occur sporadically or can be seen as a manifestation of MTS. It is important to differentiate between sporadic sebaceous tumors and sebaceous neoplasms arising in association with MTS, because the skin findings may be the primary presentation and lead to the diagnosis of MTS.

This article reviews the recent dermatopathology literature involving nonmelanocytic neoplasia, with a focus on important work done over the last 5 years. The discussion includes advances in the understanding of Merkel cell carcinoma (MCC) pathogenesis and prognosis; changes in the seventh edition of the American Joint Committee of Cancer staging manual in reference to staging of squamous cell carcinoma (SCC) and MCC; newly described or rare histopathologic patterns and entities including squamoid eccrine ductal carcinoma (SEDC), rippled-pattern adnexal neoplasms (RPAN), onychomatricoma (OM), spindle cell–predominant trichodiscoma (SCPT) and neurofollicular hamartoma, and myoepithelioma; and microsatellite instability (MSI) in sebaceous neoplasms of Muir-Torre syndrome (MTS) and other tumors.

MCC AND MERKEL CELL POLYOMAVIRUS

MCC of the skin is a rare, aggressive cutaneous malignancy that predominantly affects elderly white

Disclosures: None.
[a] Department of Pathology, Mount Sinai School of Medicine, One Gustave L Levy Place, New York, NY 10029, USA; [b] Department of Dermatology, Mount Sinai School of Medicine, One Gustave L Levy Place, New York, NY 10029, USA
* Corresponding author. 5 East 98th Street, 5th Floor, New York, NY 10029.
E-mail address: garygoldenbergmd@gmail.com

Dermatol Clin 30 (2012) 623–641
http://dx.doi.org/10.1016/j.det.2012.06.009
0733-8635/12/$ – see front matter © 2012 Elsevier Inc. All rights reserved.

men. MCC has a tendency for local recurrence and regional lymph node metastasis. Factors associated with development of MCC include ultraviolet radiation exposure, immunosuppression, and Merkel cell polyomavirus (MCPyV). MCPyV represents the first polyomavirus linked to human cancer.[1]

Feng and colleagues used a methodology known as digital transcriptome subtraction to first identify this virus. The group then confirmed the presence of MCPyV in 8 of 10 MCC tumors. Additionally, in 6 of the 10 samples, the viral genome was clonally integrated into the human genome. This integration of the viral genome not only refutes the possibility that MCpyV is merely a coincidental, passenger infection in MCC but also supports the contention that virus-associated tumors are "biologic accidents."[2] It is also important to note that this identified pattern of integration also suggests that MCPyV infection and integration occurs before the replication of tumor cells.[3]

Other researchers have identified MCPyV in MCC. In the largest retrospective case series, DNA from MCPyV was detected in 91 of 114 patients diagnosed over a 25-year period in Finland. Additionally, there was no evidence of MCPyV in 22 control samples from other tumors (glioblastoma or melanoma) or normal tissues.[4] MCPyV has also been identified in nonlesional skin of those diagnosed with MCC.[5,6]

The high incidence of MCC in the immunocompromised population first suggested the possibility of an infectious cause of MCC.[7] This tumor has an aggressive course in immunosuppressed patients with a reported mortality rate of up to 56% in this group. The mean age of diagnosis is about 10 years earlier than immunocompetent patients.[8] Chronically immunosuppressed patients are more than 15 times more likely to be diagnosed with MCC than age-matched immunocompetent individuals, especially in those who are HIV-positive.[9]

Direct causality, however, still remains a highly debated topic. Factors supporting this infectious cause include increased tumor incidence and high mortality in the immunosuppressed population, presence of viral DNA in most MCCs, large T antigen transcript presence in MCC tumor cells, and the clonal integration of MCPyV DNA in tumors. In contrast, features that argue against a viral cause of MCC include the presence of MCPyV-negative tumors, predilection for fair-skinned individuals, and lack of tumors among close contacts, all of which would be suspected with a viral infection.[3,5,7]

Thus far, only one study has explored prognosis of MCpyV presence and survival. In a Finnish study, DNA-positive MCCs were located on the extremities more frequently than those that were DNA-negative, had less frequent regional lymph node involvement, and better overall survival rates.[4] Further research is necessary to fully support this finding.[10]

MERKEL CELL POLYOMAVIRUS IN OTHER NEOPLASIA

The proposed oncogenic role of MCPyV in MCC has prompted researchers to explore its role in several human cancers, including non-Merkel skin cancers, neuroblastoma, and lung cancer. For instance, Mertz and colleagues[11] were able to establish a link between epidermodysplasia verruciformis, a rare genodermatosis in which patients are particularly susceptible to infection with specific human papillomavirus subtypes. In this study, several skin neoplasms (carcinomas in situ, invasive SCCs, and common warts) were biopsied from six patients with congenital epidermodysplasia verruciformis and one subject with acquired epidermodysplasia verruciformis secondary to immunosuppression. All specimens were found to have MCPyV DNA. In contrast, all seven normal skin samples from these subjects tested negative for MCPyV DNA. It is suggested by the authors that MCPyV and epidermodysplasia verruciformis and human papillomavirus may act as synergistic oncogenic cofactors in development of epidermodysplasia verruciformis neoplasms.[11]

Results from a recent study evaluating 72 tumors, other than MCC, have questioned an MCPyV association with other types of cancer. A study published by Ly and colleagues[12] examined 57 such lesions, consisting of 15 melanomas, 5 in situ melanomas, 15 invasive SCC, 4 basal cell carcinomas (BCC), 3 actinic keratoses, 2 seborrheic keratosis, 1 common wart, 1 verruca plana–like lesion, 1 virus-associated trichodysplasia spinulosa, and 10 benign follicular lesions. Also, 15 cases each of pulmonary and gastrointestinal neuroendocrine tumors were included in the study. All 72 tumors tested negative for MCPyV irrespective of any known MCC diagnosis or immune status. Rollison and colleagues[13] recently released the first serologic case-control study relating MCPyV and SCC. Data showed that MCPyV DNA was found in 38% of SCC cases (55 of 145). A statistically significant association was even observed between MCPyV seropositivity and MCC DNA-positive SCC (odds ratio, 2.49; 95% confidence interval, 1.03–6.04). Future research into the mechanism of the immune evasion used by MCPyV will help to establish whether causality exists among this proposed human cancer-causing virus and other tumors.

MCC PROGNOSIS AND P63

A significant correlation between expression of p63, a member of the p53 family, and the clinical course of MCC has recently been proposed.[14] The TP63 gene, which maps to chromosome 3q27–29, is expressed in basal and stem cells of the epidermis. The p63 gene can be identified, frequently amplified, and overexpressed in several different kinds of human neoplasia, including carcinoma of the head and neck, lung, skin, esophagus, mammary glands, urothelium, cervix, prostate gland, and oral SCC, and in odontogenic tumors.[15–24] Thus far, p63 is not generally a definitive indicator of poor prognosis; however, it has been correlated with poorly differentiated basaloid carcinoma.[25] Additionally, it has been reported that p63 expression can be considered a poor prognostic indicator in certain subgroups of B-cell lymphoma.[26]

An immunohistochemical analysis of close to 50 cases of MCC showed dot-like paranuclear or membranous CK20 staining in more than 80% of the cells from all cases. Reactivity was present for certain neuroendocrine markers (chromogranin and synaptophysin), whereas thyroid transcription factor-1 was nonreactive in all cases. Positivity for Ki-67 ranged from 15% to 95%. Twenty-five of the 47 cases were found to be positive for p63. It should be noted that a statistically significant association was noted between p63 and Ki-67 expression ($P = .0006$). Additionally, p63 positivity was significantly associated with an adverse overall survival compared with the absence of p63 expression ($P<.0001$). Statistics on survival analysis also demonstrated a significantly lower overall survival not only with an increase in the stage of disease ($P<.0001$) but also with those tumors demonstrating a higher proliferative index ($P = .001$). However, no link was ascertained between p63 expression and tumor site, gender, age, tumor size, stage of disease, cell size, and the presence or absence of angioinvasion, or the presence of mitotic figures. Overall, this research substantiates p63 as a marker for prognosis in MCC.[14]

The same group followed-up this initial analysis with a larger case series and found that 61% of 70 primary MCCs were p63 reactive. This was statistically significantly associated with adverse overall survival ($P<.0001$) and a decreased disease-free survival ($P<.0001$) when compared with the absence of p63 expression. In particular, those MCC cases at low stage (stage I –II) that were p63 positive exhibited a more aggressive clinical course than those that were negative ($P<.0001$). These data further support the association between p63 and prognosis in MCC. Those with p63-positive MCC showed an estimated 1-year overall survival

of 90% for stage I or stage II; 3-year overall survival of 79% for stage I and 57% for stage II; and 5-year overall survival of 66% for stage I and 57% for stage II. Taken as a whole, expression of p63 suggests worse prognosis in patients with low-stage MCC. The authors believe p63 represents a new independent marker of clinical evolution in these patients. It is thought that p63 denotes a switch toward a stem cell phenotype that might be the most consistent predictor of survival in MCC. The authors additionally suggest that the oncogenic potential of p63 may be secondary to activation of a much more lethal p53-mediated oncogenic pathway.[27]

NEW STAGING OF SCC AND MCC

For the past 20 years, the American Joint Committee of Cancer, an executive committee responsible for releasing the recommended staging criteria for all cancers, has grouped together all nonmelanoma skin cancers, including SCC. However, in the newly released seventh edition of this manual, new staging systems for MCC and SCC (with the exception of those affecting the eyelid, vulva, or penis) were separated from the existing NMSC staging system because of their increased metastatic potential.

The new MCC four-stage system is summarized in **Table 1**. Staging takes into account three variables: (1) tumor size, (2) node status, and (3) distant metastasis. Tumors of less than 2 cm in maximum dimension are pT1, those between 2 and 5 cm are pT2, and tumors larger than 5 cm are pT3. According to this system, there are two different substages for cases with pathologically confirmed lymph node metastasis. The "A" substage denotes tumors that are identified microscopically in sentinel nodes but are not clinically palpable. This substage has a more favorable prognosis. Substage "B" describes those tumors that were clinically palpable and were confirmed histologically. Therefore, pathologic examination of clinically uninvolved lymph nodes by sentinel lymph node biopsy (SLN) is now considered critical when determining MCC prognosis. Serial sectioning of SLN in conjunction with various immunohistochemical stains (CK20, CAM5.2, AE1/AE3, synaptophysin, or chromogranin, in addition to standard hematoxylin-eosin stains) are essential to provide acceptable sensitivity and specificity when diagnosing micrometastatic nodal MCC.[28,29]

Imaging studies are also being used to discover distant MCC metastasis.[30] In a retrospective review, positron-emission tomography–computed tomography exacted a change of management in 9 out of 18 patients, all with late-stage MCC.[31] Imaging may also be indicated to exclude skin metastasis

Table 1
American Joint Committee on Cancer seventh edition staging for Merkel cell carcinoma

Tumor (T)

TX: Primary tumor cannot be assessed
T0: No evidence of primary tumor (nodal/metastatic presentation without associated primary)
Tis: In situ primary tumor
T1: ≤2 cm maximum tumor dimension
T2: >2 cm but ≤5 cm maximum tumor dimension
T3: >5 cm maximum tumor dimension
T4: Primary tumor invades bone, muscle, fascia, or cartilage

Node (N)

NX: Regional lymph nodes cannot be assessed
N0: No regional lymph node metastasis
cN0: Nodes negative by clinical examination (by inspection, palpation, or imaging, but no pathologic node examination performed)
pN0: Nodes negative by pathologic examination
N1: Metastases in regional lymph node(s)
N1a: Micrometastasis (diagnosed after sentinel or elective lymphadenectomy)
N1b: Macrometastasis (clinically detectable nodal metastases confirmed by therapeutic lymphadenectomy or needle biopsy)
N2: In-transit metastasis (distinct from the primary lesion and located either between the primary lesion and draining regional lymph nodes or distal to the primary lesion)

Metastasis (M)

M0: No distant metastasis
M1: Metastases beyond regional lymph nodes
M1a: Metastases to skin, subcutaneous tissues, or distant lymph nodes
M1b: Metastasis to lung
M1c: Metastases to all other visceral sites

Stage	T	N	M
0	Tis	N0	M0
IA	T1	pN0	M0
IB	T1	cN0	M0
IIA	T2/T3	pN0	M0
IIB	T2/T3	cN0	M0
IIC	T4	N0	M0
IIIA	Any T	N1a	M0
IIIB	Any T	N1b/N2	M0
IV	Any T	Any N	M1

Data from Edge SE, Byrd DR, Compton CC, et al. AJCC Cancer Staging Manual, Springer, New York, NY, USA, 7th edition, 2010.

from a noncutaneous carcinoma. For head and neck disease, radiolabeled somatostatin receptor scintigraphy has been particularly promoted for evaluation.[5,32] Magnetic resonance imaging is reported as being useful for extremity lesions, bony metastasis, and disease at the sinonasal region, orbit, and abdominal wall by permitting better target volume planning for radiation therapy and determining response to treatment.[33]

For SCC, the seventh edition redefines T staging. No longer is there a 5-cm size cutoff for T staging. Additionally, the new edition incorporates factors other than tumor size and involvement of adjacent structures in the primary T stage (**Table 2**). The T stage is now classified by tumor diameter greater or less than 2 cm, presence of bone invasion, and high-risk features. These high-risk features include anatomic location on the ear or glabrous lip; tumor thickness of 2 mm or more; involvement of the reticular dermis (Clark level IV or higher); poor differentiation; lymphovascular invasion; or local perineural invasion.[34]

In comparison with its use in identifying occult nodal metastases in breast cancer and cutaneous melanoma, SLN biopsy is still only seen as an investigational staging tool in those with clinically

Table 2
American Joint Committee on Cancer seventh edition staging for cutaneous squamous cell carcinoma (other than eyelid, vulva, or penis)

Tumor (T)
  TX: Primary tumor cannot be assessed
  T0: No evidence of primary tumor (nodal/metastatic presentation without associated primary)
  Tis: Carcinoma in situ
  T1: ≤2 cm maximum tumor dimension with <2 high-risk features[a]
  T2: >2 cm with or without one additional high-risk feature, or any size with ≥2 high-risk features[a]
  T3: Tumor with invasion of maxilla, mandible, orbit, or temporal bone
  T4: Primary tumor invades skeleton (axial or appendicular) or perineural invasion of the skull base

Node (N)
  NX: Regional lymph nodes cannot be assessed
  N0: No regional lymph node metastasis
  N1: Metastasis in single ipsilateral lymph node, ≤3 cm in greatest dimension
  N2: Metastasis in single ipsilateral lymph node, >3 cm but not >6 cm in greatest dimension; or in multiple ipsilateral lymph nodes, none >6 cm in greatest dimension or in bilateral or contralateral lymph nodes, none >6 cm in greatest dimension
  N2a: Metastasis in a single ipsilateral lymph node, >3 cm but not >6 cm in greatest dimension
  N2b: Metastasis in a single ipsilateral lymph node, none >6 cm in greatest dimension
  N2c: Metastasis in bilateral or contralateral lymph nodes, none >6 cm in greatest dimension
  N3: Metastasis in lymph node, >6 cm in greatest dimension

Metastasis (M)
  Mx: Distant metastasis cannot be assessed
  M0: No distant metastasis
  M1: Metastases beyond regional lymph nodes

Stage	T	N	M
0	Tis	N0	M0
I	T1	N0	M0
II	T2	N0	M0
III	T3	N0	M0
	T1 or T2	N1	M0
IV	T1, T2, or T3	N1	M0
	Any T	N3	M0
	T4	Any N	M0
	Any T	Any N	M1

[a] High-risk features include depth (>2 mm thickness; Clark level ≥IV); perineural invasion; location (primary site ear; primary site nonglabrous lip); and differentiation (poorly differentiated or undifferentiated).
Data from Farasat S, Yu SS, Neel VA, et al. A new American Joint Committee on Cancer staging system for cutaneous squamous cell carcinoma: creation and rationale for inclusion of tumor (T) characteristics. J Am Acad Dermatol 2011; 64(6):1051–9.

node-negative, high-risk cutaneous SCC. Rapid growth rate, irregular borders, moderate-to-poor differentiation, and perineural invasion are considered qualities of high-risk SCC. Additionally, recurrent lesions, sites of prior radiotherapy or chronic inflammation, immunocompromised states, and genetic disorders including albinism and xeroderma pigmentosum are all considered high-risk factors for SCC.[35,36] In terms of size and location, SCC tumors are considered high-risk when measuring greater than 2 cm on the trunk and extremities. High-risk SCCs of the cheeks, forehead, scalp, and neck are larger than 1 cm. SCCs larger than 0.6 cm

on the face, genitalia, and hands and feet are now classified as high-risk. More recent studies have suggested that Clark level IV tumor thickness, desmoplastic growth, and development of nodal metastases are the strongest predictors of survival.[37,38] Until larger, prospective studies with longer follow-up are established, the integration of SLN biopsy as part of the optimal treatment of occult nodal metastasis for high-risk cutaneous SCC remains unclear.[39]

Another revision to the seventh edition involves characterization of nodal SCC metastases. Previously, nodal disease was scored as either present

(N1) or absent (N0). In the seventh edition nodal metastases is characterized by N0 to N3 by using the size and number of involved nodes.[40–42]

SQUAMOID ECCRINE DUCTAL CARCINOMA

Adnexal carcinomas of the skin are rare neoplasms that can manifest histologically in a variety of ways.[43] Carcinomas arising from the eccrine apparatus comprise less than 0.01% of all cutaneous tumors. Ductal eccrine carcinoma typically affects the scalp, trunk, arms, or legs of middle-aged or elderly individuals in the form of a nodule or plaque. Rates of metastases are much higher for eccrine tumors (up to 50%) versus SCCs (0.5%). The clinical course of these neoplasms is aggressive; characterized by multiple local recurrences, perineural invasion, and lymph node and distant organ metastasis.[44]

SEDC is exceedingly rare with only six cases reported in the English literature, which makes this a unique diagnostic challenge. Those unfamiliar with this diagnosis may erroneously diagnose SCC. This distinction is important to management because of the variable rates of recurrence and metastasis between these two carcinomas.[45–47]

SEDC has a slight male preponderance and affects those aged 30 to 90 with a mean of 69. The ear, cheek, and neck are common locations, in addition to the hand, knee, forearm, and axilla. Histologically, SEDC is an atypical squamous proliferation that lacks circumscription and infiltrates the dermis and underlying adipose tissue (**Fig. 1**). The tumor displays areas of superficial squamous differentiation, which are usually continuous with the epidermis (**Fig. 2**). Deeper portions of

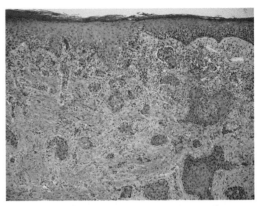

Fig. 2. Squamoid eccrine ductal carcinoma. The tumor displays areas of superficial squamous differentiation, which are usually continuous with the epidermis (hematoxylin-eosin, original magnification ×100).

the tumor may show eccrine ductal differentiation and are composed of angulated basaloid cells with tubular structures, similar to that seen in benign eccrine syringoma (**Fig. 3**). An inflammatory infiltrate is frequently seen.[48]

SEDC express CK5/6, CK903, CAM 5.2, and CK 116. EMA and CEA show positive staining in SEDC with a preference for tumor cells and ductal epithelium. However, EMA does not help determine etiopathogenesis because adnexal and epithelial neoplasms display reactivity. However, CEA staining supports an adnexal origin and assists in differentiation from SCC.[49]

The dermatopathologic differential diagnosis for SEDC includes adenosquamous carcinoma and microcystic adnexal carcinoma.[48] Adenosquamous carcinoma is a rare, malignant lesion containing mixed squamous and glandular differentiation.

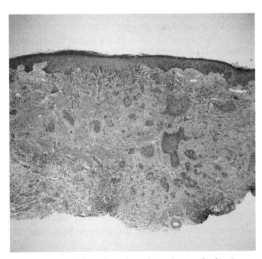

Fig. 1. Squamoid eccrine ductal carcinoma lacks circumscription and infiltrates the dermis (hematoxylin-eosin, original magnification ×40).

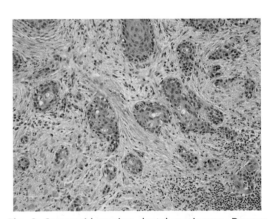

Fig. 3. Squamoid eccrine ductal carcinoma. Deeper portions of the tumor are composed of angulated aggregates of basaloid cells with tubular structures, similar to that seen in a benign syringoma (hematoxylin-eosin, original magnification ×100).

Clinically, adenosquamous carcinoma is described as a hyperkeratotic, erythematous papule or plaque occurring on sun-exposed surfaces, especially the head or neck, of older individuals.[50] On pathology, islands of squamous cells that often originate in the epidermis are seen among "keratin pearls." Intraluminal mucin may be noted.[51] Local perineural invasion is common, yet recurrence and distance metastasis rarely occur. It should be noted that adenosquamous carcinoma and SEDC can infiltrate to the subcutaneous fat. However, most tumor islands contain EMA and CEA positive ducts in SEDC.[48,49,51–53]

Patients with microcystic adnexal carcinoma most often present with erythematous papules or plaques on a sun-exposed surface of the body, especially the central face. Local invasion is commonly seen; however, distant metastasis is exceedingly rare.[54] The pathology of microcystic adnexal carcinoma often shows strands and cords of cells with pilar and glandular differentiation.[55,56] In contrast, SEDC contains more irregular, superficial squamous aggregates with focal ductal structures.[48]

SEDC is exceedingly uncommon, yet an aggressive and important eccrine neoplasm. Diagnosis is heavily determined by the tumor aggregates with ductal differentiation and focal prominent squamoid features, particularly in the most superficial areas of the neoplasm. Additionally, the CEA and EMA staining pattern can assist in histopathologic diagnosis. Currently, there is no universally accepted, standard of care for SEDC[48]; however, Mohs micrographic surgery is reported in the literature as a treatment option with high efficacy rates.[57]

ONYCHOMATRICOMA/UNGUIOBLASTIC FIBROMA

OM is a rare benign tumor of the nail matrix. Based on microscopic features, some have advocated for the name "unguioblastic fibroma" for this diagnosis. To date, only 44 cases of OM have been described in the literature. OM affects both sexes equally, more commonly in adult whites. Recent genome-wide analyses of an OM showed 34 genomic alterations, with most mutations identified on chromosome 11.[58,59]

Classic clinical findings include a longitudinal yellow band of varying thickness, proximally located splinter hemorrhages, longitudinal ridging that transverse the curvature of the nail, and with nail avulsion small fingerlike projections can be appreciated from the nail matrix.[60] The differential diagnosis of OM includes onycholemmal horn, malignant proliferating onycholemmal cyst, subungual keratoacanthoma, and subungual SCC.

Subungual and periungual warts, ungual Bowen disease, and fibrokeratoma of the nail bed might also be considered. Complete surgical excision is considered standard of care.[61]

Histopathology is a very reliable means of differentiating OM from other similar entities. Epithelial invaginations are noted with a fibrous base containing sparse fibroblasts (**Figs. 4** and **5**).[62] Immunohistochemical analyses have demonstrated the same expression of cytokeratins and integrins in OM as in the normal nail matrix. However, the AE13 antibody specific to Ha 1–4 trichocystic keratins is a uniquely useful marker.[63] Additionally, it should be noted that OM is immunoreactive with CD34, but not CD 99, EMA, or S-100.[64–77]

OM is unique because it grows within the nail plate, often making diagnosis possible just from a nail plate specimen. The thickened plate shows lacunae containing serous fluid, lined by a keratogenous portion of epithelium that represented the canals that housed the digitate epithelial projections from the nail matrix. This has been likened to a woodworm-like appearance.[64,78]

RIPPLED-PATTERN ADNEXAL NEOPLASMS

Tumors categorized as RPAN have a characteristic appearance resulting from alternating areas of epithelial cell cords and stroma. This "rippled" pattern resembles Verocay bodies of schwannoma. Rippled-pattern in a cutaneous adnexal neoplasm was first described by Hashimoto and colleagues[79] in 1989 in a trichomatricoma.

Because the components of pilosebaceous-apocrine structure have a common embryologic origin, one can expect the entire spectrum of trichoblastoma, trichoblastoma with sebaceous differentiation (sebaceous trichoblastoma), trichoblastoma with apocrine differentiation, sebaceoma,

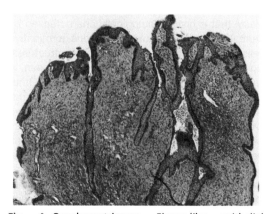

Fig. 4. Onychomatricoma. Finger-like epithelial projections with prominent connective tissue cores (hematoxylin-eosin, original magnification ×40).

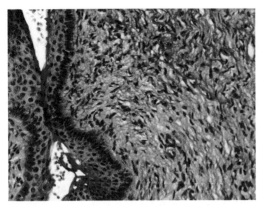

Fig. 5. Onychomatricoma. Superficial cellular stroma with fibrillary collagen (hematoxylin-eosin, original magnification ×200).

and sebaceoma with apocrine differentiation to have some similarity in their histologic patterns. Almost all tumors belonging to pilosebaceous-apocrine structure have shown a rippled-pattern.[80–82] These lesions most commonly occur on the scalp of men.[80,83–95] They usually appear after the fourth decade of life and have not been reported in the first two decades. RPAN can be skin-colored, pink, red, yellow, or yellow-red solitary, dome-shaped, and nonulcerated lesions. No association of RPAN with MTS has been reported.[80,96] One case of rippled-pattern trichoblastoma with apocrine differentiation arising in a nevus sebaceous has been reported.[97]

It can be easy to overlook focal sebaceous or apocrine differentiation in a pilosebaceous-apocrine neoplasm. This is why Ohata and Ackerman in their study concluded that all tumors that look like trichoblastoma and show a benign silhouette with a ripple-pattern or combined labyrinthine-sinusoidal pattern are sebaceomas.[98,99]

Sebaceoma, originally described by Troy and Ackerman[100] in 1984, is a benign sebaceous neoplasm that is histopathologically characterized by dermal lobules of basaloid, sebaceous germinative cells and sebaceous ductlike or cystlike structures. No atypia or atypical mitotic figures are seen. A classic sebaceoma has a lobular pattern. Other variants described include rippled pattern, carcinoid-like pattern, reticulated-cribriform pattern, and labyrinthine-sinusoidal pattern.[83,96] All of these variants likely relate to each other (ie, lobules can become carcinoid-like trabeculae/cords/rosettes/pseudorosettes when the stroma compresses them in different ways). Trabeculae-cords can either look like ripples when the relationship of stroma and epithelial cells takes the form of alternating parallel waves or a network of interconnected epithelial cords (reticulated-cribriform pattern) when the

waves are not parallel to each other. A pattern of intricate, tortuous, complex, and blind alleys is called labyrinthine-sinusoidal; when the ratio of epithelial to stromal component is greater than 1, it is called labyrinthine, and when this ratio is less than 1, it is called sinusoidal because of its resemblance to passage-like channels (sinuses).[100]

The exact pathogenesis of the classic and variant patterns is not known. Cell adhesion mechanisms, qualitative or quantitative variations in the stromal components, and extracellular signaling molecules could be involved in creating these patterns. Enhanced cell adhesion caused by overexpression of laminins and overexpression of extracellular signaling phospholipids have been postulated as possible mechanisms for the formation of Verocay bodies (which resemble rippled pattern) in schwannomas.[101,102] It has also been suggested that increased amounts of extracellular matrix deposition threaten separation of cells and the cells form palisades or Verocay bodies as an adaptive response to maintain cell-to-cell communication.[103]

Numerous markers have been studied in ripple-pattern sebaceoma. Varying studies share some overlap between the antibodies examined, but not the clones used. There was no consistent staining pattern, which could be due to the difference in clones. Basaloid cells have been reported to stain for AE1/AE3 (pancytokeratin), 34βE12, CK14, CK15, CK8/CK18/CK19, and p63 in various studies. The Ki-67 labeling index varied in one study from 10% to 20%.[81,85–87,89,91] Vacuolated cells (sebocytes) were EMA-positive in two of three studies and were adipophilin-positive in both studies that tested for its expression.[81,85,89] Vacuolated cells have stained positive for CK7/CK8/CK19 only in one case.[104] Immunohistochemical staining of ductlike structures has been commented on only in one case, which showed CK10 and CK17 positivity in the ductlike structures.[86]

Benign dermal neoplasms that form well-circumscribed collections of round or oval cells and show a rippled pattern can look like rippled-pattern sebaceoma. The entities from which rippled-pattern sebaceoma must be differentiated include trichoblastoma, BCC, schwannoma, leiomyoma, and melanocytic neoplasms. It is unlikely to have difficulty in an excision specimen of the tumor, especially when the rippled or other variant pattern is not diffuse. However, when dealing with a small biopsy of a tumor with a rippled pattern the differential diagnosis has to be considered.[105] The presence of peripheral palisading in the nodular aggregates and lack of sebocytes-ductlike structures supports the diagnosis of trichoblastoma with rippled pattern. Immunohistochemical staining for adipophilin could be a good tool to look for sebocytic differentiation in a tumor that looks like trichoblastoma with rippled pattern to rule in or out a rippled-pattern sebaceoma but the literature has been unclear. Rippled-pattern sebaceoma can be differentiated from BCC with rippled pattern by the absence of those features that are characteristic of a BCC (eg, peripheral palisading, retraction artifact, and myxoid stroma). A rippled-pattern schwannoma usually shows Antoni type A and B areas and is S-100 positive by immunohistochemical staining. A ripple-pattern leiomyoma can be diagnosed by the presence of elongated eel-like nuclei with blunt ends and immunohistochemical positivity for SMA and desmin. A melanocytic neoplasm with rippled-pattern shows positivity for S-100 and Mart-1.

SEBACEOUS NEOPLASMS, MSI, AND ASSOCIATION WITH HEREDITARY NONPOLYPOSIS COLORECTAL CANCER OR MTS

MTS is an autosomal-dominant genodermatosis characterized by the presence of cutaneous sebaceous neoplasms and visceral malignancies, initially described separately by Muir and Torre.[106,107] MTS is a phenotypic variant of the hereditary nonpolyposis colorectal cancer (HNPCC or Lynch) syndrome.[102]

Sebaceous neoplasms, including sebaceous adenomas, sebaceomas, and sebaceous carcinomas, and multiple keratoacanthomas, may occur sporadically or can be seen as a manifestation of MTS.[108,109] Sebaceous neoplasms in MTS have an inherited germline mutation in one allele of the DNA mismatch repair (MMR) genes. MMR deficiency results after a somatic loss-of-function mutation occurs in the wild-type allele.[111–113] MMR genes are responsible for fixing replication errors in DNA repeat sequences, termed "microsatellites." Microsatellite mutations accumulate if there is a lack of MMR, causing MSI. In sebaceous tumors associated with MTS immunohistochemical staining may be used to detect loss of DNA MMR proteins, most of which occur in MSH-2 and MLH-1.[113–118]

Evaluation for inherited germline mutations in MMR genes should be considered when a sebaceous lesion is diagnosed, especially when there are unusual histopathologic features seen and multiple cutaneous lesions are present.[119] In addition, work-up to rule out visceral malignancies in the patient and family members must be performed. It is important to differentiate between sporadic sebaceous tumors and sebaceous neoplasms arising in association with MTS, because the skin findings may be the primary presentation and lead to the diagnosis of MTS.

INTERNAL MALIGNANCIES ASSOCIATED WITH MTS

The visceral malignancies present most commonly in MTS are large bowel, genitourinary tract, endometrial, ovary, and breast carcinomas.[119] Approximately 61% of these internal tumors occur in the gastrointestinal tract, colorectal carcinoma being the most common, and usually located proximal to the splenic flexure.[108–121] Tumors of the urogenital tract represent 22% of cases.[119] Tumors seen in association with MTS usually have an indolent course.[119]

Germline mutations in MSH-2 and MLH-1 and less commonly MLH-3 and PMS-2 are responsible for HNPCC and MTS.[121–124] In HNPCC, 40% of the germline mutations occur in MSH-2 and 35% in MLH-1, whereas MTS most commonly is caused by mutations in MSH-2. About 25% of patients with HNPCC and MTS have no mutations detected.[120,125–127] Benign cutaneous lesions in HNPCC may also have evidence of MSI.[114]

SEBACEOUS ADENOMA

Clinically, sebaceous adenomas are tan-pink papulonodules most commonly occurring on the face of older patients, with a predilection for the nose, cheek, and scalp.[128–131] In MTS, sebaceous adenomas are seen in atypical sites and less commonly the head and neck area.[131]

Histologically, sebaceous adenomas are multilobulated, with greater than 50% of the lobule comprised of mature sebocytes, with foamy cytoplasm and hyperchromatic crenated nuclei.[132,133] The lobules have an external collagenous pseudocapsule encompassing more than two layers of basaloid cells, with oval nuclei and scant cytoplasm.[128–130] This is distinct from the two layers of germinative cells seen in sebaceous hyperplasia.[132] A lobular architecture appearing like a normal sebaceous gland is characteristic. Necrosis is not seen. Sebaceous adenomas may elevate the overlying epidermis.[128–130]

SEBACEOMA

Sebaceomas are clinically yellow or skin-colored papules, nodules, or plaques in older patients, most commonly on the face and scalp.[128–130] Histopathologically, sebaceomas are dermal tumors, but commonly elevate the epidermis. Dense eosinophilic connective tissue divides the individual lobules, consisting of basaloid cells and mature sebaceous cells.[128–130] Organized lobular architecture, peripheral palisading, and stromal-tumor clefting are absent. Small nucleoli may be seen; however, nuclear pleomorphism is absent. There are little to no mitoses present. The formation of ducts is common with sebaceous debris-filled cysts with an eosinophilic cuticle sometimes seen. Tumor necrosis in the basaloid portion is absent.[128–130]

The differential diagnosis of sebaceoma includes sebaceous adenoma or a well-differentiated sebaceous carcinoma. Sebaceous adenoma is characterized by a more organized lobular architecture. Sebaceous carcinoma exhibits greater nuclear pleomorphism, prominent nucleoli, and a higher mitotic index. BCC with sebaceous differentiation has predominant features of a BCC, such as peripheral nuclear palisading, cellular apoptosis, and stromal-tumor retraction.[134] Immunohistochemical studies may help differentiate between the two entities, because sebaceoma stains positively for EMA and D2-40 and Ber-EP4 highlights BCC.[135–137] Trichoblastoma with sebaceous differentiation may exhibit papillary mesenchymal bodies and characteristic hair germ differentiation.[97]

SEBACEOUS CARCINOMA

Sebaceous carcinoma is a rare tumor, with 75% of cases presenting in the periocular location.[138–141]

Ultraviolet radiation is thought to contribute to the pathogenesis of sebaceous carcinomas.[142]

On histology, the extraocular sebaceous carcinomas show disordered lobular patterns and less frequently may exhibit diffuse growth in the superficial dermis and continuity with the epidermis.[134] The subcutaneous fat and underlying muscle may be involved.[134] The lobules are comprised of basaloid cells and more mature sebocytes. Necrosis is commonly seen and keratin may be present.[143] In poorly differentiated sebaceous carcinomas, there is substantial nuclear and cytoplasmic pleomorphism and frequent mitoses. Perineural, lymphatic, or vascular invasion may be seen (**Fig. 6**).[134]

Immunohistochemistry plays an important role in identification of patients with MTS. A suggested immunohistochemical panel includes the MMR genes, MSH-2, MLH-1, and MLH-6. Gene inactivation of these MMR genes in tumors is present when there is a complete lack of nuclear staining of the protein produced by the MMR genes in the neoplastic cells. Other MMR proteins, such as PMS-2 and MLH-3, have rarely been found in patients with HNPCC and have not been reported in MTS.[144–147] Immunohistochemical analysis is

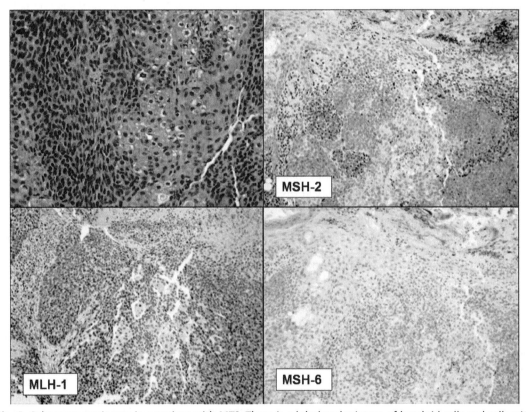

Fig. 6. Sebaceous carcinoma in a patient with MTS. There is a lobulated mixture of basaloid cells and cells with a vacuolated cytoplasm (hematoxylin-eosin, original magnification ×200). Numerous mitotic figures are seen and there is focal apoptosis. Immunohistochemistry revealed diminished staining for MSH-2 and absent staining for MSH-6. Strong staining with MLH-1 was noted.

a screening tool for MMR gene defects in sebaceous lesions to differentiate between sebaceous neoplasms seen sporadically and those associated with MTS.[145]

In MTS, the MSH-2 protein is lost in 55% to 86% of sebaceous adenomas, in 17% of sebaceous epitheliomas, and in 31% to 100% in sebaceous carcinoma. The MLH-1 protein is absent in 14% to 33% of sebaceous adenomas, in 83% of sebaceous epitheliomas, and 31% of sebaceous carcinomas. MSH-6 is lost in 50% to 78% of sebaceous adenomas, in 33% of sebaceous epitheliomas, and about 100% of sebaceous carcinoma.[112,114,146–150]

In sebaceous neoplasms in patients with MTS, the positive predicative value of lack of expression of each of the MMR proteins ranges from 33% to 88% for MLH-1, 55% to 66% for MSH-2, and is about 67% for MSH-6.[147,148] These markers can be combined to yield a positive predictive value of 55% for MTS in unselected sebaceous neoplasms with loss of MSH-2 and MSH-6, 100% for tumors with loss of MLH-1 and MSH-6, and also 100% for neoplasms demonstrating lack of all three MMRs.[147] Mutations may occur that result in an expressed but nonfunctional protein that is still detected by immunohistochemistry falsely creating the impression that there is normal expression and that they lack MTS.[151] DNA sequencing analysis of the MMR genes for MSI testing may be performed to confirm the diagnosis and has an estimated 80% sensitivity and 90% specificity for detecting MLH-1 and MSH-2 mutations.[146]

Dermatologists and dermatopathologists can play an important role in the prompt diagnosis and treatment of MTS. The diagnosis of one sebaceous neoplasm, other than sebaceous hyperplasia, should trigger MTS evaluation. Relevant family history should be elicited with subsequent referral for a screening colonoscopy in patients with a positive family history.[152]

MSI IN OTHER TUMORS

BCCs have been found to have a low frequency of MSI. Stamatelli and colleagues[153] studied MSI and B-RAF mutations in BCCs. Two out of 38 cases of BCC were positive for the exon 15 point mutations of the B-RAF gene and MSI was found in 5% of the cases.[153] There was no association found between B-RAF mutations and MSI in BCC.[153] Quinn and colleagues[154] reported less than 5% MSI in BCCs and all these patients did not have MTS. In a study conducted by Young and colleagues, there was no link found between MSI in 32 SCCs studied. Interestingly, this group noted that the MMR protein levels of MLH1, MSH2, MSH3,

MSH6, and PMS2 were actually greater in SCCs and in BCCs than in normal skin.[155,156]

It has been suggested that azathioprine, an immunosuppressive drug used in transplant recipients, may impair the MMR system causing MSI in skin malignancies.[157] However, Reuschenbach and colleagues[158] found that MSI was extremely rare in 141 nonmelanoma skin tumors studied from immunosuppressed and immunocompetent patients.

In summary, there is no conclusive evidence to support that MMR are causative in other nonmelanoma skin malignancies.

MYOEPITHELIOMA

Mixed tumors of salivary glands (pleomorphic adenomas) and cutaneous mixed tumors (chondroid syringomas) contain a ductal (epithelial) component and a variably prominent myoepithelial component. Tumors with only myoepithelial differentiation are known as "myoepitheliomas." Myoepitheliomas are classified as part of the "mixed tumor/parachordoma family" in the World Health Organization classification.

Myoepithelioma is a rare dermal and soft tissue tumor reported on the head and extremities of adults and children.[159] It has also been reported to occur in salivary glands, breast, and lung.[160] Typically histopathologic examination reveals a nodular and well-circumscribed tumor. The tumors may be solid or lobulated, consisting of epithelioid, plasmacytoid, or spindled cells. Ductal and tubular differentiation is absent. The stroma varies in amount and may be focally myxoid or chondromyxoid, occasionally with adipocytes.[160] There is a 20% chance of local recurrence; however, most low-grade myoepithelial tumors of the soft tissue do not recur.[159]

Immunohistochemical studies reveal tumor cell staining with vimentin, epithelial markers (cytokeratins, EMA), S100, calponin, and occasionally for glial fibrillary acidic protein, α-smooth muscle actin, and p63. Desmin is almost always negative.[160,161]

The differential diagnosis of myoepithelioma includes chondroid lipoma, if there is prominent myxoid stroma present; however, myoepitheliomas are usually more superficial and have myoepithelial differentiation.[162,163] Cutaneous benign mixed tumors have ducts and branching tubules, which are lined by two layers of epithelial and myoepithelial cells. Myoepithelioma is differentiated by absence of these structures.

Cutaneous myoepithelial carcinoma is histologically composed of atypical neoplastic cells with nuclear pleomorphism and prominent nucleoli. Increased mitoses and necrosis may be present.[159,160]

SPINDLE CELL PREDOMINANT TRICHODISCOMA/NEUROFOLLICULAR HAMARTOMA

Hamartomas are comprised of an abnormal mixture of tissue elements or an abnormal proportion of one element that is normal in that location.[164] Fibrofolliculomas and trichodiscomas are hamartomas, composed of epithelial and mesenchymal elements.[165] Fibrofolliculoma is an infundibulocentric papule with stromal mucin, fibrocytes, and fibrillary collagen forming a fibrous orb. The infundibulum is dilated and the epithelium forms a mantle composed of anastomotic strands and cords without fully formed follicles. Trichodiscomas predominantly consist of stroma. The stroma contains collagen bundles forming ribbons, abundant mucin, and scant fibrocytes.[166] Fibrofolliculomas and trichodiscomas have distinct histopathology, but have been reported to occur synchronously.[166] Birt-Hogg-Dube syndrome is an autosomal-dominant syndrome associated with multiple fibrofolliculomas, trichodiscomas, and acrochordons.[167]

Neurofollicular hamartomas are clinically small, dome-shaped papules, commonly seen on the face, with a predilection for the nose and nasolabial folds. Histologic examination reveals features seen in fibrofolliculoma and trichodiscoma with stroma containing fibrocytic spindle cells that are CD34 positive and focally S100 positive, arranged in short fascicles and sheets,[168–170] laterally delimited by hyperplastic folliculosebaceous units.

Sangueza and Requena[171] suggested that neurofollicular hamartomas, trichodiscomas, and fibrofolliculomas are on the same hamartomatous spectrum. On extreme ends of the same clinicopathologic spectrum are fibrofolliculomas with anastomosing strands of epithelium without fully formed follicles and on the other extreme are trichodiscomas that are stroma predominant.[166] The tumor, formerly called neurofollicular hamartoma, lies in the middle of the spectrum. It was presumed to have neural differentiation because of the spindled morphology and S100 staining, and thus was not originally included in the fibrofolliculomas/trichodiscomas spectrum. Kutzner and colleagues[165] propose that neurofollicular hamartoma is just a cellular trichodiscoma with abundant CD34-positive fibrocytic stroma, consisting of a mesenchymal component with slightly wavy nuclei that was mistaken for neural differentiation because of focal S100 positivity. They suggested the term SCPT for this variant of fibrofolliculoma-trichodiscoma (**Figs. 7–9**).[165] SCPT may contain adipocytes.[165]

It is unclear whether the CD34-positive fibrocytes in SCPT are from the dermal dendritic cell

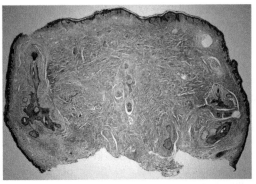

Fig. 7. Spindle cell–predominant trichodiscoma. Dome-shaped papule arranged in a fascicular pattern laterally delimited by hyperplastic folliculosebaceous units (hematoxylin-eosin, original magnification ×20).

population or from periadnexal/peri-isthmic fibrocytes.[165] A case of SCPT with focal palisading stromal cells, as seen in schwannoma, and a symplastic trichodiscoma with pseudosarcomatous-ancient features have also been reported.[172,173]

The differential diagnosis of SCPT includes well-circumscribed cellular neoplasms with CD34-positive spindle cells. A spindle cell lipoma may mimic SCPT, because both contain adipocytes, spindle cells positive for CD34-positive, and some mucin in the stroma. However, spindle cell lipoma lacks the follicular changes seen in SCPT. Angiofibroma may also resemble trichodiscoma, but angiofibromas have wiry, dense collagen in the stroma with single stellate cells, positive for vimentin and CD68, and capillaries. SCPT lacks the CD117 positive stroma seen in angiofibroma.[165]

In summary, there is a CD34-positive fibrocyte rich stroma in all fibrofolliculomas, trichodiscomas, and SCPTs with a variation in amount of

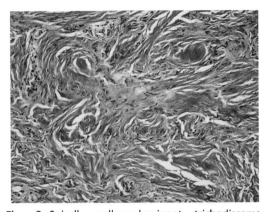

Fig. 8. Spindle cell–predominant trichodiscoma. Mesenchymal component has slightly wavy nuclei that could be mistaken for neural differentiation (hematoxylin-eosin, original magnification ×200).

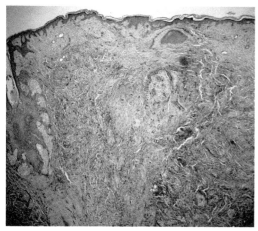

Fig. 9. Spindle cell–predominant trichodiscoma. The spindle cells in the stroma stain positively with CD34 (original magnification ×40).

stroma and range of mantle-derived follicular differentiation.[165] SCPT and neurofollicular hamartoma have not been reported to occur in association with Birt-Hogg-Dube syndrome.

SUMMARY

There have been many new discoveries in the area of nonmelanocytic neoplasia. Identification of clonally integrated MCPyV in MCC tumor cells has been an important discovery. This proposed human cancer virus produces a new model in which a common, mostly harmless member of the human viral flora can initiate cancer and it's role is being investigated in other neoplasms. Other areas that have received particular attention are MSI in sebaceous neoplasms, their association with HNPCC or MTS, and MSI in other tumors. An immunohistochemical panel including MSH-6, MSH-1, and MLH-2 can serve as a screening tool in patients with sebaceous neoplasms. Increasing numbers of cases reported of rare adnexal neoplasms of the skin, including SEDC, RPAN, and rare tumors, such as onychomatrichoma, and SCPT/neurofollicular hamartoma, and myoepithelioma, have led to better classification.

REFERENCES

1. Tai PS, Ofori AO, Robinson JK. Clinical features and diagnosis of Merkel cell (neuroendocrine) carcinoma and sebaceous cell carcinoma of the skin. 2011. Available at: http://www.uptodate.com/contents/clinical-features-and-diagnosis-of-merkel-cell-neuroendocrine-carcinoma-and-sebaceous-cell-carcinoma-of-the-skin. Accessed November 16, 2011.

2. Moore PS, Chang Y. Why do viruses cause cancer? highlights of the first century of human tumour virology. Nat Rev Cancer 2010;10(12):878–89.

3. Feng H, Shuda M, Chang Y, et al. Clonal integration of a polyomavirus in human Merkel cell carcinoma. Science 2008;319(5866):1096–100.

4. Sihto H, Kukko H, Koljonen V, et al. Clinical factors associated with Merkel cell polyomavirus infection in Merkel cell carcinoma. J Natl Cancer Inst 2009; 101(13):938–45.

5. Kassem A, Schopflin A, Diaz C, et al. Frequent detection of Merkel cell polyomavirus in human Merkel cell carcinomas and identification of a unique deletion in the VP1 gene. Cancer Res 2008;68(13):5009–13.

6. Sharp CP, Norja P, Anthony I, et al. Reactivation and mutation of newly discovered WU, KI, and Merkel cell carcinoma polyomaviruses in immunosuppressed individuals. J Infect Dis 2009;199(3): 398–404.

7. Garneski KM, DeCaprio JA, Nghiem P. Does a new polyomavirus contribute to Merkel cell carcinoma? Genome Biol 2008;9(6):228.

8. Penn I, First MR. Merkel's cell carcinoma in organ recipients: report of 41 cases. Transplantation 1999;68(11):1717–21.

9. Engels EA, Frisch M, Goedert JJ, et al. Merkel cell carcinoma and HIV infection. Lancet 2002; 359(9305):497–8.

10. Dubina M, Goldenberg G. Viral-associated nonmelanoma skin cancers: a review. Am J Dermatopathol 2009;31(6):561–73.

11. Mertz KD, Schmid M, Burger B, et al. Detection of Merkel cell polyomavirus in epidermodysplasia-verruciformis-associated skin neoplasms. Dermatology 2011;222(1):87–92.

12. Ly TY, Walsh NM, Pasternak S. The spectrum of Merkel cell polyomavirus expression in Merkel cell carcinoma, in a variety of cutaneous neoplasms, and in neuroendocrine carcinomas from different anatomical sites. Hum Pathol 2012;43(4):557–66.

13. Rollison DE, Giuliano AR, Messina JL, et al. Case-control study of MCC polyomavirus and cutaneous SCC. Cancer Epidemiol Biomarkers Prev 2012; 21(1):74–81.

14. Asioli S, Righi A, Volante M, et al. p63 expression as a new prognostic marker in Merkel cell carcinoma. Cancer 2007;110(3):640–7.

15. Urist MJ, Di Como CJ, Lu ML, et al. Loss of p63 expression is associated with tumor progression in bladder cancer. Am J Pathol 2002;161(4):1199–206.

16. Lo Muzio L, Santarelli A, Caltabiano R, et al. p63 overexpression associates with poor prognosis in head and neck squamous cell carcinoma. Hum Pathol 2005;36(2):187–94.

17. Kalhor N, Zander DS, Liu J. TTF-1 and p63 for distinguishing pulmonary small-cell carcinoma from

poorly differentiated squamous cell carcinoma in previously pap-stained cytologic material. Mod Pathol 2006;19(8):1117–23.

18. Takeuchi Y, Tamura A, Kamiya M, et al. Immunohistochemical analyses of p63 expression in cutaneous tumours. Br J Dermatol 2005;153(6):1230–2.

19. Hu H, Xia SH, Li AD, et al. Elevated expression of p63 protein in human esophageal squamous cell carcinomas. Int J Cancer 2002;102(6):580–3.

20. Koker MM, Kleer CG. p63 expression in breast cancer: a highly sensitive and specific marker of metaplastic carcinoma. Am J Surg Pathol 2004; 28(11):1506–12.

21. Comperat E, Camparo P, Haus R, et al. Immunohistochemical expression of p63, p53 and MIB-1 in urinary bladder carcinoma. A tissue microarray study of 158 cases. Virchows Arch 2006;448(3): 319–24.

22. Wang TY, Chen BF, Yang YC, et al. Histologic and immunophenotypic classification of cervical carcinomas by expression of the p53 homologue p63: a study of 250 cases. Hum Pathol 2001;32(5): 479–86.

23. Signoretti S, Waltregny D, Dilks J, et al. p63 is a prostate basal cell marker and is required for prostate development. Am J Pathol 2000;157(6): 1769–75.

24. Lo Muzio L, Santarelli A, Caltabiano R, et al. p63 expression correlates with pathological features and biological behaviour of odontogenic tumours. Histopathology 2006;49(2):211–4.

25. Marucci G, Betts CM, Liguori L, et al. Basaloid carcinoma of the pancreas. Virchows Arch 2005; 446(3):322–4.

26. Fukushima N, Satoh T, Sueoka N, et al. Clinicopathological characteristics of p63 expression in B-cell lymphoma. Cancer Sci 2006;97(10):1050–5.

27. Asioli S, Righi A, de Biase D, et al. Expression of p63 is the sole independent marker of aggressiveness in localised (stage I-II) Merkel cell carcinomas. Mod Pathol 2011;24(11):1451–61.

28. McCardle TW. Merkel cell carcinoma: pathologic findings and prognostic factors. Curr Probl Cancer 2010;34(1):47–64.

29. Su LD. Immunostaining for cytokeratin 20 improves detection of micrometastatic Merkel cell carcinoma. J Am Acad Dermatol 2002;46(5):661–6.

30. National Comprehensive Cancer Network. Clinical practice guidelines in oncology. Merkel cell carcinoma, vol.1. Fort Washington, PA: NCCN; 2010.

31. Concannon R. The impact of (18)F-FDG PET-CT scanning for staging and management of MCC. J Am Acad Dermatol 2010;62(1):76–84.

32. Anderson SE, Beer KT, Banic A, et al. MRI of Merkel cell carcinoma: histologic correlation and review of the literature. AJR Am J Roentgenol 2005;185(6):1441–8.

33. Nicolaidou E, Mikrova A, Antoniou C, et al. Advances in Merkel cell carcinoma pathogenesis and management: a recently discovered virus, a new international consensus staging system and new diagnostic codes. Br J Dermatol 2012;166(1):16–21.

34. Farasat S, Yu SS, Neel VA, et al. A new American Joint Committee on Cancer staging system for cutaneous squamous cell carcinoma: creation and rationale for inclusion of tumor (T) characteristics. J Am Acad Dermatol 2011;64(6):1051–9.

35. Rowe DE, Carroll RJ, Day CL Jr. Prognostic factors for local recurrence, metastasis, and survival rates in squamous cell carcinoma of the skin, ear, and lip. Implications for treatment modality selection. J Am Acad Dermatol 1992;26:976–90.

36. North JH Jr, Spellman JE, Driscoll D, et al. Advanced cutaneous squamous cell carcinoma of the trunk and extremity: analysis of prognostic factors. J Surg Oncol 1997;64:212–7.

37. Brantsch KD, Meisner C, Schonfisch B, et al. Analysis of risk factors determining prognosis of cutaneous squamous-cell carcinoma: a prospective study. Lancet Oncol 2008;9:713–20.

38. Mullen JT, Feng L, Xing Y, et al. Invasive squamous cell carcinoma of the skin: defining a high-risk group. Ann Surg Oncol 2006;13:902–9.

39. Kwon S, Dong ZM, Wu PC, et al. Sentinel lymph node biopsy for high-risk cutaneous squamous cell carcinoma: clinical experience and review of literature. World J Surg Oncol 2011;9:80.

40. Lardaro T. Improvement in the staging of cutaneous SCC. Mounting evidence suggests that increase nodal burden corresponds with decreased survival. Ann Surg Oncol 2010;17:1979–80.

41. Andruchow JL. Implication for clinical staging of metastatic cutaneous carcinoma. Studies also suggest that those with increased nodal burden may also benefit from more aggressive therapy. Cancer 2006;106:1078–83.

42. Audet N. Cutaneous metastatic squamous cell carcinoma to the parotid gland. Head Neck 2004; 26:727–32.

43. Nakhleh RE, Swanson PE, Wick MR. Cutaneous adnexal carcinomas with divergent differentiation. Am J Dermatopathol 1990;12(4):325–34.

44. Wong TY, Suster S, Mihm MC. Squamoid eccrine ductal carcinoma. Histopathology 1997;30(3): 288–93.

45. Chhibber V, Lyle S, Mahalingam M. Ductal eccrine carcinoma with squamous differentiation: apropos a case. J Cutan Pathol 2007;34(6):503–7.

46. Urso C, Paglierani M, Bondi R. Histologic spectrum of carcinomas with eccrine ductal differentiation (sweat-gland ductal carcinomas). Am J Dermatopathol 1993;15(5):435–40.

47. Swanson PE, Cherwitz DL, Neumann MP, et al. Eccrine sweat gland carcinoma: an histologic and

immunohistochemical study of 32 cases. J Cutan Pathol 1987;14(2):65–86.

48. Terushkin E, Leffell DJ, Futoryan T, et al. Squamoid eccrine ductal carcinoma: a case report and review of the literature. Am J Dermatopathol 2010;32(3):287–92.

49. Herrero J, Monteagudo C, Jorda E, et al. Squamoid eccrine ductal carcinoma. Histopathology 1998; 32(5):478–80.

50. Fu JM, McCalmont T, Yu SS. Adenosquamous carcinoma of the skin: a case series. Arch Dermatol 2009;145(10):1152–8.

51. Weidner N, Foucar E. Adenosquamous carcinoma of the skin. An aggressive mucin- and gland-forming squamous carcinoma. Arch Dermatol 1985;121(6):775–9.

52. Banks ER, Cooper PH. Adenosquamous carcinoma of the skin: a report of 10 cases. J Cutan Pathol 1991;18(4):227–34.

53. Kavand S, Cassarino DS. "Squamoid eccrine ductal carcinoma": an unusual low-grade case with follicular differentiation. Are these tumors squamoid variants of microcystic adnexal carcinoma? Am J Dermatopathol 2009;31(8):849–52.

54. Pugh TJ, Lee NY, Pacheco T, et al. Microcystic adnexal carcinoma of the face treated with radiation therapy: a case report and review of the literature. Head Neck 2012;34(7):1045–50.

55. Chiller K, Passaro D, Scheuller M, et al. Microcystic adnexal carcinoma: forty-eight cases, their treatment, and their outcome. Arch Dermatol 2000; 136(11):1355–9.

56. Snow S, Madjar DD, Hardy S, et al. Microcystic adnexal carcinoma: report of 13 cases and review of the literature. Dermatol Surg 2001;27(4): 401–8.

57. Kim YJ. Mohs micrographic surgery for SEDC. Dermatol Surg 2005;31:1462–4.

58. Chang Y, Moore PS. Merkel cell carcinoma: a virus-induced human cancer. Annu Rev Pathol 2012;7: 123–44.

59. Canueto J, Santos-Briz A, Garcia JL, et al. Onychomatricoma: genome-wide analyses of a rare nail matrix tumor. J Am Acad Dermatol 2011;64(3): 573–8, 578.e1.

60. Perrin C, Baran R. Onychomatricoma with dorsal pterygium: pathogenic mechanisms in 3 cases. J Am Acad Dermatol 2008;59(6):990–4.

61. Van Holder C, Dumontier C, Abimelec P. Onychomatricoma. J Hand Surg Br 1999;24(1):120–1.

62. Perrin C, Goettmann S, Baran R. Onychomatricoma: clinical and histopathologic findings in 12 cases. J Am Acad Dermatol 1998;39(4 Pt 1):560–4.

63. Perrin C, Baran R, Pisani A, et al. The onychomatricoma: additional histologic criteria and immunohistochemical study. Am J Dermatopathol 2002;24(3): 199–203.

64. Perrin C. Onychomatricoma: new clinical and histological features. Am J Dermatopathol 2010;32:1–8.

65. Rothko K, Farmer ER, Zeligman I. Superficial epithelioma with sebaceous differentiation. Arch Dermatol 1980;116:329–31.

66. Friedman KJ, Boudreau S, Farmer ER. Superficial epithelioma with sebaceous differentiation. J Cutan Pathol 1987;14:193–7.

67. Vaughn TK, Sau P. Superficial epithelioma with sebaceous differentiation. J Am Acad Dermatol 1990;23:760–2.

68. Steffen C, Ackerman AB, editors. Reticulated acanthoma with sebaceous differentiation. Neoplasms with sebaceous differentiation. Philadelphia: Lea & Febiger; 1994. p. 449–67.

69. Akasaka T, Imamura Y, Tomichi N, et al. A case of superficial epithelioma with sebaceous differentiation. J Dermatol 1994;21:264–7.

70. Lee MJ, Kim YC, Lew W. A case of superficial epithelioma with sebaceous differentiation. Yonsei Med J 2003;44:347–50.

71. Fukai K, Sowa J, Ishii M. Reticulated acanthoma with sebaceous differentiation. Am J Dermatopathol 2006;28:158–61.

72. Kato N, Ueno H. Superficial epithelioma with sebaceous differentiation. J Dermatol 1992;19:190–4.

73. Haake DL, Minni JP, Nowak M, et al. Reticulated acanthoma with sebaceous differentiation: lack of association with Muir-Torre syndrome. Am J Dermatopathol 2009;31:391–2.

74. Chen TL, Tsai TF. Superficial epithelioma with sebaceous differentiation. Dermatol Sinica 2000;18: 250–4. Available at: http://www.dermatol-sinica. com/web/backissues_2.php?y=2000&n=3&k=538. Accessed July 7, 2011.

75. Sanchez Yus E, Requena L, Simon P, et al. Complex adnexal tumor of the primary epithelial germ with distinct patterns of superficial epithelioma with sebaceous differentiation, immature trichoepithelioma and apocrine adenocarcinoma. Am J Dermatopathol 1992;14:245–52.

76. Shuweiter M, Boer A. Spectrum of follicular and sebaceous differentiation induced by dermatofibroma. Am J Dermatopathol 2009;31:778–85.

77. Shuweiter M. New quandary: superficial epithelioma with sebaceous differentiation. Dermatopathology Practical and Conceptual 2010;16. Available at: Derm101.Com. Accessed November 20, 2011.

78. Miteva M, de Farias DC, Zaiac M, et al. Nail clipping diagnosis of onychomatricoma. Arch Dermatol 2011;147(9):1117–8.

79. Hashimoto K, Prince C, Kato I, et al. Rippled pattern trichomatricoma: histological, immunohistological and ultrastructural studies of an immature hair matrix tumor. J Cutan Pathol 1989;16:19–30.

80. Akasaka T, Imamaura Y, Mori Y, et al. Trichoblastoma with rippled pattern. J Dermatol 1997;24:174–8.

81. Misago N, Narisawa Y. Ripple/carcinoid pattern sebaceoma with apocrine differentiation. Am J Dermatopathol 2011;33:94–7.

82. Manabe T, Inagaki Y, Nakagawa S, et al. Ripple pigmentation of the neck in atopic dermatitis. Am J Dermatopathol 1987;9:301–7.

83. Yamamoto O, Hisaoka M, Yasuda H, et al. A rippled-pattern trichoblastoma: an immunohistochemical study. J Cutan Pathol 2000;27:460–5.

84. Requena L, Barat A. Giant trichoblastoma on the scalp. Am J Dermatopathol 1993;15:497–502.

85. Graham BS, Barr RJ. Rippled pattern sebaceous trichoblastoma. J Cutan Pathol 2000;27:455–9.

86. Ansai S, Kimura T. Rippled-pattern sebaceoma: a clinicopathological study. Am J Dermatopathol 2009;31:364–6.

87. Kazakov DV, Kutzner H, Rütten A, et al. Carcinoid-like pattern in sebaceous neoplasms. Another distinctive, previously unrecognized pattern in extraocular sebaceous carcinoma and sebaceoma. Am J Dermatopathol 2005;27:195–203.

88. Kurokawa I, Nishimura K, Hakamada A, et al. Rippled-pattern sebaceoma with an immunohistochemical study of cytokeratins. J Eur Acad Dermatol Venereol 2007;21:104–43.

89. Akira I, Masataka S, Yoshifumi K, et al. A case of rippled pattern sebaceoma on the scalp. J Jap Dermatohistopathol Soc 2004;20:22–5. Available at: http://sciencelinks.jp/j-east/article/200506/000020050605A0077959.php. Accessed August 10, 2011.

90. Kawakami Y, Ansai S, Nakamura-Wakatsuki T, et al. Case of rippled-pattern sebaceoma with clinically yellowish surface and histopathological paucity of lipid-containing neoplastic cells. J Dermatol 2011;38:1–2.

91. Nielson TA, Maia-Cohen S, Hessel AB, et al. Sebaceous neoplasm with reticulated and cribriform features: a rare variant of sebaceoma. J Cutan Pathol 1998;25:233–5.

92. Misago N, Narisawa Y. Rippled-pattern sebaceoma. Am J Dermatopathol 2001;23:437–43.

93. Kiyohara T, Kumakiri M, Kuwahara H, et al. Rippled pattern sebaceoma: a report of a lesion on the back and review of the literature. Am J Dermatopathol 2006;28:446–8.

94. Sakaguchi M, Ashida M, Ueda M, et al. A case of rippled-pattern sebaceoma. Rinsho Derma (Tokyo) 2008;50:1113–6.

95. Yasuda M, Kiyohara T, Kumakiri M, et al. A case of rippled-pattern sebaceoma on the thigh. Rinsho Derma (Tokyo) 2008;50:1707–9 [in Japanese].

96. Miyamoto S, Ito T, Nakagawa N, et al. Rippled-pattern sebaceoma. Rinsho Hifuka 2010;64:493–6 [in Japanese]. Available at: http://sciencelinks.jp/j-east/article/200506/000020050605A0077959.php. Accessed August 10, 2011.

97. Swick BL, Baum CL, Walling HW. Rippled-pattern trichoblastoma with apocrine differentiation arising in a nevus sebaceous: report of a case and review of the literature. J Cutan Pathol 2009;36:1200–5.

98. Ohata C, Ackerman AB. Ripple-pattern signifies sebaceoma (not trichoblastoma or trichomatricoma). Dermatopathol: Prac Conc 2001;7:355–62. Available at: http://www.derm101.com/content/32016. Accessed August 12, 2011.

99. Ackerman AB, Ball E, Guo Y. Labyrinthine/sinusoidal pattern in sebaceoma. Dermatopathol: Prac Conc 2002;8. Accessed November 20, 2011.

100. Troy JL, Ackerman AB. Sebaceoma: a distinctive benign neoplasm of adnexal epithelium differentiating toward sebaceous cells. Am J Dermatopathol 1984;6:7–13.

101. Reibel J, Wewer U, Albrechtsen R. The pattern of distribution of laminin in neurogenic tumors, granular cell tumors, and nevi of the oral mucosa. Acta Pathol Microbiol Immunol Scand A 1985;93:41–7.

102. Weiner JA, Fukushima N, Contos JJ, et al. Regulation of Schwann cell morphology and adhesion by receptor-mediated lysophosphatidic acid signaling. J Neurosci 2001;21:7069–78.

103. Llatjós R, Fernández-Figueras MT, Díaz-Cascajo C, et al. Palisading and verocay body-prominent dermatofibrosarcoma protuberans: a report of three cases. Histopathology 2000;37:452–5.

104. Nomura M, Tanaka M, Nunomura M, et al. Dermoscopy of rippled-pattern sebaceoma. Dermatol Res Pract 2010;27:140486.

105. Biswas A, Setia N, Bhawan J. Cutaneous neoplasms with prominent verocay body-like structures: the so-called "rippled-pattern." Am J Dermatopathol 2011;33:539–50.

106. Muir EG, Yates Bell AJ, Barlow KA. Multiple primary carcinomata of the colon, duodenum, and larynx associated with keratoacanthomata of the face. Br J Surg 1967;54:191–5.

107. Torre D. Multiple sebaceous tumors. Arch Dermatol 1968;98:549–51. PMID: 5684233.

108. Ackerman B, Nussen S. New concept: sebaceous "adenoma" is sebaceous carcinoma. Dermatopathol: Pract Concep 1998;4. Available at: http://www.derm101.com/content/31654. Accessed August 12, 2011.

109. Ackerman B, Nussen S. New Concept: Neoplasms in allorgans of Muir-Torre syndrome are carcinomas: sebaceous carcinomas and squamous-cell carcinomas (keratoacanthomas) in skin and adenocarcinomas, squamous-cell carcinomas, and transitional-cell carcinomas in internal organs. Dermatopathol Pract Concept 1999;5. Available at: http://www.derm101.com/content/31827. Accessed August 12, 2011.

110. Kruse R, Rütten A, Hosseiry-Malayeri HR, et al. "Second hit" in sebaceous tumors from Muir-Torre patients with germ-line mutations in MSH-2: allele loss is not the preferred mode of inactivation. J Invest Dermatol 2001;116:463–5.

111. Zhang J, Lindroos A, Ollila S, et al. Gene conversion is a frequent mechanism of inactivation of the wild-type allele in cancers from MLH1/MSH2 deletion carriers. Cancer Res 2006;66: 659–64.

112. Machin P, Catasus L, Pons C, et al. Microsatellite instability and immunostaining for MSH-2 and MLH-1 in cutaneous and internal tumors for patient of Muir-Torre syndrome. J Cutan Pathol 2002;29:415.

113. Marcus VA, Madlensky L, Gryfe R, et al. Immunohistochemistry for hMLH1 and hMSH2: a practical test for DNA mismatch repair-deficient tumors. Am J Surg Pathol 1999;23:1248–55.

114. Mathiak M, Rütten A, Mangold E, et al. Loss of DNA mismatch repair proteins in skin tumors from patients with Muir-Torre syndrome and MSH2 or MLH1 germline mutations: establishment of immunohistochemical analysis as a screening test. Am J Surg Pathol 2002;26:338–43.

115. Ponti G, Ponz de Leon M, Losi L, et al. Different phenotypes in Muir-Torre syndrome: clinical and biomolecular characterization in two Italian families. Br J Dermatol 2005;152:1335–8.

116. Southey M, Young MA, Whitty J, et al. Molecular pathologic analysis enhances the diagnosis and management of Muir-Torre syndrome and gives insight its underlying molecular pathogenesis. Am J Surg Pathol 2001;25:936–41.

117. Kruse R, Rütten A, Schweiger N, et al. Frequency of microsatellite instability in unselected sebaceous gland neoplasias and hyperplasias. J Invest Dermatol 2003;120:858–64.

118. Marazza G, Masouyé I, Taylor S, et al. An Illustrative case of Muir-Torre syndrome. Arch Dermatol 2006;142:1039–42.

119. Curry ML, Eng W, Lund K, et al. Muir-Torre syndrome: role of the dermatopathologist in diagnosis. Am J Dermatopathol 2004;26(3):217–21.

120. Akhtar S, Oza K, Khan S, et al. Muir-Torre syndrome: case report of a patient with concurrent jejunal and ureteral cancer and a review of literature. J Am Acad Dermatol 1999;41:681–6.

121. Cohen P, Kohn S, Kurzrock R. Association of sebaceous gland tumors and internal malignancy: the Muir-Torre syndrome. Am J Med 1991;90:606–13.

122. Ponti G, Losi L, Pedroni M, et al. Value of MLH1 and MSH2 Mutations in the appearance of Muir-Torre syndrome phenotype in HNPCC patients presenting sebaceous gland tumors or keratoacanthomas. J Invest Dermatol 2006;126:2302–7.

123. Fernandez-Flores A. Considerations on the performance of immunohistochemistry for mismatch repair gene proteins in cases sebaceous neoplasms and keratoacanthomas with reference to Muir-Torre syndrome. Am J Dermatopathol 2012; 34(4):416–22.

124. Tanyi M, Olasz J, Lukacs G, et al. A new mutation in Muir-Torre syndrome associated with familial transmission of different gastrointestinal adenocarcinomas. Eur J Surg Oncol 2009;35:1128–30.

125. Lynch H, Fusaro R. The Muir-Torre syndrome in kindreds with hereditary nonpolyposis colorectal cander (Lynch syndrome): a classic obligation in preventive medicine. J Am Acad Dermatol 1999; 41:797–9.

126. Lynch H, Leibowitz R, Smyrk T, et al. Colorectal cancer and the Muir-Torre syndrome in a gypsy family: a review. Am J Gastroenterol 1999;95: 575–80.

127. Kubota T, Dakeishi M, Nozaki J, et al. Probable involvement of a germline mutation of an unknown mismatch repair gene in a Japanese Muir-Torre syndrome phenotype. J Dermatol Sci 2000;23: 117–25.

128. Lever WF. Sebaceous adenoma, review of the literature and report of a case. Arch Derm Syphilol 1948;57:102–11.

129. Rulon DB, Helwig EB. Cutaneous sebaceous neoplasms. Cancer 1974;33:82–102.

130. Mehregan AH, Rahbari H. Benign epithelial tumors of the skin II: benign sebaceous tumors. Cutis 1977;19:317–20.

131. Lazar AJ, Lyle S, Calonje E. Sebaceous neoplasia and Torre-Muir syndrome. Curr Diagn Pathol 2007;13:301–19.

132. Brownstein MH, Shapiro L. The pilosebaceous tumors. Int J Dermatol 1977;16:340–52.

133. Essenhigh DM, Jones D, Rack JH. A sebaceous adenoma: histological and chemical studies. Br J Dermatol 1964;76:330–40.

134. Calonje JE, Brenn T, Lazar AJ, et al. Mckee's pathology of the skin. 4th edition. Philadelphia: Saunders; 2011.

135. Yang HM, Cabral E, Dadras SS, et al. Immunohistochemical expression of D2–40 in benign and malignant sebaceous tumors and comparison to basal and squamous cell carcinomas. Am J Dermatopathol 2008;30:549–54.

136. Fan YS, Carr RA, Sanders DS, et al. Characteristic Ber-EP4 and EMA expression in sebaceoma is immunohistochemically distinct from basal cell carcinoma. Histopathology 2007;51:80–6.

137. Prioleau PG, Santa Cruz DJ. Sebaceous gland neoplasia. J Cutan Pathol 1984;11:396–414.

138. Graham RH, McKee PH, McGibbon DH. Sebaceous carcinoma. Clin Exp Dermatol 1984;9: 466–71.

139. Rulon DB, Helwig EB. Cutaneous sebaceous tumors. Cancer 1974;33:82–102.

140. Ausidio RA, Lodeville O, Quaglivolo V, et al. Sebaceous carcinoma arising from the eyelid and from extra-ocular sites. Tumori 1987;73:531–5.

141. Akhtar S, Oza KK, Roulier RG. Multiple sebaceous adenomas and extraocular sebaceous carcinoma in a patient with multiple sclerosis: case report and review of literature. J Cutan Med Surg 2001;5: 490–5.

142. Wick MR, Goellner JR, Wolfe JT, et al. Adnexal carcinomas of the skin. II Extraocular sebaceous carcinomas. Cancer 1985;56:1163–72.

143. Loeffler M, Hornblass A. Characteristics and behavior of eyelid carcinoma (basal cell, squamous cell sebaceous gland, and malignant melanoma). Ophthalmic Surg 1990;21:513–8.

144. Kruse R, Ruzicka T. DNA mismatch repair and the significance of a sebaceous skin tumor for visceral cancer prevention. Trends Mol Med 2004;10:136.

145. Morales-Burgos A, Sánchez JL, Figueroa LD, et al. MSH-2 and MLH-1 protein expression in Muir Torre syndrome-related and sporadic sebaceous neoplasms. P R Health Sci J 2008;27(4):3227.

146. Chao EC, Velasquez JL, Witherspoon MS, et al. Accurate classification of MLH1/MSH2 missense variants with multivariate analysis of protein polymorphisms-mismatch repair (MAPP-MMR). Hum Mutat 2008;29(6):852–60.

147. Popnikolov NK, Gatalica Z, Colome-Grimmer MI, et al. Loss of mismatch repair proteins in sebaceous gland tumors. J Cutan Pathol 2003;30:178.

148. Chhibber V, Dresser K, Mahalingam M. MSH-6: extending the reliability of immunohistochemistry as a screening tool in Muir-Torre syndrome. Mod Pathol 2008;21:159–64.

149. Cesinaro AM, Ubiali A, Sighinolfi P, et al. Mismatch repair proteins expression and microsatellite instability in skin lesions with sebaceous differentiation: a study in different clinical subgroups with and without extracutaneous cancer. Am J Dermatopathol 2007;29:351.

150. Entius MM, Keller JJ, Drillenburg P, et al. Microsatellite instability and expression of hMLH-1 and hMSH-2 in sebaceous gland carcinomas as markers for Muir-Torre syndrome. Clin Cancer Res 2000;6:1784.

151. Kariola R, Hampel H, Frankel WL, et al. MSH6 missense mutations are often associated with no or low cancer susceptibility. Br J Cancer 2004; 91(7):1287–92.

152. Ang JM, Alai NN, Ritter KR, et al. Muir-Torre syndrome: case report and review of the literature. Cutis 2011;87(3):125–8.

153. Stamatelli A, Saetta AA, Bei T, et al. B-Rafmutations, microsatellite instability and p53 protein expression in sporadic basal cell carcinomas. Pathol Oncol Res 2011;17(3):633–7.

154. Quinn GA, Healy E, Rehman I, et al. Microsatellite instability in human non-melanoma and melanoma skin cancer. J Invest Dermatol 1995;104: 309–12.

155. Young LC, Listgarten J, Trotter MJ, et al. Evidence that dysregulated DNA mismatch repair characterizes human nonmelanoma skin cancer. Br J Dermatol 2008;158:59–69.

156. Santos DC, Zaphiropoulos PG, Neto CF, et al. PTCH1 gene mutations in exon 17 and loss of heterozygosity on D9S180 microsatellite in sporadic and inherited human basal cell carcinomas. Int J Dermatol 2011;50(7):838–43.

157. Karran P, Attard N. Thiopurines in current medical practice: molecular mechanisms and contributions to therapy-related cancer. Nat Rev Cancer 2008;8: 24–36.

158. Reuschenbach M, Sommerer C, Hartschuh W, et al. Absence of mismatch repairdeficiency-related microsatellite instability in non-melanoma skin cancer. J Invest Dermatol 2012;132(2):491–3.

159. Patrizi A, Tabanelli M, Misciali C, et al. Benign myoepithelioma in the interdigital space of the foot. Am J Dermatopathol 2008;30(1):86–7.

160. Mentzel T, Requena L, Kaddu S, et al. Cutaneous myoepithelial neoplasms: clinicopathologic and immunohistochemical study of 20 cases suggesting a continuous spectrum ranging from benign mixed tumor of the skin to cutaneous myoepithelioma and myoepithelial carcinoma. J Cutan Pathol 2003;30(5):294–302.

161. Hornick JL, Fletcher C. Cutaneous myoepithelioma: a clinicopathologic and immunohistochemical study of 14 cases. Hum Pathol 2004;35:14–24.

162. Petit T, Wechsler J, Arigon V. Mixoid tumor or myoepithelioma of the skin? histologic andimmunohistochemical features. Ann Pathol 2004;24:50–3.

163. Hornick JL, Fletcher CD. Myoepithelial tumors of soft tissue: a clinicopathologic and immunohistochemical study of 101 cases with evaluation of prognostic parameters. Am J Surg Pathol 2003; 27:1183–96.

164. Stedman's Medical Dictionary. 28th edition. Baltimore, MD: Williams & Wilkins; 2000.

165. Kutzner H, Requena L, Rütten A, et al. Spindle cell predominant trichodiscoma: a fibrofolliculoma/trichodiscoma variant considered formerly to be a neurofollicular hamartoma: a clinicopathological and immunohistochemical analysis of 17 cases. Am J Dermatopathol 2006;28(1):1–8.

166. Ackerman AB, Reddy VB, Soyer HP. Neoplasms with follicular differentiation. New York: Ardor Scribendi Publishers; 2001.

167. Collins GL, Somach S, Morgan MB. Histomorphologic and immunophenotypic analysis of

fibrofolliculomas and trichodiscomas in Birt-Hogg-Dube syndrome and sporadic disease. J Cutan Pathol 2002;29(9):529–33.

168. Barr RJ, Goodman MM. Neurofollicular hamartoma: a light microscopic and immunohistochemical study. J Cutan Pathol 1989;16:336–41.

169. Nova MP, Zung M, Halperin A. Neurofollicular hamartoma. A clinicopathological study. Am J Dermatopathol 1991;13:459–62.

170. Xie DL, Nielsen TA, Pellegrini AE, et al. Neurofollicular hamartoma with strong diffuse S-100 positivity: a case report. Am J Dermatopathol 1999;21:253–5.

171. Sangueza OP, Requena L. Neurofollicular hamartoma. A new histogenetic interpretation. Am J Dermatopathol 1994;16(2):150–4.

172. Kacerovska D, Kazakov DV, Michal M. Spindle-cell predominant trichodiscoma with a palisaded arrangement of stromal cells. Am J Dermatopathol 2010;32(7):743–4.

173. Battistella M, Van Eeckhout P, Cribier B. Symplastic trichodiscoma: a spindle-cell predominant variant of trichodiscoma with pseudosarcomatous/ancient features. Am J Dermatopathol 2011; 33(7):e81–3.

Fibrous and Fibrohistiocytic Neoplasms: An Update

Loren E. Clarke, MD[a,b],*

KEYWORDS

- Myxofibrosarcoma • Atypical fibroxanthoma • CD10 • Solitary fibrous tumor • Neurothekeoma
- Nerve sheath myxoma • Desmoid tumor (desmoid fibromatosis)
- Dermatofibrosarcoma protuberans (DFSP)

KEY POINTS

- The recognition that myxofibrosarcoma is a distinct entity that often presents in skin.
- CD10 is not specific for atypical fibroxanthoma (AFX).
- Evidence that 'neurothekeomas' are likely fibroblastic/fibrohistiocytic tumors, while S100+ myxoid variants are better classified as 'nerve sheath myxomas'.
- The recognition of primary cutaneous solitary fibrous tumors.
- The limitations of beta-catenin immunohistochemistry in desmoid tumors.
- Prognostic utility of clinical and histopathologic features in dermatofibrosarcoma protuberans, and the effects of imatinibmesylate therapy.

INTRODUCTION

Recent advances in fibroblastic and fibrohistiocytic tumors have led to the following conclusions: (1) myxofibrosarcoma is a distinct entity with a propensity to present in the skin; (2) CD10 is not at all specifc for atypical fibroxanthoma; (3) nerve sheath myxomas are distinct from neurothekeomas; (4) solitary fibrous tumors may be primary to the skin, and most appear to be indolent; (5) beta-catenin immunohistochemistry is of only limited value in the diagnosis of desmoid tumors; and (6) metastasis remains the only relevant predictor of survival in dermatofibrosarcoma protuberans; imatinib mesylate therapy may complicate margin interpretation.

MYXOFIBROSARCOMA: A DISTINCTIVE SARCOMA THAT COMMONLY ARISES IN SKIN

The myxofibrosarcoma is not new. What is new is its recognition as a distinctive sarcoma that commonly presents in the skin. Angervall and colleagues[1] characterized myxofibrosarcomas

Key points

- Most myxofibrosarcomas arise within the dermis, subcutis, or fascia, and presentation as a cutaneous nodule is common.
- The skin nodule is often merely the tip of the proverbial iceberg, because myxofibrosarcoma has a marked tendency to spread diffusely along the fascia, in some cases with little or no connection to the remainder of the overlying skin. Surgeons frequently underestimate the tumor's true extent. Positive margins are common, as are recurrences.
- Many myxofibrosarcomas may be partially or entirely low-grade at initial biopsy. Even those that ultimately prove to be high-grade often contain low-grade regions at their surface and periphery. As a result, what the histopathologist sees in a superficial biopsy may be easily misinterpreted as a benign tumor or even a cutaneous mucinosis.
- Recurrence is common for the reasons mentioned earlier, and the recurrences may be of increasingly higher grade.

[a] Department of Pathology, Penn State Hershey Medical Center, 500 University Drive, Hershey, PA 17033, USA;
[b] Department of Dermatology, Penn State Hershey Medical Center, 500 University Drive, Hershey, PA 17033, USA
* Department of Pathology, Penn State Hershey Medical Center, 500 University Drive, Hershey, PA 17033.
E-mail address: lclarke@hmc.psu.edu

Dermatol Clin 30 (2012) 643–656
http://dx.doi.org/10.1016/j.det.2012.06.005
0733-8635/12/$ – see front matter © 2012 Published by Elsevier Inc.

Table 1
A comparison of myxofibrosarcoma and MFH/UPS

Feature	Myxofibrosarcoma	MFH/UPS
Sites of involvement	Dermis, subcutis, fascia	Deep (subfascial) soft tissue
Histopathologic features	A broad spectrum from low-grade to high-grade Low-grade: low cellularity, mild atypia High-grade: dense cellularity and atypia indistinguishable from other high-grade sarcomas	Densely cellular tumors with marked cytologic atypia
Growth	Diffuse, often deceptively extensive horizontal growth along fascial planes; slow growth relative to MFH/UPS	Deep, bulky, vertical growth Rapid enlargement common
Clinical course	Metastasis uncommon except in high-grade cases Recurrences are common Histologic grade may progress with each recurrence	5% have metastatic disease at presentation (often to lung)
Survival	60%–70% 5-y survival	50% 5-y survival

more than 35 years ago, but the study was largely ignored and most pathologists considered this tumor merely a myxoid variant of so-called malignant fibrous histiocytoma (MFH).

During the past decade, however, several sarcoma experts have challenged the concept of fibrohistiocytic tumors in general, because no common line of fibrohistiocytic differentiation has been defined.[2] Instead, several studies showed that many tumors traditionally classified as MFH have genetic aberrations commonly encountered in other high-grade sarcomas, such as liposarcoma or leiomyosarcoma.[3] Some experts believe that with diligent study, most high-grade sarcomas can be classified as something other than MFH. As a result, some recommend abandoning the term MFH in favor of "undifferentiated pleomorphic sarcoma" (UPS) for these tumors.[4]

Much of the debate is academic, but a practical by-product is the increasing awareness that myxofibrosarcoma is not myxoid MFH. Myxofibrosarcomas and MFH/UPS actually differ in many ways (**Table 1**).[5] The most distinct differences are:

- Myxofibrosarcomas arise within the dermis, subcutis, or fascia and have a propensity to grow horizontally along the fascia. Myxoid MFH, however, arises deep to the fascia. Only rarely (and late in their course) do they penetrate the fascia and extend into the subcutis or dermis.

- Myxofibrosarcomas are often low-grade at initial presentation or contain low-grade areas. High-grade features are usually encountered in longstanding tumors or in

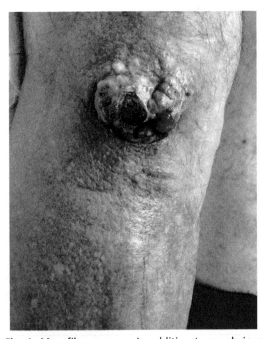

Fig. 1. Myxofibrosarcoma. In addition to an obvious tumor, often deceptively widespread extension of the neoplasm is present along the fascia beneath skin that appears uninvolved. This tumor infiltrated the subcutis and fascia more than 20 cm distal to the clinically evident mass.

those that recur. In MFH/UPS, by contrast, high-grade atypia from the outset is the rule.

A common presentation of myxofibrosarcoma is an obvious cutaneous nodule or tumor that appears relatively localized (**Fig. 1**). Beneath the obvious tumor, however, deceptively broad extension of the neoplasm is often present along the underlying fascia without overt involvement of the skin. Tumor often involves the dermis, but even in intermediate- or high-grade tumors, the dermal component is frequently sparsely cellular with banal cytomorphology (**Fig. 2**). The deeper regions are composed of pleomorphic cells within a myxoid stroma (**Fig. 3**).

CD10: SENSITIVE BUT NOT SPECIFIC FOR ATYPICAL FIBROXANTHOMA

Differentiating atypical fibroxanthoma (AFX), melanoma, leiomyosarcoma, poorly differentiated squamous cell carcinoma, and other assorted dermal neoplasms composed of spindled or pleomorphic cells is a task familiar to all dermatopathologists. Among these, AFX is generally considered a diagnosis of exclusion. Although one generally expects S-100 expression in melanomas, desmin

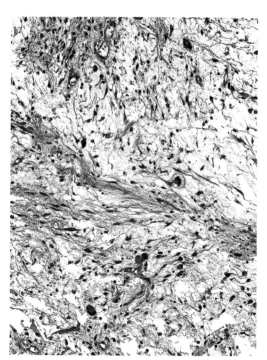

Fig. 3. Myxofibrosarcoma. This tumor is best classified as intermediate-grade. The features include pleomorphic cells within a myxoid stroma. Cells resembling lipoblasts are often present and are sometimes referred to as *pseudolipoblasts*. Unlike a genuine lipoblast, their cytoplasm contains acid polysaccharides rather than lipid (hematoxylin and eosin stain, original magnification ×400).

in leiomyosarcomas, and cytokeratin in squamous cell carcinomas, most atypical fibroxanthomas label only with antibodies directed against the very nonspecific vimentin. The lack of a positive marker for AFX was much lamented. In 2005, however, Weedon and colleagues[6] announced their serendipitous discovery that CD10 was consistently expressed in AFX in a letter to the editor of the *American Journal of Dermatopathology*. This very letter actually emphasized the nonspecificity of CD10 (to the extent of suggesting it might be the "vimentin of the 21st century"). Nonetheless, additional studies quickly confirmed the finding,[7,8] and soon CD10 was touted as a critical component of

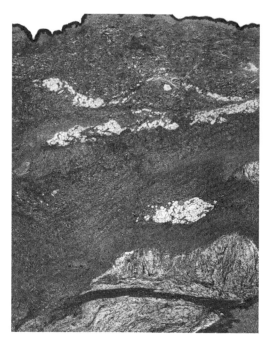

Fig. 2. Myxofibrosarcoma. Even when intermediate- or high-grade tumor is present in the deep dermis or subcutis, the superficial dermis may show only low-grade features. In this case, cellular density and cytologic atypia were minimal within the upper reticular dermis, despite obvious sarcoma immediately beneath it. Deep biopsies are crucial to diagnosis in these cases (hematoxylin and eosin stain, original magnification ×40).

Key points

- CD10 is expressed in most AFXs but is also expressed in many other cutaneous tumors, including spindle cell squamous carcinomas, melanomas, and other tumors that may simulate AFX.

- Using a panel of immunohistochemical markers remains the best approach to establishing a firm diagnosis of AFX.

immunohistochemistry panels for AFX. The ability of CD10 to label most AFXs strongly and diffusely is not in question (**Figs. 4** and **5**), and several studies have concluded that it is useful within the proper context.[7,9] Others, however, emphasized its poor specificity and the potential pitfalls that invariably arise with overreliance on immunohistochemical markers.[10] CD10 expression in melanoma has been well documented,[11,12] and a recent study[13] showed CD10 positivity in 50% of spindle cell squamous cell carcinomas[14] (**Table 2**). Clearly, CD10 is sensitive but not at all specific for AFX.

NEUROTHEKEOMAS: MORE FIBROBLASTIC/ FIBROHISTIOCYTIC THAN NEURAL

The term *neurothekeoma* has been applied to a clinically and morphologically heterogeneous group of tumors. Traditionally, three variants were recognized: (1) myxoid neurothekeomas; (2) cellular neurothekeomas; and (3) mixed neurothekeomas. "Nerve sheath myxomas" was a term reserved for the myxoid variants that expressed S100 protein.

In 2005 Fetsch and colleagues[15] reported a clinicopathologic analysis of 57 "myxoid neurothekeomas." Based on morphology, consistent S100 protein and glial fibrillary acidic protein (GFAP) expression, and a predilection for certain anatomic sites, they concluded that these neoplasms were a distinct type of peripheral nerve sheath tumor unrelated to other neurothekeomas, and averred that only these were genuine nerve sheath myxomas.[15]

Two years later, Fetsch and colleagues[16] produced an analysis of 178 cellular neurothekeomas, emphasizing features that differentiated them

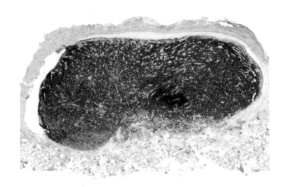

Fig. 5. AFX (CD10). Strong CD10 expression of the tumor cells is characteristic of AFX but not specific (CD10, original magnification ×20).

from nerve sheath myxomas. These cellular neurothekeomas (which from here on will be referred to simply as *neurothekeomas*) lacked evidence of peripheral nerve differentiation and seemed more closely related to dermatofibromas, plexiform fibrohistiocytic tumors, and other fibrohistiocytic or fibroblastic tumors than to tumors of peripheral nerve. In 2011, Sheth and coauthors[17] reported microarray gene expression profiles of neurothekeomas and nerve sheath myxomas, suggesting

Table 2	
Partial list of cutaneous tumors that may express CD10	
Tumor Type	**Approximate Percentage that Express CD10**
AFX	>90%
Melanoma	0%–60%[a]
Squamous cell carcinoma	14%
MFH/UPS	70%
Dermatofibrosarcoma protuberans	60%
Dermatofibroma	70%
Fibrosarcoma	100%
Myxofibrosarcoma	70%

[a] The frequency of CD10 expression by malignant melanomas varies considerably within the literature and may differ between primary and metastatic lesions.[12]

Data from Clarke LE, Frauenhoffer E, Fox E, et al. CD10-positive myxofibrosarcomas: a pitfall in the differential diagnosis of atypical fibroxanthoma. J Cutan Pathol 2010;37(7):737–43; and Kanner WA, Brill LB 2nd, Patterson JW, et al. CD10, p63 and CD99 expression in the differential diagnosis of atypical fibroxanthoma, spindle cell squamous cell carcinoma and desmoplastic melanoma. J Cutan Pathol 2010;37(7):744–50.

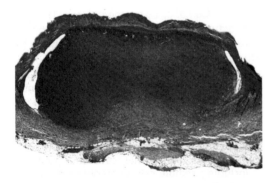

Fig. 4. AFX. These tumors characteristically arise on sun-damaged skin, mostly on the head and neck of older adults, but the same is true of spindle cell/poorly differentiated squamous carcinomas and other tumors with similar histopathologic features (hematoxylin and eosin stain, original magnification ×20).

that nerve sheath myxomas are more closely related to schwannomas than to the other neurothekeomas. Tumors with overlapping features remain a source of contention, but many fit well into the categories proposed by Fetsch and colleagues[16] Despite the apparent lack of neural differentiation, *neurothekeoma* is still used to refer to the nonmyxoid tumors. As more is learned about them, a more appropriate name will likely be adopted.

According to current criteria, then, neurothekeomas are rare tumors of uncertain origin. They affect both genders and almost every age group, but it has a predilection for women and for those in the second decade of life (median age, 17 years). Favored sites are the head (particularly the nose, cheeks, and orbital region), the upper extremities, and the shoulder girdle. A firm, solitary, slow-growing nodule in the skin or subcutis is a typical presentation.[16]

Histopathologically, neurothekeomas are dermal or subcutaneous tumors composed of nodules of spindled cells (**Fig. 6**). Some are densely cellular with a collagenous stroma. Many others exhibit low cellularity, however, and abundant myxoid stroma (one of the features that suggested a relationship to nerve sheath myxoma) (**Fig. 7**). Scattered multinucleated giant cells are common. The neoplastic cells typically express vimentin,

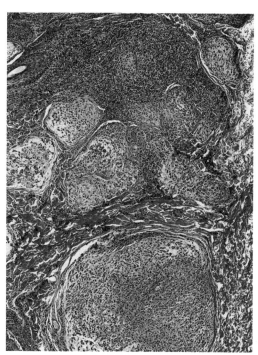

Fig. 7. Neurothekeoma. Many neurothekeomas have at least some myxoid stroma, a feature that initially suggested a relationship to what are now referred to as *nerve sheath myxomas* (hematoxylin and eosin stain, original magnification ×200).

NKI/C3, CD10, smooth muscle actin, factor 13a, protein gene product 9.5, and microphthalmia transcription factor.[16] They are negative for S100, Melan-A, and GFAP.

The histopathologic differential diagnosis may include nerve sheath myxoma, plexiform fibrohistiocytic tumor (PFT), perivascular epithelioid cell tumors, and melanocytic tumors. Nerve sheath myxomas and melanocytic tumors are usually easily excluded, because neurothekeomas are negative for S100. PFTs may closely simulate neurothekeomas in both appearance and immunoprofile, although PFTs are more common in the deep subcutis and are more often located on the extremities. Nevertheless, PFTs and neurothekeomas may be closely related.[16]

Mitotic activity and cytologic atypia may be conspicuous in some cases of neurothekeoma. The significance of atypical features is unknown, partly because of the rarity of the tumor and the lack of consistent terminology, but no convincing evidence shows that they confer a worse prognosis. Neurothekeomas occurring on the face seem more likely to recur.[16] No well-documented cases of metastasis exist.

Nerve sheath myxomas, by contrast, have a strong predilection for the extremities, particularly the fingers, hands, knees, ankles, and feet.[15]

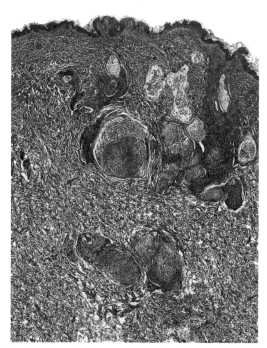

Fig. 6. Neurothekeoma. Most neurothekeomas are composed of nodules of epithelioid and spindled cells distributed irregularly within the dermis (hematoxylin and eosin stain, original magnification ×100).

Peak incidence is in the fourth decade, and the tumors typically present as slow-growing, solitary, superficial masses from 0.5 to 2.0 cm. Most nerve sheath myxomas are multinodular dermal and/or subcutaneous tumors composed of spindled and epithelioid cells within a myxoid stroma. In most cases a rim of compressed collagen and fibrous septa divides the tumor into distinct lobules (Fig. 8).[15] The epithelioid cells are often arranged in cords or nests (Fig. 9). Spindled and stellate cells are distributed haphazardly or in loosely formed fascicles. The neoplastic cells express S100 protein (Fig. 10), vimentin, GFAP, neuron-specific enolase, and CD57. Epithelial membrane antigen often labels a small population of perineurial cells at the periphery of the myxoid lobules. CD34 highlights a sparse population of intralobular fibroblasts, and collagen IV is expressed by the rim of compressed connective tissue.[15]

Histopathologically, nerve sheath myxomas may closely resemble myxoid variants of neurothekeoma, of course (Table 3). Other simulators are myxomas,[4] myxofibrosarcomas, myxoid schwannomas, and myxoid neurofibromas. Neither myxofibrosarcomas nor myxomas express S100 protein. Myxoid variants of schwannomas usually have a thicker, more conspicuous capsule, and neurofibromas generally have a more diffuse growth pattern, but nerve sheath myxomas have many similarities to schwannomas and some variants of neurofibroma, and may be closely related to these tumors. Recurrence of nerve sheath myxomas is common if incompletely excised.[15] Recurrence is also theoretically possible if satellite lesions are undetected at excision, but satellites seem to be a rare phenomenon.

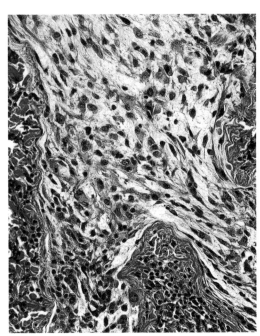

Fig. 9. Nerve sheath myxoma. Most cases contain at least a few epithelioid cells that are arranged in cords or syncytial aggregates. This finding is uncommon in neurothekeoma (hematoxylin and eosin stain, original magnification ×400).

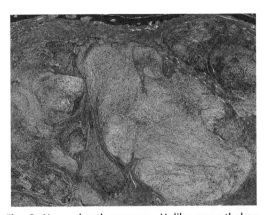

Fig. 8. Nerve sheath myxoma. Unlike neurothekeomas, these tumors have a predilection for the distal extremities. The neoplastic cells are often arranged in lobules, but the lobules tend to be closely packed and well demarcated by intervening fibrous bands (hematoxylin and eosin stain, original magnification ×40).

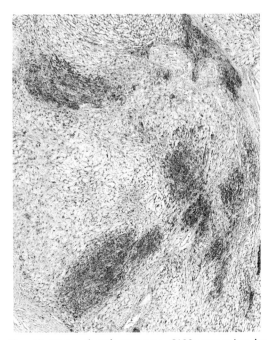

Fig. 10. Nerve sheath myxoma. S100 expression by most of the neoplastic cells is characteristic (S100, original magnification ×200).

Table 3
A comparison of nerve sheath myxoma and neurothekeoma (cellular neurothekeoma)

Feature	Nerve Sheath Myxoma	Neurothekeoma
Common sites	Hands Knees Ankles	Face Upper extremities Shoulder girdle
Gender	M = F	F > M
Age	4th decade	2nd decade
Morphology		
Capsule	Present	Absent
Septa	Present	Absent or ill-defined
Syncytial epithelioid cells	Present	Absent
Immunophenotype		
S100	+	−
GFAP	+	−
Epithelial membrane antigen	+	−
Neuron-specific enolase	+	−
Recurrence	>40%	<10%

Key points

- Nerve sheath myxomas are distinct from other types of nerve sheath myxoma and seem to be closely related to schwannomas and neurofibromas.
- Expression of S100 and GFAP is present in nerve sheath myxomas but generally absent in neurothekeomas; immunohistochemical panels that include these markers seem to be useful in distinguishing these groups.
- When nerve sheath myxomas are excluded, neurothekeomas constitute a group of neoplasms that have more similarities to fibroblastic or fibrohistiocytic tumors than to nerve sheath; some are myxoid, however, hence the confusion.
- Neurothekeomas may actually be a heterogeneous group of neoplasms with overlapping morphologic features.

CUTANEOUS SOLITARY FIBROUS TUMOR: AN INDOLENT CD34-POSITIVE NEOPLASM NOT TO BE MISTAKEN FOR DERMATOFIBROSARCOMA PROTUBERANS

Solitary fibrous tumors (SFTs) have been studied extensively over the past decade.[18] The realization that these tumors were not unique to the pleura prompted reevaluation of an entire group of neoplasms, and many authors now consider SFTs part of a spectrum of tumors that includes hemangiopericytomas and giant cell angiofibroma.[4] Because these tumors have been described in virtually every anatomic site, it is not surprising that a cutaneous variant exists.[19] However, based on the number of cases reported to date (<40 well-documented examples), they seem to be rare.[19,20] Given some overlapping histopathologic features, it is possible that before their recognition in the skin, some cutaneous SFTs were misinterpreted as dermatofibrosarcoma protuberans (DFSP), spindle cell lipomas, or the unusual CD34-positive variant of dermatofibroma. Firm conclusions about biologic potential should not be drawn, because so few cases have been studied and follow-up data are scarce, but thus far it seems that most cutaneous SFTs behave in a benign or relatively indolent manner. Only a few cases have recurred, and metastasis has not been reported.[19]

Most cutaneous SFTs are well demarcated (**Fig. 11**). Typically they are cellular and composed of ovoid or plump spindled cells that are cytologically banal (**Fig. 12**). Elongated vessels with angular, tapered contours ("staghorn vessels") are common (**Fig. 13**) but not specific to SFT. What is most crucial is to simply be aware that SFTs exist and that they can be mistaken for DFSPs and other CD34-positive tumors. Most

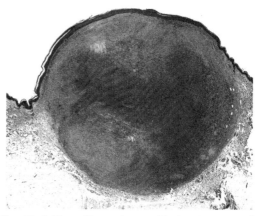

Fig. 11. Solitary fibrous tumor. Most cutaneous solitary fibrous tumors are well circumscribed and do not encircle adnexal structures (hematoxylin and eosin stain, original magnification ×20).

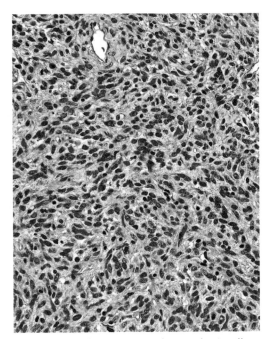

Fig. 12. Solitary fibrous tumor. The neoplastic cells are usually uniform in size and nuclear detail. Some appear spindled, but many are more ovoid or fusiform (hematoxylin and eosin stain, original magnification ×200).

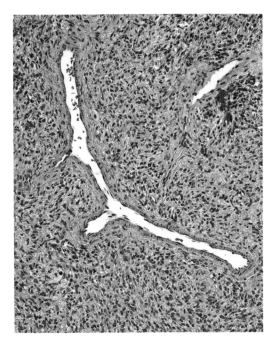

Fig. 13. Solitary fibrous tumor. Elongated vessels with tapered angular ends ("staghorn vessels") are common but not specific to solitary fibrous tumor (hematoxylin and eosin stain, original magnification ×200).

dermatopathologists are aware that many cutaneous tumors may express CD34, but a pathologist that only rarely encounters cutaneous spindle cell tumors may mistakenly equate CD34-positive spindle cells in skin with DFSP. Occasionally this may even pose a problem for experienced dermatopathologists, because some SFTs have areas that resemble DFSP. Reliable differentiation can usually be made by careful attention to the overall architecture, however, because the neoplastic cells of DFSPs infiltrate the dermis diffusely, encircling or entrapping adnexal structures. SFTs, on the other hand, are usually well demarcated and do not infiltrate diffusely around adnexa.[21]

Key points

- SFTs are rare cutaneous CD34-positive spindle cell tumors.
- Of the few reported cases, recurrence has been infrequent and metastasis has not occurred.
- The differential diagnosis can include various CD34-positive spindle cell tumors, most notably DFSP and intradermal spindle cell lipoma.

β-CATENIN IMMUNOHISTOCHEMISTRY FOR DESMOID TUMORS: NOT AS HELPFUL AS HOPED

The recent elucidation of the Wnt pathway produced detailed insights into the pathogenesis of Gardner syndrome and desmoid tumors. Upregulated signaling in the Wnt pathway from abnormal persistence of β-catenin drives the growth of most desmoid tumors. In patients with Gardner syndrome and familial adenomatous polyposis (FAP), germline mutations in the adenomatous polyposis coli (APC) gene produce a faulty APC protein that fails to inhibit or degrade β-catenin. Sporadic desmoid tumors, however, carry activating mutations of β-catenin itself. The end result of both abnormalities was β-catenin stabilization and accumulation, so it seemed that immunohistochemical detection of β-catenin would be a valuable aid in distinguishing desmoid tumors from other fibroblastic proliferations. Although initial studies suggested that this was the case,[22] results from larger series were less impressive. Carlson and Fletcher[23] found nuclear immunoreactivity for β-catenin in 80% of sporadic desmoids and in only 67% of those in patients with FAP. At the same time, positivity was also evident in superficial fibromatoses, low-grade myofibroblastic sarcomas, and SFTs, among others.[23]

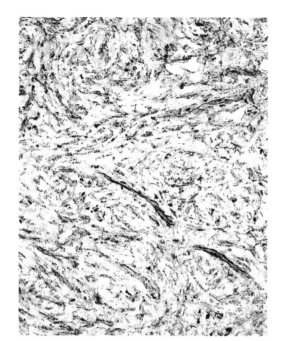

Fig. 14. Desmoid tumor. β-Catenin immunoreactivity within the nuclei of neoplastic cells is supportive of the diagnosis but its sensitivity and specificity are poor. In addition, staining of the cytoplasm of both lesional cells and nonlesional cells can complicate interpretation. In this field, some of the strongest reactivity is actually within the cytoplasm of endothelial cells (Beta-catenin, original magnification ×200).

Complicating matters further is the fact that only nuclear accumulation of β-catenin is indicative of dysregulated Wnt signaling (**Fig. 14**); staining may be indistinct, focal, or weak in some tumors[22,23]; and nonneoplastic cells (eg, endothelial cells) routinely show cytoplasmic reactivity. At best, therefore, it seems that immunohistochemistry for β-catenin plays a supportive role. Its presence does not exclude other tumors, and its absence does not preclude the diagnosis of a desmoid tumor. However, β-catenin may be useful in assessing margin status in resection specimens of tumors known to express the antigen. The low cellular density and banal cytology of desmoids can make them difficult to differentiate from scar

Key points

- β-Catenin accumulates within the nucleus in desmoid tumors; this occurs in sporadic cases and those associated with Gardner syndrome and FAP.

- β-Catenin can be detected immunohistochemically within the neoplastic cells of desmoids tumors, but it is not specific and its sensitivity may be as low as 65%.

tissue or even normal connective tissue (**Fig. 15**), but clusters of spindled cells with nuclear immunoreactivity for β-catenin may make this otherwise difficult distinction straightforward (**Fig. 16**).

DFSP: WHAT IS USEFUL AND WHAT IS NOT IN PREDICTING WHICH WILL RECUR, WHICH WILL METASTASIZE, AND WHICH WILL RESPOND TO TARGETED THERAPY

DFSP can frustrate dermatopathologists in many ways. On biopsy, they can simulate several other tumors, including benign ones such as SFTs, intradermal spindle cell lipomas, cellular dermatofibromas, and diffuse neurofibromas. Within excisions, their banal spindled cells often blend imperceptibly with scar tissue or even normal collagen at their borders, making margin assessment difficult in many cases and virtually impossible in some. Even when margins seem negative, up to 20% will recur; and although very few metastasize, those that do can cause death rather quickly. However, because of their rarity, clinical and pathologic prognostic determinants have remained obscure. It is well-known that some DFSPs harbor areas indistinguishable from standard fibrosarcoma, but the clinical impact of this finding has been unclear.[24] The same was true of mitotic

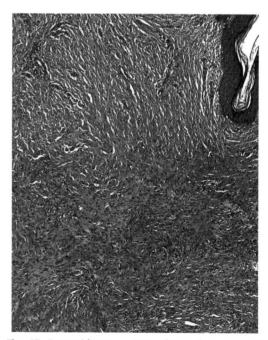

Fig. 15. Desmoid tumor. Some desmoids tumors are difficult to differentiate from scars. In this case, spindled cells were present at the margin of a desmoid tumor excision, but whether the area was scar or residual tumor was unclear (hematoxylin and eosin stain, original magnification ×200).

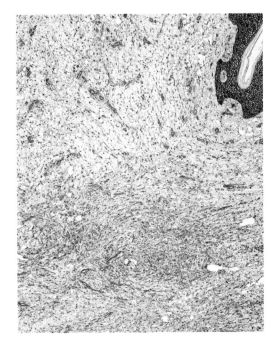

Fig. 16. Desmoid tumor. β-Catenin was useful in this setting, because the tumor was known to express the antigen, and the numerous spindled cells with nuclear positivity supported interpretation as residual neoplasm at the margin (Beta-catenin, original magnification ×40).

index, cellular density, necrosis, and other parameters. Moreover, patients with extensive or metastatic disease had few options except continued reexcision and radiotherapy.

Recent efforts have provided new prognostic data and new therapeutic options, however. To assess the impact of clinical and pathologic features on recurrence and overall survival, Erdem and colleagues[25] evaluated a group of 122 patients with DFSP treated and followed up at a single institution. On multivariate analysis, decreased overall survival was associated with only one factor: the presence of metastatic disease. No other histopathologic variable, including fibrosarcomatous change, impacted survival.

However, DFSPs with fibrosarcomatous change and those on acral sites did have shorter recurrence-free intervals after wide local excision.[25] The reported frequency and significance[26] of fibrosarcomatous change within DFSP have varied widely,[24,25,27,28] perhaps because the frequency of detection depends on how it is defined and how thoroughly one searches for it. In the study by Erdem and colleagues,[25] it was defined as areas with a densely cellular fascicular herringbone architecture, a mitotic index of greater than 2 per mm^2 (range, 2–20 per mm^2, median, 6 per mm^2), and increased nuclear atypia that

occupied greater than 5% of the tumor (mean, 13%). According to these criteria, fibrosarcomatous change was present in more than 20% of the 122 cases. Therefore, careful search for areas of fibrosarcomatous change in DFSP seems warranted (**Fig. 17**), because in addition to wide local excision, more aggressive therapy may benefit patients with tumors on acral sites and those with fibrosarcomatous change.

Until recently, more aggressive therapy meant wider excision and/or radiotherapy, because conventional chemotherapeutic agents were ineffective for DFSP. In 2006, however, the U.S. Food and Drug Administration approved imatinib mesylate for use in metastatic or unresectable DFSP. Although it was originally developed to target the Abl/Bcr-Abl tyrosine kinase receptor, researchers quickly discovered that imatinib was also an effective inhibitor of the tyrosine kinase receptors KIT and platelet-derived growth factor (PDGF). In the mid-1990s, supernumerary ring chromosomes containing the chromosome 22 centromere along with interstitial sequences from chromosomes 17 and 22 were shown to be common in DFSP, and this was found to lead to low-level genomic amplification of selected

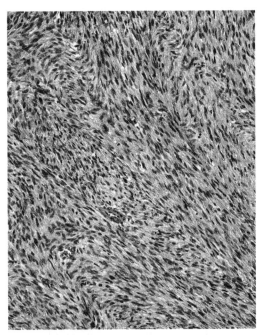

Fig. 17. Fibrosarcomatous change in a DFSP. Increased cellular density with a herringbone architecture, a mitotic index of greater than 2 per mm^2, and increased nuclear atypia occupied greater than 5% of this otherwise typical DFSP. Recent evidence suggests that up to 20% of DFSPs may harbor this finding (hematoxylin and eosin stain, original magnification ×200).

sequences.[29,30] It was ultimately demonstrated that the specific translocation, t(17;22)(q22;q13), fuses exon 2 of the *PDGFβ* gene to exons of the collagen type 1 α1 gene (*COL1A1*). This fusion places the *PDGFβ* gene under control of the highly active *COL1A1* promoter, leading to *PDGFβ* overexpression and, therefore, overactivation of the PDGF receptor.[31–33] This sequence then drives the growth of fibroblasts in DFSP. Imatinib mesylate blocks PDGF receptor (PDGFR) signaling, and imatinib therapy can produce shrinkage or regression in DFSPs that harbor this specific translocation. Multiple studies have shown that imatinib therapy is associated with tumor shrinkage,[34–43] and it has been touted as a neoadjuvant therapy capable of making unresectable tumors amenable to surgery.[40]

Several important caveats exist, however. First, although detection of the *COL1A1-PDGFβ* fusion can help confirm the diagnosis of DFSP (particularly when a rare CD34-negative case is encountered), a small percentage of DFSPs are driven by other chromosomal aberrations.[41] Second, molecular techniques are subject to the same inherent false-negative phenomenon as other diagnostic tests. False-negative results in this situation have several potential causes, but common among them are a failure to obtain sufficient RNA from a sample for reverse transcription polymerase chain reaction (RT-PCR) or a failure of the amplification reaction itself.[41] Third, even if the *COL1A1-PDGFβ* fusion is present, it may not be producing a viable transcript.[41] In other words, defective DNA does not always produce a defective protein that will respond to targeted therapy. Many tumors harbor multiple genetic aberrations; which of them are responsible for the unregulated growth is not always clear.

Although imatinib treatment may make excision of some DFSPs easier for the surgeon, for the dermatopathologist it can make an already challenging specimen even more difficult to evaluate. Many of the tumors that shrink miraculously in response to imatinib have a dramatically reduced number of tumor cells (**Figs. 18** and **19**).[44,45] This reduction, however, makes determining whether a few scattered CD34-positive spindle cells at the margin are merely normal dendritic fibroblasts or residual tumor even more difficult. Whether a small amount of residual tumor at a margin affects recurrence after imatinib therapy and surgical excision is not known, but it can affect the confidence of the dermatopathologist tasked with declaring whether those margins are free of tumor.

Even worse is the fact that imatinib-treated DFSPs may contain areas of diminished or entirely regressed tumor directly adjacent to pockets of

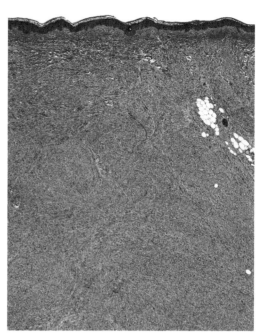

Fig. 18. DFSP. Most DFSP tumors exhibit dense and uniform cellularity (hematoxylin and eosin stain, original magnification ×40).

residual tumor that seem completely unaffected by the therapy.[41,45] Obviously, this further complicates assessment of residual tumor burden and margin status (**Figs. 20** and **21**).

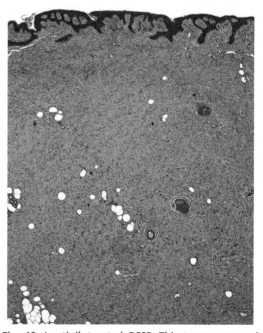

Fig. 19. Imatinib-treated DFSP. This tumor, resected after imatinib therapy, had much lower cellularity and a more hyalinized collagenous stroma (hematoxylin and eosin stain, original magnification ×40).

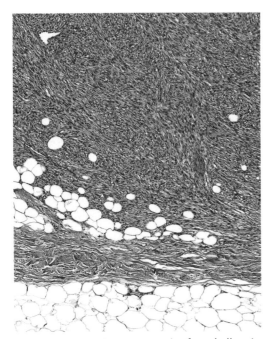

Fig. 20. DFSP. Margin assessment is often challenging in DFSP. In this case (not treated with imatinib), an abrupt change in cellularity helps distinguish tumor from normal tissue (hematoxylin and eosin stain, original magnification ×100).

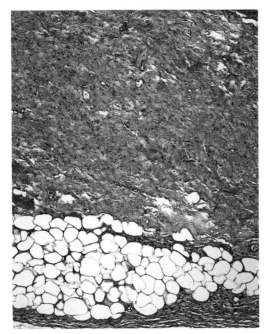

Fig. 21. DFSP. This tumor was treated with imatinib before resection, and the marked reduction in cellularity made margin assessment more difficult (hematoxylin and eosin stain, original magnification ×200).

Key points

- In DFSP, only the presence of metastasis impacts overall survival.

- DFSPs with fibrosarcomatous change and those on acral sites have shorter recurrence-free intervals after wide local excision.

- Detection of the *COL1A1-PDGFβ* fusion can help confirm the diagnosis of DFSP.

- Most, but not all, tumors with this fusion will respond to imatinib mesylate therapy. A small number of DFSPs lack this aberration. Also, some contain the fusion but seem to lack abnormal expression of PDFGβ.

- Treatment with imatinib often results in DFSPs with areas that are sclerotic, hypocellular, or even devoid of viable tumor. However, these same tumors may harbor pockets of fully viable tumor, and sometimes these areas are discontiguous and widespread throughout the tumor.

SUMMARY

1. Myxofibrosarcoma is a distinct entity that should be recognized by dermatologists and dermatopathologists because most present in the skin and subcutis. Dermatopathologists must be aware that superficial and peripheral areas of these tumors are often deceptively banal and may simulate benign tumors or even reactive dermatoses.

2. CD10 has been touted as a useful marker for AFX. Although it is sensitive, it is not at all specific and can be expressed by spindle cell squamous cell carcinomas, melanomas, myxofibrosarcomas, pleomorphic sarcomas, dermatofibromas, and DFSP, among others.

3. Despite their name, no convincing evidence exists that so-called cellular neurothekeomas are neural tumors. Myxoid neurothekeomas, however, express S100 and GFAPs and seem to be a distinct type of peripheral nerve sheath tumor. For these tumors, the term *nerve sheath myxoma* is now preferred.

4. Primary cutaneous SFTs are a distinct entity to be distinguished from the many other CD34-positive cutaneous tumors. Long-term follow-up data are limited, but thus far most of these tumors have behaved in a benign or indolent manner.

5. β-Catenin is central to the pathogenesis of desmoid tumors (deep fibromatoses), whether sporadic or associated with FAP. Its immunohistochemical detection in the nucleus of the neoplastic cells may aid in margin assessment,

but its sensitivity and specificity limit its use as a diagnostic aid.

6. In DFSPs, only the presence of metastasis confers a decreased overall survival. Those with fibrosarcomatous change or acral location have a shorter disease-free interval after wide local excision. The *COL1A1-PDGFβ* fusion product is detected in approximately 95% of DFSPs, and these may be amenable to treatment with imatinib mesylate. Not all contain this translocation, however, and even some that do may not respond. Tumors resected after neoadjuvant imatinib therapy can have pockets of viable residual tumor interspersed among sclerotic zones, complicating margin assessment.

REFERENCES

1. Angervall L, Kindblom LG, Merck C. Myxofibrosarcoma. A study of 30 cases. Acta Pathol Microbiol Scand A 1977;85(2):127–40.

2. Hollowood K, Fletcher CD. Malignant fibrous histiocytoma: morphologic pattern or pathologic entity? Semin Diagn Pathol 1995;12(3):210–20.

3. Fletcher CD. Pleomorphic malignant fibrous histiocytoma: fact or fiction? A critical reappraisal based on 159 tumors diagnosed as pleomorphic sarcoma. Am J Surg Pathol 1992;16(3):213–28.

4. Fletcher CD. The evolving classification of soft tissue tumours: an update based on the new WHO classification. Histopathology 2006;48(1):3–12.

5. Mentzel T, Calonje E, Wadden C, et al. Myxofibrosarcoma. Clinicopathologic analysis of 75 cases with emphasis on the low-grade variant. Am J Surg Pathol 1996;20(4):391–405.

6. Weedon D, Williamson R, Mirza B. CD10, a useful marker for atypical fibroxanthomas. Am J Dermatopathol 2005;27(2):181.

7. de Feraudy S, Mar N, McCalmont TH. Evaluation of CD10 and procollagen 1 expression in atypical fibroxanthoma and dermatofibroma. Am J Surg Pathol 2008;32(8):1111–22.

8. Hultgren TL, DiMaio DJ. Immunohistochemical staining of CD10 in atypical fibroxanthomas. J Cutan Pathol 2007;34(5):415–9.

9. Kanner WA, Brill LB 2nd, Patterson JW, et al. CD10, p63 and CD99 expression in the differential diagnosis of atypical fibroxanthoma, spindle cell squamous cell carcinoma and desmoplastic melanoma. J Cutan Pathol 2010;37(7):744–50.

10. Clarke LE, Frauenhoffer E, Fox E, et al. CD10-positive myxofibrosarcomas: a pitfall in the differential diagnosis of atypical fibroxanthoma. J Cutan Pathol 2010;37(7):737–43.

11. Bilalovic N, Sandstad B, Golouh R, et al. CD10 protein expression in tumor and stromal cells of malignant melanoma is associated with tumor progression. Mod Pathol 2004;17(10):1251–8.

12. Kanitakis J, Narvaez D, Claudy A. Differential expression of the CD10 antigen (neutral endopeptidase) in primary versus metastatic malignant melanomas of the skin. Melanoma Res 2002;12(3):241–4.

13. Carrel S, Zografos L, Schreyer M, et al. Expression of CALLA/CD10 on human melanoma cells. Melanoma Res 1993;3(5):319–23.

14. Wieland CN, Dyck R, Weenig RH, et al. The role of CD10 in distinguishing atypical fibroxanthoma from sarcomatoid (spindle cell) squamous cell carcinoma. J Cutan Pathol 2011;38(11):884–8.

15. Fetsch JF, Laskin WB, Miettinen M. Nerve sheath myxoma: a clinicopathologic and immunohistochemical analysis of 57 morphologically distinctive, S-100 protein- and GFAP-positive, myxoid peripheral nerve sheath tumors with a predilection for the extremities and a high local recurrence rate. Am J Surg Pathol 2005;29(12):1615–24.

16. Fetsch JF, Laskin WB, Hallman JR, et al. Neurothekeoma: an analysis of 178 tumors with detailed immunohistochemical data and long-term patient follow-up information. Am J Surg Pathol 2007;31(7):1103–14.

17. Sheth S, Li X, Binder S, et al. Differential gene expression profiles of neurothekeomas and nerve sheath myxomas by microarray analysis. Mod Pathol 2011;24(3):343–54.

18. Smith KJ, Skelton HG. Solitary fibrous tumor. Am J Dermatopathol 2001;23(1):81–2.

19. Erdag G, Qureshi HS, Patterson JW, et al. Solitary fibrous tumors of the skin: a clinicopathologic study of 10 cases and review of the literature. J Cutan Pathol 2007;34(11):844–50.

20. Soldano AC, Meehan SA. Cutaneous solitary fibrous tumor: a report of 2 cases and review of the literature. Am J Dermatopathol 2008;30(1):54–8.

21. Wood L, Fountaine TJ, Rosamilia L, et al. Cutaneous CD34+ spindle cell neoplasms: histopathologic features distinguish spindle cell lipoma, solitary fibrous tumor, and dermatofibrosarcoma protuberans. Am J Dermatopathol 2010;32(8):764–8.

22. Bhattacharya B, Dilworth HP, Iacobuzio-Donahue C, et al. Nuclear beta-catenin expression distinguishes deep fibromatosis from other benign and malignant fibroblastic and myofibroblastic lesions. Am J Surg Pathol 2005;29(5):653–9.

23. Carlson JW, Fletcher CD. Immunohistochemistry for beta-catenin in the differential diagnosis of spindle cell lesions: analysis of a series and review of the literature. Histopathology 2007;51(4):509–14.

24. Stacchiotti S, Pedeutour F, Negri T, et al. Dermatofibrosarcoma protuberans-derived fibrosarcoma: clinical history, biological profile and sensitivity to imatinib. Int J Cancer 2011;129(7):1761–72.

25. Erdem O, Wyatt AJ, Lin E, et al. Dermatofibrosarcoma protuberans treated with wide local excision and followed at a cancer hospital: prognostic significance of clinicopathologic variables. Am J Dermatopathol 2012;34(1):24–34.

26. Hamada M, Hirakawa N, Fukuda T, et al. A progression to dermatofibrosarcoma protuberans with a fibrosarcomatous component: a special reference to the chromosomal aberrations. Pathol Res Pract 1999;195(7):451–60.

27. Diaz-Cascajo C, Weyers W, Borrego L, et al. Dermatofibrosarcoma protuberans with fibrosarcomatous areas: a clinico-pathologic and immunohistochemic study in four cases. Am J Dermatopathol 1997; 19(6):562–7.

28. Goldblum JR, Reith JD, Weiss SW. Sarcomas arising in dermatofibrosarcoma protuberans: a reappraisal of biologic behavior in eighteen cases treated by wide local excision with extended clinical follow up. Am J Surg Pathol 2000;24(8):1125–30.

29. Pedeutour F, Simon MP, Minoletti F, et al. Translocation, t(17;22)(q22;q13), in dermatofibrosarcoma protuberans: a new tumor-associated chromosome rearrangement. Cytogenet Cell Genet 1996; 72(2–3):171–4.

30. Pedeutour F, Simon MP, Minoletti F, et al. Ring 22 chromosomes in dermatofibrosarcoma protuberans are low-level amplifiers of chromosome 17 and 22 sequences. Cancer Res 1995;55(11):2400–3.

31. Kikuchi K, Soma Y, Fujimoto M, et al. Dermatofibrosarcoma protuberans: increased growth response to platelet-derived growth factor BB in cell culture. Biochem Biophys Res Commun 1993;196(1):409–15.

32. Macarenco RS, Zamolyi R, Franco MF, et al. Genomic gains of COL1A1-PDFGB occur in the histologic evolution of giant cell fibroblastoma into dermatofibrosarcoma protuberans. Genes Chromosomes Cancer 2008;47(3):260–5.

33. Minoletti F, Miozzo M, Pedeutour F, et al. Involvement of chromosomes 17 and 22 in dermatofibrosarcoma protuberans. Genes Chromosomes Cancer 1995; 13(1):62–5.

34. Han A, Chen EH, Niedt G, et al. Neoadjuvant imatinib therapy for dermatofibrosarcoma protuberans. Arch Dermatol 2009;145(7):792–6.

35. Handolias D, McArthur GA. Imatinib as effective therapy for dermatofibrosarcoma protuberans: proof of concept of the autocrine hypothesis for cancer. Future Oncol 2008;4(2):211–7.

36. Johnson-Jahangir H, Ratner D. Advances in management of dermatofibrosarcoma protuberans. Dermatol Clin 2011;29(2):191–200, viii.

37. Johnson-Jahangir H, Sherman W, Ratner D. Using imatinib as neoadjuvant therapy in dermatofibrosarcoma protuberans: potential pluses and minuses. J Natl Compr Canc Netw 2010;8(8):881–5.

38. Labropoulos SV, Fletcher JA, Oliveira AM, et al. Sustained complete remission of metastatic dermatofibrosarcoma protuberans with imatinib mesylate. Anticancer Drugs 2005;16(4):461–6.

39. Labropoulos SV, Razis ED. Imatinib in the treatment of dermatofibrosarcoma protuberans. Biologics 2007;1(4):347–53.

40. Lemm D, Muegge LO, Hoeffken K, et al. Remission with Imatinib mesylate treatment in a patient with initially unresectable dermatofibrosarcoma protuberans—a case report. Oral Maxillofac Surg 2008; 12(4):209–13.

41. Llombart B, Sanmartin O, Lopez-Guerrero JA, et al. Dermatofibrosarcoma protuberans: clinical, pathological, and genetic (COL1A1-PDGFB) study with therapeutic implications. Histopathology 2009; 54(7):860–72.

42. Rutkowski P, Debiec-Rychter M, Nowecki Z, et al. Treatment of advanced dermatofibrosarcoma protuberans with imatinib mesylate with or without surgical resection. J Eur Acad Dermatol Venereol 2011;25(3):264–70.

43. Rutkowski P, Van Glabbeke M, Rankin CJ, et al. Imatinib mesylate in advanced dermatofibrosarcoma protuberans: pooled analysis of two phase II clinical trials. J Clin Oncol 2010;28(10):1772–9.

44. Thomison J, McCarter M, McClain D, et al. Hyalinized collagen in a dermatofibrosarcoma protuberans after treatment with imatinib mesylate. J Cutan Pathol 2008;35(11):1003–6.

45. Kerob D, Porcher R, Verola O, et al. Imatinib mesylate as a preoperative therapy in dermatofibrosarcoma: results of a multicenter phase II study on 25 patients. Clin Cancer Res 2010;16(12):3288–95.

Update on Vascular Neoplasms

Omar P. Sangüeza, MD

KEYWORDS

- Wilms tumor • Kaposi sarcoma • Infantile hemangioma • Acquired elastotic hemangioma

KEY POINTS

- Wilms tumor 1 (WT1) is a tumor suppressor gene (map locus 11p13).
- *Myc* amplification is found in angiosarcomas secondary to radiation and chronic lymphedema but not in atypical vascular proliferations secondary to radiotherapy.
- ERG is also useful in separating angiosarcomas and epithelioid hemangioendotheliomas from their histologic mimics, such as nonendothelial tumors with corded, myxohyaline, and hemorrhagic, highly vascular patterns.

NEW IMMUNOHISTOCHEMICAL MARKERS FOR THE DIAGNOSIS OF VASCULAR NEOPLASMS
Wilms Tumor 1

Wilms tumor 1(*WT1*) is a tumor suppressor gene (map locus 11p13). The gene product, WT1/Wilms tumor protein, is a transcription factor that contains 4 epidermal growth factor (EGR)–family C2H2-type zinc fingers at 323–347, 353–377, 383–405, and 414–438 and a 57 amino acid, proline-rich region, which recognizes and binds the DNA sequence 5′-CGCCCCGC-3′. This gene plays an essential role in the normal development of the urogenital system but is also involved in hematopoiesis and angiogenesis.[1] The expression of WT1 is maintained during the differentiation of the various bone marrow stem cells into endothelial cells.[2] WT1 has been detected in acute leukemias, breast carcinomas, melanomas, non–small cell lung cancer, and carcinomas of the genitourinary tract.[3–7]

WT1 immunostaining has been used to discriminate between vascular neoplasms and most vascular malformations. A study by Lawley and colleagues[8] showed WT1 expression in infantile hemangiomas (8 of 9), pyogenic granulomas (2 of 2), angiosarcomas (9 of 9), epithelioid hemangioendothelioma (1 of 1), and hobnail hemangiomas (1 of 1). A single case of malignant hemangioendothelioma was negative for WT1. However, vascular malformations (2 port-wine stains, 10 venous malformations, and 8 lymphatic malformations) did not show any positive endothelial staining. More recently Trindade and colleagues,[9] confirmed these results and expanded these findings. They found expression of WT1 in arteriovenous malformations (AVMs), noninvoluting congenital hemangiomas (NICHs) (**Fig.** 1A and B), rapidly involuting congenital hemangiomas (RICHs), tufted angiomas, and spindle cell hemangiomas. They also confirmed the absence of *WT1* expression in anomalous vessels in capillary, lymphatic, and venous malformations. All AVMs showed positivity for *WT1* in the lesional endothelia; this could be related to the proliferative stage of the AVM, because all their cases were in stage II, with arteriovenous shuntings and clinical enlargement.

Claudins

Claudins are a family of proteins that are components of the tight junctions and are part of the cellular barrier that controls the flow of molecules in the intercellular space between epithelial cells. They have 4 transmembrane domains, with the *N*-terminus and the *C*-terminus in the cytoplasm. They are expressed in various endothelia and in some, especially juxtaluminal, glandular and

Departments of Pathology and Dermatology, Wake Forest University School of Medicine, Winston Salem, NC 27157, USA
E-mail address: osanguez@wakehealth.edu

Dermatol Clin 30 (2012) 657–665
http://dx.doi.org/10.1016/j.det.2012.06.013
0733-8635/12/$ – see front matter © 2012 Elsevier Inc. All rights reserved.

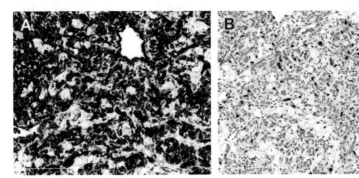

Fig. 1. (*A*) NICH staining strongly positive for *WT1*. (*B*) NICH-negative staining for GLUT1 (original magnification ×40).

ductal epithelial cells.[10] Claudin-5 is also required in cardiovascular development, and monoallelic loss of a chromosome 22 segment including claudin-5 locus causes velocardiofacial syndrome, including cardiac malformations.[11]

Miettinen and colleagues[12] found that claudin-5 is a sensitive marker for angiosarcoma and hemangioendothelioma but is not very specific, considering its widespread expression in carcinomas. Claudin-5 is significantly expressed in most angiosarcomas, indicating that this cell junction protein is generally conserved in endothelia with malignant transformation. Claudin-5 is very specific for angiosarcomas. Only synovial sarcomas are positive for this antibody. Claudin-5 is useful to differentiate from mimics of angiosarcoma, such as epithelioid sarcoma, and melanoma, which are consistently claudin-5–negative.

Avian V-Ets Erythroblastosis Virus E26 Oncogene Homolog

Avian v-ets erythroblastosis virus E26 oncogene homolog (ERG) is a transcription factor of the erythroblast transformation–specific family. It is expressed in the nuclei of endothelial cells and in normal lymphatics. It is also expressed in subsets of prostatic carcinoma, acute myeloid leukemia, and Ewing sarcoma.[13]

ERG stain is a highly specific endothelial marker for vascular neoplasms. It can be useful in differentiating hemangiomas, which have a dual cell population (ERG-positive endothelial cells and ERG-negative nonendothelial components, especially pericytes) from angiosarcomas, which generally have only ERG-positive endothelial components.

ERG is also expressed in malignant vascular endothelial neoplasms (hemangioendotheliomas, angiosarcomas, and Kaposi sarcomas). The staining is usually seen in most tumor cells, indicating that the expression of the ERG transcription factor in endothelial cells and angiosarcomas is an all-or-

none phenomenon. ERG is also useful in separating angiosarcomas and epithelioid hemangioendotheliomas from their histologic mimics, such as nonendothelial tumors with corded, myxohyaline, and hemorrhagic, highly vascular patterns.[13]

ERG is more specific than other endothelial markers, such as CD31, the current gold standard in the definition of angiosarcoma. ERG immunoreactivity is highly endothelium-restricted and straightforward to interpret, whereas interpretation of CD31 can be problematic, because it also stains histiocytes and plasma cells, which can lead to an overdiagnosis of angiosarcoma. CD31 also stains platelets.

c-Myc

c-*Myc* is a regulator gene that codes for a transcription factor. A mutated version of *Myc* is found in many cancers, which causes *Myc* to be constitutively (persistently) expressed. This function leads to the unregulated expression of many genes, some of which are involved in cell proliferation and results in the formation of cancer.

A common translocation involving *Myc* is t(8;14). This translocation is found in some malignant neoplasms, including secondary but not primary angiosarcomas. This is the most frequent recurrent alteration on chromosome 8q24.21 (50%), followed by 10p12.33 (33%) and 5q35.3 (11%).[14]

Myc amplification is found in angiosarcomas secondary to radiation and chronic lymphedema (**Fig. 2**A–C), but not in atypical vascular proliferations secondary to radiotherapy.[15]

INFANTILE HEMANGIOMAS

Infantile hemangioma (IH) is the most common benign vascular proliferation, and traditionally has been considered a neoplasm. This classification may be true for a minority of these proliferations, but most IHs are better considered as hyperplasias. Classical IHs, after an initial proliferative

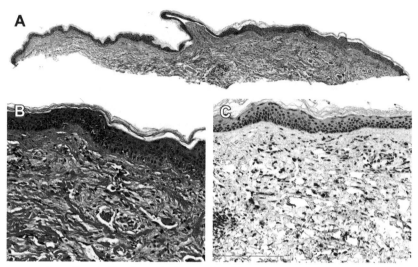

Fig. 2. Angiosarcoma in radiated skin. (*A* and *B*) Irregular dilated spaces lined by prominent endothelial cells (hematoxylin and eosin stain, original magnification *A* ×20, *B* ×40). (*C*) Positive staining for *c-Myc* of the endothelial cells.

phase, undergo complete regression, through a process of fibrosis, even in the absence of therapy. The histopathologic composition of IHs varies with the age of the lesion. Early hemangiomas are highly cellular and are characterized by plump endothelial cells aligned to vascular spaces with small inconspicuous lumina. As the lesions mature, blood flow increases, endothelium flattens, and the lumina of the vessels enlarge and become more obvious. During this interval, the vessels convey a "cavernous" appearance that can be misinterpreted as a venous malformation. Regression is portrayed as progressive interstitial fibrosis and adipose metaplasia, a process without known stimulus.[16]

The other 2 types of IH include NICH and RICH. NICH is a rare true vascular tumor that is fully formed at birth, grows proportionally with the patient or expands slightly over time, and does not regress.[17] RICH is also fully formed at birth but completely regresses within the first 6 months to 1 year of life. NICH is characterized by the presence of lobular collections of small, thin-walled vessels with large, often stellate, central lumina, separated by variable amounts of fibrous tissue richly supplied with normal and abnormal veins and arteries (**Fig. 3**).

These vascular proliferations differ from IH in their growth patterns and lack of immunoreactivity for the glucose transporter-1 protein (GLUT1), which is a sensitive and specific marker for IH (see **Fig. 1**B). This protein is not detectable in the blood vessels of normal skin or in most other types of vascular tumors but is highly expressed in endothelia at sites of blood-tissue barriers, which include the brain and placenta.

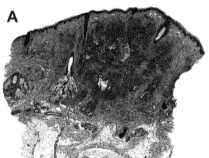

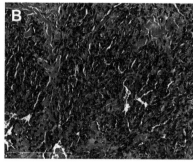

Fig. 3. (*A*) NICH. Low-power view shows a large vascular neoplasm showing an admixture of large dilated vessels and lobular collections of small, thin-walled vessels (hematoxylin and eosin stain, original magnification *A* ×20). (*B*) Higher magnification of the lobular areas showing thin-walled vessels lined with uniform endothelial cells (hematoxylin and eosin stain, original magnification *B* ×40).

MYOPERICYTOMAS

Myopericytomas are a group of neoplasms that originate from perivascular myoid cells (myopericytes), which share features of both smooth muscle cells and glomus cells.[18]

Clinically, myopericytoma arises most commonly in the dermis or subcutaneous tissue, with a predilection for distal extremities; however, it can affect other sites. They are more common in younger adults, although other age groups also can be affected.[19] The skin lesions may have a purplish hue, whereas others present as white nodules or fixed masses. Larger skin lesions can cause ulceration. The lesions tend to be generally painless and slow growing. They are usually solitary in adults, but can be multiple, especially in children. Recurrence has been reported to occur in 10% to 20% of patients.

Histopathologically, myopericytomas show a broad range of histologic growth patterns. Malignant transformation may also occur.

Myopericytomas are circumscribed but unencapsulated tumors composed of relatively monomorphic oval- to spindle-shaped myoid-like cells with cytoplasm that may be eosinophilic to amphophilic, and which share overlapping morphologic features with myofibromas. Classically, 3 growth patterns have been described (classic myopericytoma, myofibroma-like, and glomangiopericytoma), although Mentzel and colleagues[20] recently described other histologic patterns, including hypocellular, fibroma-like, angioleiomyoma-like, and hemangiopericytoma-like neoplasms, and immature and cellular lesions (**Fig. 4**). Lesions with focal glomoid features and intravascular growth have been also reported.[21] Features of all these patterns may be present in a lesion, although one pattern may predominate. Most cases had low mitotic rates of less than 1/10 per high-power fields, and necrosis was not usually seen. Immunohistochemically, myopericytomas are uniformly positive for smooth muscle antigen (SMA), h-caldesmon, and vimentin, and are sometimes weakly positive for desmin.

PERIVASCULAR EPITHELIOID CELL TUMORS

Perivascular epithelioid cell tumors (PEComas) are a group of rare mesenchymal neoplasms that show perivascular epithelioid differentiation. They include angiomyolipoma, lymphangiomyomatosis, clear cell "sugar" tumor of the lung, and a group of rare, morphologically, and immunophenotypically similar lesions arising at a variety of visceral and soft tissue sites. These tumors all share a distinctive cell type, the perivascular epithelioid cell.[22]

PEComas show a marked female predominance and seem to arise most commonly at visceral (especially gastrointestinal and uterine), retroperitoneal, and abdominopelvic sites, with a subset occurring in somatic soft tissue and skin.[23]

PEComas are composed of nests and sheets of usually epithelioid but occasionally spindled cells with clear to granular eosinophilic cytoplasm and a focal association with blood vessel walls. So far, most of the skin cases have presented as an ill-defined dermal neoplasm, with extension into the subcutis composed of perivascularly arranged clear and pale eosinophilic tumor cells surrounding numerous blood vessels with a lace-like pattern and slightly thickened walls (**Fig. 5A, B**). Nearly all PEComas show immunoreactivity for both melanocytic (HMB-45 or melan-A, tyrosinase, microphthalmia transcription factor, and NKIC3) (see **Fig. 5C**) and muscle markers, such as SMA, muscle actin, muscle myosin, and calponin, whereas desmin is expressed less frequently. In contrast, S100 protein and pancytokeratin are usually absent. Some PEComas may behave in a malignant fashion.[24,25] Although clear criteria for malignancy are still lacking, the combination of infiltrative growth, hypercellularity, cellular atypia, increased proliferative activity, and tumor

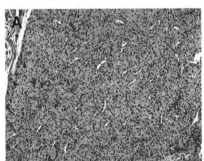
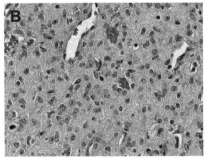

Fig. 4. Myopericytoma. (*A*) Monomorphic oval- to spindle-shaped myoid-like cells with an eosinophilic cytoplasm and a centrally placed nuclei (hematoxylin and eosin stain, original magnification ×20). (*B*) Detail of the cells present in a myopericytoma (hematoxylin and eosin stain, original magnification *B* ×40).

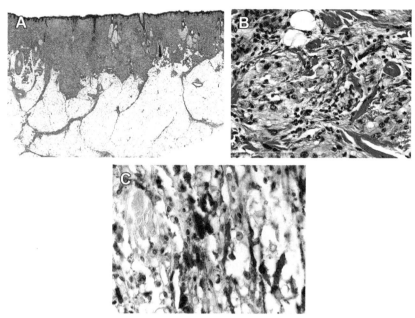

Fig. 5. PEComa. (*A*) Ill-defined neoplasm composed of nests of epithelioid and spindle cell with clear cytoplasm (hematoxylin and eosin stain, original magnification ×20). (*B*) Detail of the clear cells (hematoxylin and eosin stain, original magnification ×40). (*C*) Positive staining for HMB-45.

necrosis seem to be associated with a malignant clinical course.

ACQUIRED ELASTOTIC HEMANGIOMA

Acquired elastotic hemangioma is a recently described variant of cutaneous hemangioma. These lesions develop during adulthood on chronic sun-damaged skin on the extensor surface of the forearms or the lateral aspects of the neck. It mainly affects middle-aged and elderly women.[26]

Acquired elastotic hemangioma presents as a slightly elevated, irregularly shaped, solitary lesion with violaceous coloration. The lesions are usually well-demarcated plaques that range from 2 to 5 cm in diameter. The lesions blanch under diascope pressure. Clinically, these lesions are confused with basal cell carcinoma, hemangioma, or Bowen disease. In most cases no evidence of previous trauma is seen at the site of the lesion.

Histopathologically, acquired elastotic hemangioma consists of a proliferation of capillaries involving the superficial dermis in a band-like arrangement parallel to the epidermis. A narrow band of noninvolved papillary dermis separates the newly formed capillaries from the normal or flattened epidermis. The capillary proliferation involves the papillary and upper reticular dermis, but the deep reticular dermis is characteristically spared. The neoformed capillaries show small cleft-like or round lumina and contain few erythrocytes (**Fig. 6**). The endothelial cells in many cases have a hobnail appearance, but cellular atypia of endothelial cells is absent and very few mitotic figures are identified. Papillary projections are also present in some cases. No hemosiderin deposits or extravasated erythrocytes are seen. The connective tissue surrounding or intermingled with the newly formed capillaries show intense solar elastosis, which is seen as basophilic degeneration or amorphous basophilic granular material replacing the normal superficial dermis.[27,28]

Immunohistochemically, the neoplastic endothelial cells of acquired elastotic hemangioma strongly express CD31, CD34, and D2-40. A continuous rim of α-SMA–positive pericytes surrounds most of the neoplastic vascular channels. Proliferating markers Ki-67 and MPM2 stain only a few of the nuclei of the endothelial cells of the newly formed blood vessels.

VASCULAR PROLIFERATIONS IN RADIATED SKIN

Vascular proliferations are well recognized in previously irradiated areas of the skin. The nomenclature in the literature is complex, compounded by terms such as *lymphangiectases*, *benign lymphangiomatous papules*, *lymphangiomas*, *atypical vascular lesions*, and *benign lymphangioendothelioma*. The vascular lesions appear within the field

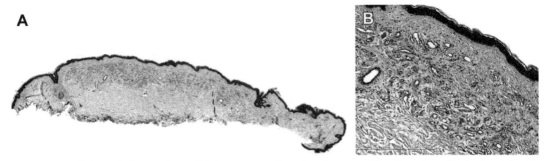

Fig. 6. Acquired elastotic hemangioma. (*A*) Low-power view showing a proliferation of capillaries involving the superficial dermis (hematoxylin and eosin stain, original magnification ×20). (*B*) Detail of the capillaries, which are lined by uniform endothelial cells. The stroma shows solar elastosis (hematoxylin and eosin stain, original magnification ×40).

of radiation. The interval between the application of radiotherapy and the appearance of the cutaneous lesions spans several years.[29–31]

Assessment of these lesions is problematic, because sometimes they can be difficult to differentiate from well-differentiated angiosarcomas. In a few cases, lesions initially diagnosed as benign vascular proliferations have evolved into angiosarcomas.

Clinically, benign vascular proliferations present as papules, small vesicles, and erythematous plaques (**Fig. 7**A). Lymphangiomatous papules and plaques are the most common. These lesions are the lymphatic counterpart of telangiectases. They result from acquired permanent dilatation of lymphatic capillaries having appeared in areas of the skin affected by obstruction or destruction of the lymphatics. It is conjectured that they result from interference in the drainage of lymphatic vessels secondary to radiotherapy or surgery. Benign lymphangiomatous papules and plaques, however, may also appear in the skin of the elderly without any evidence of primary lymphatic injury.[31]

Histologically, at low magnification, the lesions appear as well-circumscribed vascular proliferations centered in the dermis, without extension

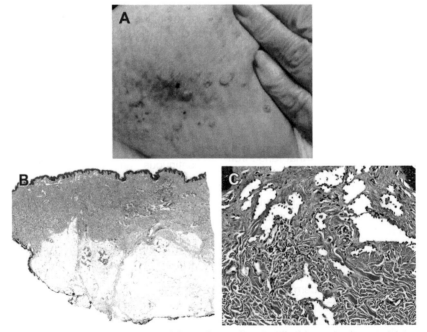

Fig. 7. Vascular proliferation in radiated skin. (*A*) Small translucent papules on the breast. (*B*) Low-power view showing several irregularly dilated lymphatics present in the upper part of the dermis (hematoxylin and eosin stain, original magnification ×20). (*C*) Higher magnification showing prominent uniform endothelial cells (hematoxylin and eosin stain, original magnification ×40).

into the subcutaneous fat. The epidermis is usually spared. Most lesions show irregularly dilated lymphatic spaces that branch and anastomose within the superficial dermis. The vascular spaces most often devoid of content; however, in some cases lymph is present (see **Fig. 7B**). They are lined by a discontinuous single layer of endothelial cells with flattened nuclei (see **Fig. 7C**). Commonly, adjacent vascular channels lie "back-to-back," separated only by a thin layer of endothelial cells. Multiple papillary projections, covered by a single layer of endothelium, project into the lumina of the dilated lymphatic. The stroma consists of fibrillary collagen rich with spindle or stellate fibroblasts. Nodular infiltrates of lymphocytes with germinal centers are occasionally present in the vicinity of the dilated vascular channels. Rarely, vascular proliferations are poorly circumscribed and focally intermingled with irregular jagged vascular spaces that may permeate the entire dermis. Endothelial cells line the latter inconspicuously. Irregular slit-like vascular spaces may be between collagen bundles of the dermis together with tufts of endothelial cells that protrude into the lumens of the newly formed vessels.

The endothelial cells that line the vascular spaces express immunoreactivity for CD31, but they do so only focally or not at all for CD34. The lymphatic marker podoplanin (D2-40) is also expressed by the neoplastic cells. Although a minority of newly formed vessels show an attenuated muscle layer, external to the endothelial cells, that occasionally is immunoreactivity for α-SMA antibody, this marker is usually nonreactive. The immunohistochemical profile substantiates the lymphatic nature of these newly formed vessels.

Some dermal vascular proliferations in irradiated skin, such as the benign lymphangioendothelioma or an atypical angiomatous proliferation, may mimic the histopathologic appearance of the patch stage of Kaposi sarcoma or even a well-differentiated angiosarcoma. Contrastingly with the patch stage of Kaposi sarcoma, atypical benign vascular proliferations, as induced by radiation, do not contain erythrocytes, hemosiderin deposits, or stromal plasma cells. The striking tufts of endothelial cells and the intravascular papillary projections, evidenced in the vascular proliferations of irradiated skin, are absent in the lesions of Kaposi sarcoma. Benign vascular proliferations are negative for human herpesvirus 8 (HHV8).

In contrast with well-differentiated angiosarcoma, atypical dermal vascular proliferations in irradiated skin do not involve the subcutaneous tissues. Distinctively, they each have cytologic atypia. The nuclei of the endothelial cells are monomorphous, have inconspicuous nucleoli, and lack mitotic figures. Contrastingly, the endothelial cells of an angiosarcoma may form stratified layers that irregularly line anastomotic channels in a manner and to a degree not seen in the atypical vascular proliferations of irradiated skin (see **Fig. 2A, B**). Recently, the use of the marker *c-Myc* has been advocated to differentiate these processes. Angiosarcomas usually express the marker *c-Myc*, which is absent in benign vascular proliferations (see **Fig. 2C**).[14,15]

NEW HISTOPATHOLOGIC VARIANTS OF AIDS-RELATED KAPOSI SARCOMA

Kaposi sarcoma is an endothelial lymphatic proliferation induced by HHV8. Cutaneous lesions of Kaposi sarcoma evolve through different stages; patch, plaque, and tumor. Histologically, lesions of Kaposi sarcoma may show a marked variation and simulate other vascular lesions. Immunohistochemically, lesions of Kaposi sarcoma stain positive for the latent nuclear antigen-1 (LNA-1), which identifies HHV8 infection in lesions of Kaposi sarcoma. This stain has proven valuable in identifying different variants of Kaposi sarcoma.

The spectrum of Kaposi sarcoma includes anaplastic (pleomorphic) Kaposi sarcoma, lymphedematous variants (lymphangioma-like, lymphangiectatic, and bullous Kaposi sarcoma), and hyperkeratotic (verrucous), keloidal, micronodular, pyogenic granuloma–like, and intravascular Kaposi sarcoma. More recently, O'Donnell and colleagues[32] described 5 new histologic variants of cutaneous Kaposi sarcoma, including glomeruloid, telangiectatic, ecchymotic, pigmented, and Kaposi sarcoma with myoid nodules.

Glomeruloid Kaposi Sarcoma

Clinically, these lesions present as plaques of Kaposi sarcoma, and microscopically they show areas of plaque-stage Kaposi sarcoma with a prominent vascular proliferation involving the full thickness of the dermis accompanied by conspicuous spindle-shaped cells, vascular clefts, and a mild lymphoplasmacytic inflammatory infiltrate. The deep dermis at the periphery of the lesion is punctuated by circumscribed, congested, microscopic glomeruloid vascular structures resembling the glomeruli of the kidney.

Telangiectatic Kaposi Sarcoma

These lesions consist of dark, hemorrhagic lesions, and histologically they show large, congested, ectatic vascular spaces admixed with areas that show characteristic nodular-stage Kaposi sarcoma.

Ecchymotic Kaposi Sarcoma

This variant presents with widespread violaceous macules, patches, and plaques. Microscopically, the lesions exhibit an intradermal vascular proliferation accompanied by extensive extravasation of red blood cells.

Kaposi Sarcoma with Myoid Nodules

This variant can present with ulcerated nodules, which microscopically consist of nodules of Kaposi sarcoma involving the deep dermis and subcutaneous tissue. Within the nodules are aggregates of bland spindle cells with abundant eosinophilic cytoplasm and tapered nuclei reminiscent of smooth muscle.

Pigmented Kaposi Sarcoma

These lesions microscopically consist of nodules of Kaposi sarcoma containing spindle and epithelioid cells with marked cytologic atypia, increased mitotic figures, and prominent brown pigment deposition limited to admixed dendritic-appearing cells. This pigment was shown to be melanin (Fontana-Masson–positive), and not hemosiderin (iron; Prussian blue–negative).

REFERENCES

1. Moore MA. Putting the neo into neoangiogenesis. J Clin Invest 2002;109:313–5.
2. Ellisen LW, Carlesso N, Cheng T, et al. The Wilms tumor suppressor WT1 directs stage-specific quiescence and differentiation of human hematopoietic progenitor cells. EMBO J 2001;20:1897–909.
3. Nowakowska-Kopera A, Sacha T, Florek I, et al. Wilms': tumor gene 1 expression analysis by real-time quantitative polymerase chain reaction for monitoring of minimal residual disease in acute leukaemia. Leuk Lymphoma 2009;50:1326–32.
4. Gupta S, Joshi K, Wig JD, et al. High frequency of loss of allelic integrity at Wilms': tumor suppressor gene-1 locus in advanced breast tumors associated with aggressiveness of the tumor. Indian J Cancer 2009;46:303–10.
5. Perry BN, Cohen C, Govindarajan B, et al. Wilms tumor 1 expression present in most melanomas but nearly absent in nevi. Arch Dermatol 2006;142:1031–4.
6. Oji Y, Kitamura Y, Kamino E, et al. WT1 IgG antibody for early detection of nonsmall cell lung cancer and as its prognostic factor. Int J Cancer 2009;125:381–7.
7. Ohno S, Dohi S, Ohno Y, et al. Immunohistochemical detection of WT1 protein in endometrial cancer. Anticancer Res 2009;29:1691–5.
8. Lawley LP, Cerimele F, Weiss SW, et al. Expression of Wilms tumor 1 gene distinguishes vascular malformations from proliferative endothelial lesions. Arch Dermatol 2005;141:1297–300.
9. Trindade F, Tellechea O, Torrelo A, et al. Wilms tumor 1 expression in vascular neoplasms and vascular malformations. Am J Dermatopathol 2011;33:569–72.
10. Heiskala M, Peterson PA, Yang Y. The roles of claudin superfamily proteins in paracellular transport. Traffic 2001;2:92–8.
11. Moll R, Sievers E, Hammerling B, et al. Endothelial and virgultar cell formations in the mammalian lymph node sinus: endothelial differentiation morphotypes characterized by a special kind of junction (complexus adherens). Cell Tissue Res 2009;335:109–41.
12. Miettinen M, Sarlomo-Rikala M, Wang ZF. Claudin-5 as an immunohistochemical marker for angiosarcoma and hemangioendotheliomas. Am J Surg Pathol 2011;35:1848–56.
13. Miettinen M, Wang ZF, Paetau A, et al. ERG transcription factor as an immunohistochemical marker for vascular endothelial tumors and prostatic carcinoma. Am J Surg Pathol 2011;35:432–41.
14. Manner J, Radlwimmer B, Hohenberger P, et al. MYC high level amplification is a distinctive feature of angiosarcomas after irradiation or chronic lymphedema. Am J Pathol 2010;176:34–9.
15. Guo T, Zhang L, Chang NE, et al. Consistent MYC ad FLT4 gene amplification in radiation-induced angiosarcoma but not in other radiation-associated atypical vascular lesions. Genes Chromosomes Cancer 2011;50:25–33.
16. Requena I, Sanguenza OP. Cutaneous vascular proliferations. II. Hyperplasia and benign neoplasms. J Am Acad Dermatol 1997;37:887–919.
17. Enroljas O, Mulliken JB, Boon LM, et al. Noninvoluting congenital hemangioma: a rare cutaneous vascular anomaly. Plast Reconstr Surg 2001;107:1647–54.
18. Dray MS, McCarthy SW, Palmer AA, et al. Myopericytoma: a unifying term for a spectrum of tumours that show overlapping features with myofibroma. A review of 14 cases. J Clin Pathol 2006;59(1):67–73.
19. Gengler C, Guillou L. Solitary fibrous tumour and haemangiopericytoma: evolution of a concept. Histopathology 2006;48(1):63–74.
20. Mentzel T, Tos AP, Sapi Z, et al. Myopericytoma of skin and soft tissues: clinicopathologic and immunohistochemical study of 54 cases. Am J Surg Pathol 2006 Jan;30(1):104–13.
21. McMenamin ME, Calonje E. Intravascular myopericytoma. J Cutan Pathol 2002 Oct;29(9):557–61.
22. Bonetti F, Pea M, Martignoni G, et al. Clear cell ('sugar') tumor of the lung is a lesion strictly related to

angiomyolipoma—the concept of a family of lesions characterized by the presence of the perivascular epithelioid cells (PEC). Pathology 1994;26:230–6.

23. Folpe AL, McKenney JK, Li Z, et al. Clear cell myomelanocytic tumor of the thigh: report of a unique case. Am J Surg Pathol 2002;26:809–12.

24. Pea M, Bonetti F, Zamboni G, et al. Clear cell tumor and angiomyolipoma. Am J Surg Pathol 1991;15:199–202.

25. Mentzel T, Reisshauer S, Rutten A, et al. Cutaneous clear cell myomelanocytic tumour: a new member of the growing family of perivascular epithelioid cell tumours (PEComas). Clinicopathological and immunohistochemical analysis of seven cases. Histopathology 2005;46:498–504.

26. Requena L, Kutzner H, Mentzel T. Acquired elastotic hemangioma: a clinicopathologic variant of hemangioma. J Am Acad Dermatol 2002;47(3):371–6.

27. Martorell-Calatayud A, Balmer N, Sanmartín O, et al. Definition of the features of acquired elastotic hemangioma reporting the clinical and histopathological characteristics of 14 patients. J Cutan Pathol 2010; 37(4):460–4.

28. Brenn T, Fletcher CD. Postradiation vascular proliferations: an increasing problem. Histopathology 2006; 48:106–14.

29. Sener SF, Milos S, Feldman JL, et al. The spectrum of vascular lesions in the mammary skin, including angiosarcoma, after breast conservation treatment for breast cancer. J Am Coll Surg 2001;193:22–8.

30. Diaz-Cascajo C, Borghi S, Weyers W, et al. Benign lymphangiomatous papules of the skin following radiotherapy: a report of five new cases and review of the literature. Histopathology 1999;35:319–27.

31. Requena L, Kutzner H, Mentzel T, et al. Benign vascular proliferations in irradiated skin. Am J Surg Pathol 2002;26:328–37.

32. O'Donnell PJ, Pantanowitz L, Grayson W. Unique histologic variants of cutaneous Kaposi sarcoma. Am J Dermatopathol 2010;32:244–50.

Current Knowledge in Inflammatory Dermatopathology

Maxwell A. Fung, MD*, Keira L. Barr, MD

KEYWORDS

- Inflammatory skin disorders • Dermatitis • Dermatopathology • Histopathology • Dermatology
- Pathology

KEY POINTS

- Clinical correlation maximizes diagnostic accuracy in the histologic interpretation of inflammatory skin disease.
- Variations from the classic histopathologic features are increasingly recognized. Examples include sarcoid, Sweet syndrome, and paraneoplastic pemphigus.
- The clinical differential diagnosis for nonspecific histologic reaction patterns is increasingly recognized. Examples include interstitial granulomatous infiltrates, flame figures, and dermal hypersensitivity.

Since the last dermatopathology update in *Dermatologic Clinics* in 1999,[1] practicing dermatopathologists interpret most cases of inflammatory skin disease much the same as they did in previous decades: primarily if not solely, based on hematoxylin and eosin (H&E)–stained sections of formalin-fixed tissue specimens, with judicious use of histochemical stains such as the periodic acid Schiff for dermatophytes, and with mindfulness of the clinical context. If anything, only greater emphasis on the importance of clinical correlation at dermatopathology conferences has been observed over the past several years. The current transformation in pathology and laboratory medicine is toward a place at which inflammatory dermatopathology has always rested: the best dermatopathologists are talented microscopists who are conversant in the relevant aspects of clinical dermatology, not just experts of histomorphology within a microscopic vacuum.[2,3]

During the first decade of the 21st century, numerous advances in the understanding of inflammatory disease mechanisms have occurred,[4,5] particularly in psoriasis and atopic dermatitis.

Continuation of this trend will assure a future in which molecular tests for biomarkers of immediate clinical relevance are used in routine patient care, not only for diagnosis but also for prognosis and management.

This article is organized from the perspective of one approaching a new case at the microscope and follows the traditional pattern-based approach used in many dermatopathology textbooks and in the authors' institution's training program (www.ucdermpath.org/detail/TrainingProgUCD. htm). However, out of necessity, the authors assume that the reader possesses baseline knowledge of the basic clinical and histopathologic features of the most common disorders. The emphasis is focused on selected recent or noteworthy developments that are clinically relevant for the histologic diagnosis of inflammatory skin diseases.

SPONGIOTIC DERMATITIS

Spongiotic dermatitis remains one of the more commonly biopsied inflammatory dermatoses, yet distinction among nummular, atopic, irritant contact,

The authors have nothing to disclose.
UC Davis Dermatopathology Service, Department of Dermatology, University of California Davis School of Medicine, 3301 C Street, Suite 1400, Sacramento, CA 95816, USA
* Corresponding author.
E-mail address: maxwell.fung@ucdmc.ucdavis.edu

allergic contact, dyshidrotic dermatitis, id reactions, spongiotic drug reactions, and rare paraneoplastic reactions[6] continues to require clinical correlation.

Spongiotic Dermatitis Versus Mycosis Fungoides

The differential diagnosis of early patch-stage mycosis fungoides versus spongiotic dermatitis remains a challenge, clinically and histologically. Clinical correlation reveals that some of these cases may be classified as lymphomatoid drug reactions or lymphomatoid contact dermatitis,[7,8] with a range of implicated allergens, including nickel,[9] antioxidants, cosmetic-grade preservatives in baby wipes,[10] and even teakwood toilet seats.[11] In contrast to the epidermotropism that is a hallmark of mycosis fungoides, lymphomatoid reactions tend to exhibit appearances that may be characterized more descriptively as exocytosis, characterized by greater spongiosis (even if mild), mild or absent cytologic atypia, and a more randomly scattered pattern of lymphocytes throughout all levels of the epidermis (the epidermotropic lymphocytes in mycosis fungoides tend to collect in the basilar epidermis).[12] When additional diagnostic analysis is required, demonstration of a clonal T-cell receptor (TCR) gene rearrangement provides additional support for lymphoma. However, clonality has been documented in some cases of nonneoplastic disorders (spongiotic dermatitis, pemphigoid, lichen planus, lichen sclerosus, psoriasis, pityriasis lichenoides, chronic cutaneous lupus erythematosus, and lymphomatoid drug reactions).[13] Demonstrating the presence of an identical clone in two specimens ("dual TCR") or more offers greater diagnostic specificity in support of lymphoma.[14,15]

Prurigo Pigmentosa (Nagashima's Disease)

Reports of this rare but clinically distinctive disorder originated in Japan, with rare subsequent reports from America and Europe.[16] Prurigo pigmentosa presents as highly pruritic inflamed papules that coalesce into a reticulate pattern on the trunk and neck, perhaps appearing clinically as an inflammatory variant of confluent and reticulated papillomatosis. Histopathologic features have been regarded as nonspecific, but early lesions show combined spongiotic and interface features with neutrophilic spongiosis, necrotic keratinocytes, and papillary dermal edema (Fig. 1). Established lesions may exhibit a patchy lichenoid mixed infiltrate with neutrophils and eosinophils, nuclear debris "dust," reticular alteration and necrosis of the epidermis, and neutrophilic crust.[16] Rare reports have associated Helicobacter pylori infection with prurigo pigmentosa,[17] including a

recent report in which H pylori was immunohistochemically confirmed within the stratum corneum of prurigo pigmentosa.[18]

PSORIASIFORM DERMATITIS

The differential diagnosis for psoriasiform dermatitis typically includes psoriasis, psoriasiform drug reactions, chronic spongiotic/eczematous dermatitis, lichen simplex chronicus, and pityriasis rubra pilaris. Secondary syphilis and patch/plaque mycosis fungoides tend to have a superimposed lichenoid infiltrate, creating a psoriasiform lichenoid pattern.

Deficiency Dermatitis

Necrolytic migratory erythema (glucagonoma syndrome) remains a notorious mimic of psoriasis and should be considered in the appropriate clinical setting (hyperglycemia, anemia, glossitis) for any adult with an unusually eroded or refractory psoriasiform dermatitis (Fig. 2).[19] Compared with classic psoriasis, necrolytic migratory erythema exhibits confluent parakeratosis, hypogranulosis with pallor of the superficial epidermis, and eventual necrolysis (a term that encompasses vacuolization, ballooning degeneration, and subsequent confluent necrosis of keratinocytes within the superficial stratum spinosum and stratum granulosum). Nonspecific findings may also be seen, including mild spongiosis, single necrotic keratinocytes, and eosinophils; these features may be present to a limited extent in psoriasis but are nevertheless not classic for psoriasis. Necrolytic acral erythema exhibits similar histopathologic features to other forms of deficiency dermatitis but is confined to acral skin and is highly associated with hepatitis C virus (HCV) infection. Although HCV-associated leukocytoclastic vasculitis is well recognized, necrolytic acral erythema seems to develop in a different subset of patients who are HCV-positive, because vasculitis and necrolytic acral erythema have not been documented simultaneously in the same patient to date.[20,21] Overlapping features of necrolytic acral erythema and necrolytic migratory erythema have been described, suggesting a common pathogenesis.[22,23] The differential diagnosis for deficiency dermatitis also includes other nutritional deficiency states, the best characterized being zinc transporter protein (ZIP4/SLC39A4) mutation–associated zinc deficiency (acrodermatitis enteropathica, OMIM 201100),[24] acquired zinc deficiency, and vitamin B_3 (niacin) deficiency (pellagra). Necrolytic acral erythema is often associated with hypozincemia and responds to zinc supplementation.[25,26]

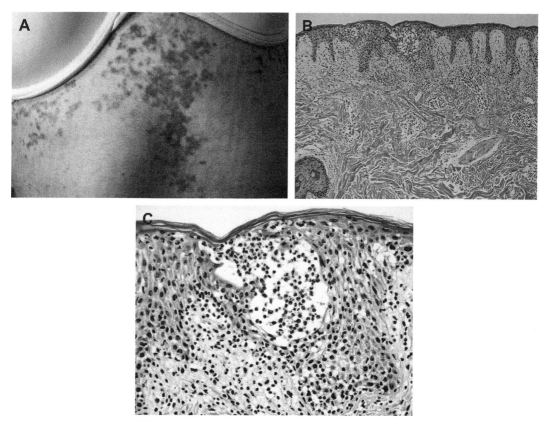

Fig. 1. Prurigo pigmentosa. (A) Pruritic reticulated erythematous papules on the trunk; (B, C) Neutrophilic spongiosis. Eosinophils are also prominent (hematoxylin and eosin stain, original magnification: B ×40; C ×400). (*Courtesy of* Errol Craig, MD, and William Liss, MD, Walnut Creek, CA.)

Pityriasis Rubra Pilaris

Biopsies from patients with pityriasis rubra pilaris (PRP) are characterized by psoriasiform hyperplasia, classic "checkerboard" parakeratosis, and sparse superficial perivascular lymphocytes. Comprehensive reviews of histopathologic features in PRP have confirmed additional features that may assist in the distinction between PRP and psoriasis, including the presence in PRP of hypergranulosis, acantholysis, and areas of atrophy amidst a background of psoriasiform hyperplasia, and eosinophils and denser lichenoid infiltrates in some cases.[27–29] One case exhibited superficial acantholysis resembling pemphigus foliaceus.[30]

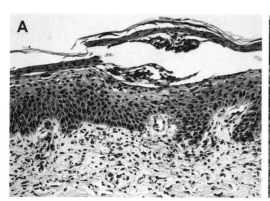
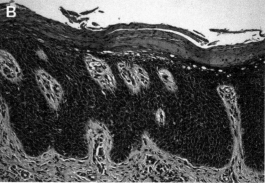

Fig. 2. Necrolytic migratory erythema. (A) Neutrophilic spongiosis, which may also be seen in psoriasis. (B) Psoriasiform hyperplasia with hypogranulosis and pallor, features that may also be seen in psoriasis (hematoxylin and eosin stain, original magnification: A, B ×400).

Actinic Prurigo

Actinic prurigo (hereditary polymorphous light eruption, Hutchinson summer prurigo) shares many features with polymorphous light eruption (PMLE). Some classifications include actinic prurigo as a severe variant of PMLE, although consistent clinical and histologic differences have been documented that permit separation of actinic prurigo as a distinct disorder.[31] Actinic prurigo usually arises in childhood and is more common in women. Strong HLA-associated susceptibility has been documented. Most cases in the United States have been reported in native North Americans, but actinic prurigo also affects Mestizos (mixed Native Indian and European) in Central and South America and has also been reported in the United Kingdom. As a clinically polymorphous eruption, actinic prurigo exhibits variable histopathologic features. Characteristic histopathologic features include psoriasiform epidermal hyperplasia, papillary dermal edema, and perivascular dermatitis (often dense, lichenoid, and/or deep) with eosinophils. More variable findings include solar elastosis, orthokeratosis or parakeratosis, spongiosis, vacuolar interface changes, and plasma cells. Reactive lymphoid follicles are a variable but distinctive finding.[32] Thus, although it is expected that some cases of actinic prurigo will be clinically and histologically indistinguishable from PMLE, the presence of psoriasiform hyperplasia, eosinophils, and lymphoid follicles favors actinic prurigo (**Fig. 3**). Specific clinical features of actinic prurigo include conjunctivitis and cheilitis, and the typical ethnicity/ancestry.

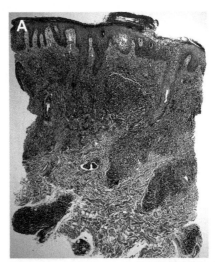
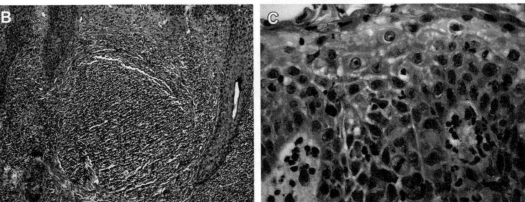

Fig. 3. Actinic prurigo. This young Native American female presented with associated conjunctivitis and cheilitis. (A) Biopsy of a papulovesicular lesion on the cheek showed psoriasiform hyperplasia with spongiosis, and dense dermal perivascular and periadnexal infiltrates. (B, C) The additional presence of reactive lymphoid follicles and eosinophils favors actinic prurigo over polymorphous light eruption (hematoxylin and eosin stain, original magnification: A ×20; B ×200; C ×600).

INTERFACE DERMATITIS

Interface dermatitis may be subclassified based on the density of the associated inflammatory infiltrate—vacuolar (sparse) versus lichenoid (dense, band-like)—or based on the pattern of associated epidermal changes. LeBoit[33] proposed the following five epidermal patterns: erythema multiforme–like (necrotic keratinocytes present in clusters and above the basal layer), lichen planus–like (basilar squamatization), irregular epidermal hyperplasia (eg, hypertrophic lichen planus), psoriasiform hyperplasia (eg, lichen striatus, lichen aureus), and atrophic (eg, poikilodermatomyositis).

A recently recognized pitfall in the interpretation of lichenoid dermatitis is the rare presence of small junctional nests of Melan-A immunopositive cells, thus presumed to be melanocytes. Clinical correlation is required to avoid an incorrect diagnosis of melanoma in situ in cases with these pseudonests. Final clinical-pathologic diagnoses have included lupus erythematosus, lichen planus, lichenoid phototoxic dermatitis, and lichenoid keratosis.[34,35]

Cutaneous Lupus Erythematosus

Lupus erythematosus (LE) may exhibit sparse vacuolar change (usually acute or subacute cutaneous LE) or lichenoid change with denser deep perivascular and periadnexal extension of lymphocytes, including plasma cells, and follicular plugging (discoid variant of chronic cutaneous LE). Although perieccrine lymphocytes are distinctive, perineural involvement has also been documented.[36] Marked papillary edema resembling polymorphous light eruption may rarely occur.[37] Eosinophils are generally rare or absent in acute, subacute, and chronic cutaneous LE (with the exception of lupus profundus), and in dermatomyositis, graft-versus-host disease (GVHD),[38] and pityriasis lichenoides.[39]

Nonbullous neutrophilic variants of LE have been documented that exhibit dermal perivascular and interstitial neutrophils and leukocytoclastic nuclear debris (nuclear "dust"), without vasculitis or blister formation.[40,41] Clinically, these lesions are more likely to present as pruritic urticarial papules and plaques compared with conventional cases of LE.

One potential diagnostic pitfall is the recognition of LE-like interface dermatitis induced by topical imiquimod therapy.[42–44] Curiously, imiquimod also has been rarely reported to induce LE[45] and its remission.[46]

Paraneoplastic Dermatitis

Paraneoplastic dermatitis is not a defined clinical-pathologic entity but, rather, is a phrase that has been used by some clinicians to describe rare paraneoplastic reactions that are not readily classified. To date, the documented spectrum of paraneoplastic reactions includes paraneoplastic pemphigus (see next section) but also disorders that lack vesiculobullous lesions or mucositis clinically and acantholysis histologically. For example, unexplained spongiotic/eczematous dermatitis and "dermal hypersensitivity" reactions have been associated with systemic lymphoma.[6,47]

Several recent reports have highlighted the presence of interface dermatitis in patients with thymoma, not only in humans but also in rabbits, cats, and dogs.[48–50] A recent human case characterized as thymoma-associated multiorgan autoimmunity (TAMA) exemplifies the clinical and histologic resemblance to GVHD.[51] In TAMA, a history of thymoma is definitional, and GVHD and drug reactions must be excluded by the clinical history. Gastrointestinal involvement has been a feature in all reported cases to date, with variable hepatic and cutaneous involvement.[52,53] The skin lesions have been characterized as maculopapular (morbilliform), confluent nummular, or erythema multiforme–like. Oral involvement suggestive of paraneoplastic pemphigus may occur but, in contrast to paraneoplastic pemphigus, is not a hallmark of TAMA. Histologically, involvement of adnexal epithelium through an interface reaction with prominent necrotic/apoptotic keratinocytes represents an overlapping feature with GVHD, TAMA, and the lichenoid variant of paraneoplastic pemphigus (paraneoplastic autoimmune multiorgan syndrome) (Fig. 4). Single-cell apoptosis is a common feature in TAMA-associated colitis and GVHD-associated colitis. A loss of T-regulatory function, as reflected by the loss of expression of transcription factor FOXP3 and autoimmune

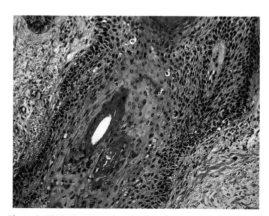

Fig. 4. TAMA. Prominent involvement of adnexal epithelium resembles GVHD. GVHD-like features and thymoma may also fall within the spectrum of the lichenoid variant of paraneoplastic pemphigus (paraneoplastic autoimmune multiorgan syndrome).[158] However, this patient had an exfoliative dermatitis without blisters, crusting, or mucocutaneous involvement (hematoxylin and eosin stain, original magnification ×200).

regular (AIRE) within intratumoral thymic T cells, might be indicative of a loss of tolerance to self-antigens in the pathogenesis of TAMA.[54,55]

Histiocytic Necrotizing Lymphadenitis

Most individuals who develop histiocytic necrotizing lymphadenitis (Kikuchi-Fujimoto disease, Kikuchi disease) are young women who present with fever, pancytopenia, and lymphadenopathy, and in whom no skin lesions arise. However, the clinical and histologic spectrum of cutaneous lesions can be dramatic and have been better characterized over the past several years.[56–58] The clinical course is generally benign and self-limited, but clinical correlation is required to exclude lupus erythematosus. Cases initially diagnosed as histiocytic necrotizing lymphadenitis have rarely evolved to systemic LE.[59] Skin lesions may be maculopapular/morbilliform, nodular, or vesiculobullous. The mechanism of blister formation may be secondary to interface dermatitis or marked papillary dermal edema, and is accompanied by the distinctive presence of leukocytoclastic nuclear debris (leukocyte nuclear dust) without vasculitis or neutrophils (**Fig. 5**). In both lymph node and skin, CD68-positive mononuclear cells (resembling plasmacytoid lymphocytes on H&E) were originally classified as plasmacytoid T cells or plasmacytoid monocytes. More recently, these lesional cells in the lymph node have been identified immunophenotypically as two populations of immature dendritic cells: plasmacytoid dendritic cells and myeloid dendritic cells.[60]

VASCULITIS AND VASCULOPATHY
Levamisole-Induced Vasculopathy

Levamisole-induced vasculopathy with ecchymosis and necrosis (LIVEN) has received a great deal of attention in the past couple of years after reports from multiple centers in North America attributing LIVEN to recreational use of cocaine intentionally contaminated with the veterinary antihelminthic agent, levamisole.[61–64] The clinical presentation consists of necrosis and retiform purpura most commonly affecting the ears, cheeks, nose, digits, trunk, and proximal extremities, with

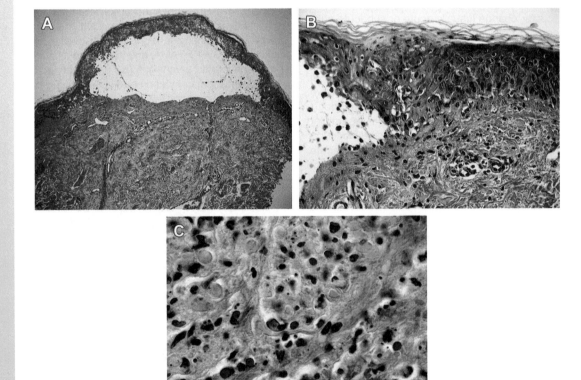

Fig. 5. Cutaneous involvement in histiocytic necrotizing lymphadenitis (Kikuchi disease). (*A, B*) Subepidermal vesiculation secondary to interface dermatitis. (*C*) The presence of karyorrhectic/leukocytoclastic nuclear fragments (nuclear dust) without vasculitis or neutrophils is distinctive (hematoxylin and eosin stain, original magnification: *A* ×20; *B* ×400; *C* ×600).

variable progression to ulceration and eventual remission. Patients have a history of recreational cocaine use (sniffed, snorted, or smoked) and present with associated neutropenia, positive antineutrophil cytoplasmic antibody (ANCA) serologies (both p-ANCA and c-ANCA), and hypocomplementemia. Antibodies against neutrophil granules (neutrophil elastase, myeloperoxidase, lactoferrin, cathepsin G, proteinase 3) are also present.[65] In particular, the presence of human neutrophil elastase antibodies has been proposed to be a sensitive and specific feature of LIVEN that distinguishes it from autoimmune vasculitis.[61,66] Agranulocytosis with associated myeloid hypoplasia in the bone marrow may be associated with potentially fatal secondary systemic bacterial or fungal infection. Histologically, small vessel thrombosis with or without leukocytoclastic vasculitis is characteristic (**Fig. 6**). In patients with vasculitis, direct immunofluorescence demonstrates vascular immune complex deposition. Extensive perivascular and interstitial neovascularization may be seen.[63] These clinical and histologic features are not specific for LIVEN, and therefore additional clinical and laboratory evaluation may be required to definitively assess for other causes of coagulopathy (eg, antiphospholipid antibody syndrome, cryoglobulinemia, warfarin-induced skin necrosis) or other causes of vasculitis. LIVEN

manifesting as purpura on the earlobes and cheeks has been documented in children receiving levamisole as adjuvant therapy for nephrotic syndrome.[67]

Macular Lymphocytic Arteritis and Lymphocytic Thrombophilic Arteritis

Macular lymphocytic arteritis (MLA)[68] and lymphocytic thrombophilic arteritis (LTA)[69,70] are designations that seem to reflect nearby points along the spectrum of a single rare but distinctive clinical-pathologic entity whose relationship, if any, to cutaneous polyarteritis or autoimmune connective tissue disorders remains uncertain.[71,72] Most patients to date have been young or middle-aged adult women, with macular, livedoid, or minimally indurated nonulcerated lesions usually on the lower extremities bilaterally. The clinical course is chronic and benign, and the clinical evaluation, by definition, falls short of a connective tissue disorder or coagulopathy, such as antiphospholipid antibody syndrome, although low-titer anticardiolipin antibodies are frequently documented in these individuals. The histologic common denominator is a lymphocytic arteritis centered at the dermal-subcutaneous junction associated with a thick fibrin ring (resembling a strawberry donut) partly occluding the lumen of the arteriole (endarteritis obliterans). A sparse to moderately dense

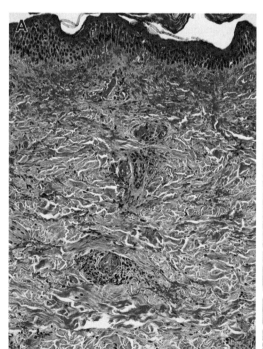
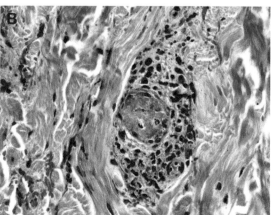

Fig. 6. Levamisole-induced vasculopathy. (*A, B*) Fibrin occluding small dermal vessels, with sparse associated neutrophils and nuclear "dust" (hematoxylin and eosin stain, original magnification: *A* ×40; *B* ×400). (*Courtesy of* Tammie Ferringer, MD, Danville, PA.)

lymphocytic infiltrate with nuclear dust is present, but neutrophils and eosinophils are minimal or absent. Elastin stains usually demonstrate an intact elastic lamina.

VESICULOBULLOUS DISORDERS
Grover Disease (Transient Acantholytic Dermatosis)

Histologic variants of Grover disease may resemble Darier disease (acantholytic dyskeratosis), pemphigus vulgaris (suprabasilar acantholysis), pemphigus foliaceus (intragranular acantholysis), Hailey-Hailey disease (full-thickness acantholysis), or spongiotic dermatitis. Grover disease may rarely coexist with herpes simplex virus (HSV); the viral cytopathic changes may be obscured, particularly by acantholytic dyskeratosis (**Fig. 7**). The demonstration of HSV-I immunohistochemical positivity in a case of Grover disease, and in rare cases of Darier disease, pemphigus vulgaris, and bullous pemphigoid, suggests the possibility of occult colonization by herpesvirus in some examples of these diseases.[73] Clinical superinfection analogous to eczema herpeticum may also occur in Grover disease.[74]

Papular Genitocrural Acantholysis

Papular genitocrural acantholysis (papular acantholytic dyskeratosis of the vulva) is included in the 2006 International Society for the Study of Vulvar Dermatoses (ISSVD) Classification for Vulvar Dermatoses for papular lesions confined to the genitocrural region that show the epidermal reaction pattern of acantholytic dyskeratosis.[75] Immunofluorescence studies are negative. This benign disorder may occur in adults[76,77] or

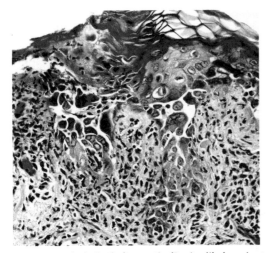

Fig. 7. Acantholytic dyskeratotic (Darier-like) variant of transient acantholytic dyskeratosis (Grover disease) with superimposed HSV infection (hematoxylin and eosin stain, original magnification ×400).

children,[78] and is believed to represent cases reported in the past as Darier disease (keratosis follicularis) localized to the vulva.

Paraneoplastic Pemphigus

Paraneoplastic pemphigus was the subject of a recent review in *Dermatologic Clinics*,[79] but selected aspects are also reviewed here. Since its original description by Anhalt and coworkers[80] in 1990, the spectrum of paraneoplastic pemphigus subsequently expanded to include lichenoid variants. The additional recognition of systemic involvement (often pulmonary) resulted in a broader classification under the heading of paraneoplastic autoimmune multiorgan syndrome proposed by Grando and coworkers.[81,82] This broadened disease spectrum encompassed under the heading of paraneoplastic pemphigus/paraneoplastic autoimmune multiorgan syndrome may explain the elusive nature of diagnosis. Classic cases of paraneoplastic pemphigus present with oral involvement, an associated internal malignancy, biopsies that show combined acantholytic and interface changes, perilesional direct immunofluorescence (DIF) showing concomitant intercellular (cell surface) and basement membrane zone (BMZ) deposition of IgG and C3, and confirmatory serum studies (indirect immunofluorescence, enzyme-linked immunosorbent assay [ELISA], immunoblotting, immunoprecipitation) for IgG antibodies directed against many or all of the recognized components of the antigen complex that contain the self-targets in paraneoplastic pemphigus: desmoplakin I (250-kd), bullous pemphigoid antigen 1 (230-kd), desmoplakin II-envoplakin (210-kd), periplakin (190-kd), and a 170-kd protein. The existence of several reports of nonclassical presentations of paraneoplastic pemphigus emphasizes the need for careful correlation between the clinical, H&E, DIF, and serum studies in the evaluation of patients with pemphigus. Nonclassical examples include cases with negative serum studies,[83,84] no malignancy,[85] either pure acantholytic or pure lichenoid histology, and negative or nonclassic DIF findings.[84,86–88]

GRANULOMATOUS DERMATITIS

Granulomatous dermatitis is traditionally subclassified into sarcoidal, tuberculoid, palisaded, interstitial, and foreign body types. During medical school, the first author reported a novel finding of "granuloma initiation factor" using a *Schistosoma mansoni*–murine model[89]; in retrospect, this was a very focused and relatively narrow concept of a diverse spectrum of diseases with granulomatous inflammation. The past decade saw an ever-broadening spectrum of granulomatous reactions that sometimes seems intent on teaching more by breaking the established rules. At the same time, the increasing use of immunosuppressive therapy has resulted in a resurgence of opportunistic infections, of which fungi, mycobacteria, and protozoa stereotypically induce a suppurative neutrophilic granulomatous host response.

Sarcoid

Cutaneous sarcoid is clinically protean but characterized histologically by sarcoidal granulomas composed of nodules of epithelioid histiocytes and sparse lymphocytes ("naked granulomas"). However, Ball and coworkers[90] showed a significantly broader spectrum of findings in clinically confirmed cases, including tuberculoid granulomas, interstitial granulomatous infiltrates, and associated lichenoid interface reactions. Perineural granulomas have been documented,[36] as has evolution from palisaded neutrophilic and granulomatous dermatitis (see next section).[91] Perigranulomatous fibroplasia has been reported to be a distinctive feature of subcutaneous sarcoid.[92]

Immunodeficiency Syndrome–Associated Granulomatous Dermatitis

Granulomatous dermatitis may occur in a variety of immunodeficiency syndromes, including ataxia telangiectasia, chronic granulomatous disease, severe combined immunodeficiency, common variable immunodeficiency, X-linked hypogammaglobulinemia, and familial hemophagocytic lymphohistiocytosis (**Fig. 8**).[93–95] The pattern may be sarcoidal, tuberculoid, necrotizing, or palisaded.

Metastatic Crohn Disease

Crohn disease only rarely involves the skin, but may develop at sites discontiguous from the gastrointestinal orifices, so-called metastatic Crohn disease. The legs, genitalia, and face are most commonly involved, and the clinical presentation is varied, ranging from papules (including perifollicular), nodules, and lichenoid plaques. Histologically, the granulomas are sarcoidal, often with prominent eosinophils. More variable features include ulceration, a lichenoid interface component, marked dermal edema, and subcutaneous involvement.[96]

Palisaded Neutrophilic and Granulomatous Dermatitis and Interstitial Granulomatous Dermatitis

Whether palisaded neutrophilic and granulomatous dermatitis (PNGD) and interstitial granulomatous dermatitis (IGD; IGD with cutaneous cords

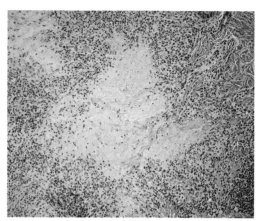

Fig. 8. Immunodeficiency-associated granulomatous dermatitis in familial hemophagocytic lymphohistiocytosis (FHL). FHL may be associated with multiple mutations; in this case, a *MUNC13-4* mutation was identified in this infant boy who presented with a papular eruption on the extremities (hematoxylin and eosin stain, original magnification ×200). (*Courtesy of* Michael J. Murphy, MD, Farmington, CT.)

and arthritis, Ackerman's disease) reflect a single disease spectrum[97,98] versus two unrelated disorders with overlapping histopathologic findings is still uncertain.[99] The histologic common denominator is a palisaded and interstitial granulomatous dermatitis with collagen degeneration (necrobiosis). The additional presence of neutrophils and leukocytoclastic vasculitis are typical of PNGD, not IGD. In PNGD, the clinical presentation is that of papules on the extremities and associated connective tissue disease, most commonly rheumatoid arthritis. IGD may also be associated with connective tissue disease, but classically presents on the trunk or proximal extremities, most distinctively as cutaneous cord-like or rope-like plaques. Moreover, some cases of IGD seem to represent drug reactions,[100] including lymphomatoid variants.[101] In contrast to the interstitial variant of granuloma annulare (IGA), IGD typically exhibits diffuse involvement of the upper dermis, whereas IGA exhibits patchy dermal involvement that includes the deep dermis. Interstitial granulomatous drug reactions may additionally exhibit superimposed interface changes (**Fig. 9**).

Granulomatous Pigmented Purpura

The classic variants of pigmented purpuric dermatosis include progressive pigmented purpura (Schamberg disease), lichenoid purpura (Gougerot-Blum syndrome), lichen aureus, itching or eczematid-like purpura (Doucas and Kapetanakis), and the annular telangiectatic Majocchi variant. Kaplan and coworkers[102] described the

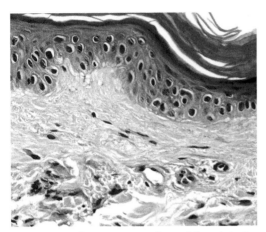

Fig. 9. IGD. The presence of overlying interface changes suggests the possibility of an interstitial granulomatous drug reaction. Diffuse involvement of the upper dermis is typical of IGD, whereas the interstitial/incomplete histologic variant of granuloma annulare typically exhibits patchy involvement of the papillary and reticular dermis (hematoxylin and eosin stain, original magnification ×400).

most recently published case of granulomatous pigmented purpuric dermatosis, a rare variant that has mostly been reported in Asians and exhibits a superficial palisaded or noncaseating granulomatous infiltrate in concert with extravasated erythrocytes and siderophages. An associated lichenoid component may be present. Involvement of the lower extremities (particularly the legs and dorsal feet) is typical, although involvement of the upper extremities and trunk has rarely been reported. Many cases are associated with hyperlipidemia.[102–105]

NEUTROPHILIC DERMATITIS
Neutrophilic Dermatosis of the Dorsal Hands

Acute febrile neutrophilic dermatosis, also known as Sweet syndrome (SS) was first described in 1964 by Robert Sweet[106] as a reactive skin eruption characterized by abrupt onset of painful, erythematous, pseudovesicular plaques, and nodules occurring on the face, neck, and limbs, accompanied by fever and peripheral blood leukocytosis. The condition may be idiopathic, although it often follows a viral infection, especially of the upper respiratory tract, and has been associated with systemic diseases of an inflammatory or neoplastic nature, both visceral and hematologic malignancies, medications (mostly granulocyte colony-stimulating factor), and pregnancy. In 1986, Su and Liu[107] established clinical criteria they deemed necessary to establish a diagnosis of classical SS (**Table 1**). These criteria remain relevant today, although various interpretations and modifications have been reported.[108] Histopathologically, SS is categorized as a neutrophilic dermatosis and shares overlapping features with other entities in this category, including pyoderma gangrenosum (PG), erythema elevatum diutinum, and subcorneal pustular dermatosis (Sneddon-Wilkinson disease). The usual histopathologic findings in SS consist of prominent papillary dermal edema; a dense dermal inflammatory infiltrate composed primarily of mature neutrophils with leukocytoclasis, admixed eosinophils, lymphocytes, and histiocytes[109]; and the absence of a primary vasculitis. Features of leukocytoclastic vasculitis have been reported in typical lesions of SS,[110] although the vasculitis is believed to occur

Table 1
Diagnostic criteria for Sweet syndrome[a] **include the presence of both major and two minor clinical findings**

Major Criteria	Minor Criteria
Abrupt onset of tender or painful erythematous plaques or nodules, occasionally with vesicles, pustules, or bullae	Preceding respiratory or gastrointestinal tract infection, associated inflammatory disease, hemoproliferative disorder, solid malignant tumor, pregnancy, or vaccination
Predominantly neutrophilic infiltration in the dermis without leukocytoclastic vasculitis	Periods of general malaise and pyrexia (body temperature >38°C) Three of four of the following must be fulfilled: 1. Laboratory values at onset exhibiting an erythrocyte sedimentation rate >20 mm 2. Positive C-reactive protein 3. Neutrophils >70% in peripheral blood smear 4. Leukocytosis (count >8000/μL) Excellent response to treatment with systemic corticosteroids or potassium iodide

[a] Proposed by Su and Liu[107] and revised by von den Driesch.[108]

secondary to the significant inflammation surrounding the vessels and has been interpreted as an epiphenomenon.[111]

Since the initial report by Sweet, additional clinical variants of SS including bullous and subcutaneous, have been recognized.[112] Neutrophilic dermatosis of the dorsal hands (NDDH) is a recently described entity that is considered a localized variant of SS. The presentation of violaceous papulonodules on the radial aspect of the dorsal hands was originally reported in 1995 by Strutton and colleagues[113] as sharing morphologic and clinical features with Sweet syndrome, but because of the severe leukocytoclastic vasculitis changes on histology, the term *pustular vasculitis of the hands* was preferred. Galaria and colleagues[114] presented three similar cases in 2000 and, because of the absence of leukocytoclastic vasculitis, *neutrophilic dermatosis of the dorsal hands* was the preferred term to represent this localized variant of SS.

Subsequent cases have been reported, with commentary on the similarity between NDDH and SS.[115–117] In 2006, Walling and colleagues[118] took the commentary a step further when they reported an additional nine cases in a review of the existing literature. Their assimilation of reported cases highlighted a female preponderance, and the presence of associated systemic disease, laboratory abnormalities, and a response to systemic corticosteroid therapy similar to SS. The presence or absence of vasculitis within the specimens did not deter from the diagnosis because, although rare, vasculitic changes have been reported in classic SS.[110,119] Favoring the designation of NDDH, Walling and colleagues[118,120] proposed that when cases of atypical PG occur on the upper extremity, they are clinically and histopathologically indistinguishable from NDDH. Drawing on conclusions from other reports detailing the similarities between atypical PG and bullous SS, they further opined that pustular vasculitis of the hands, bullous SS, and atypical PG are best categorized as variations of a single disease entity, most appropriately designated as NDDH. A recent report regarding the discovery of the same HLA-B54 haplotype[121] in both SS and NDDH further supports regarding these entities as overlapping variants along the spectrum of neutrophilic dermatoses, and perhaps may provide additional diagnostic tools to aid in further defining these entities in the future.

Histiocytoid SS

The recent report by Requena and colleagues[122] expanded the histopathologic spectrum of SS. In this report, they detailed 41 patients with SS whose biopsy specimens showed a predominance of histiocytoid mononuclear cells in the infiltrate, in contrast to mature polymorphonuclear cells in classical SS, which they designated as histiocytoid SS (HSS). Although these cells may be misinterpreted as histiocytes, immunohistochemical studies showed that they were consistent with immature neutrophils. Initially, the intense myeloperoxidase activity coupled with the morphology of the cells suggested myeloid lineage and raised suspicion that these cells could represent leukemia cutis. Therefore, fluorescent in situ hybridization studies were performed ruling out the presence of *bcr/abl* gene fusion (also known as the Philadelphia chromosome), which, if present, would have defined the lesions as leukemia cutis. Requena and colleagues[122] opined that these lesions likely result from the release of immature myeloid cells by the bone marrow in early acute stages of the disease, and that mature neutrophils replace the immature myeloid cells in later stages of evolution.

Despite the novel histopathologic findings, the clinical presentation of erythematous plaques and nodules, accompanied by leukocytosis with neutrophilia, elevated sedimentation rate, and a prompt response to oral steroids supported that these findings represent a histologic variant of SS.

Subsequent reports of HSS have detailed cases associated with subacute cutaneous lupus,[123] medications including trimethoprim-sulfamethoxazole and bortezomib,[124,125] and inflammatory bowel disease.[126]

The diagnosis of HSS rests on the histopathologic findings, and exclusion of entities that share either morphologic or immunohistochemical features, including interstitial granuloma annulare; interstitial granulomatous dermatitis (see previous section); methotrexate-induced rheumatoid papules; in the appropriate clinical context, palisaded neutrophilic and granulomatous dermatitis[97]; and malignancy, specifically leukemia cutis and subcutaneous T-cell lymphoma.[127,128] However, if clinical-pathologic correlation renders HSS the correct diagnosis, the implications for the associated disorders, management, and follow-up are the same as those for classical SS.[129]

Cryopyrin-Associated Periodic Syndromes

When neutrophilic infiltrates are encountered in neonates, the differential diagnosis includes the rare monogenic hereditary periodic fever syndromes, including cryopyrin (NLRP3/NALP3)-associated periodic syndromes (CAPS), which include familial cold autoinflammatory syndrome, Muckle-Wells syndrome, and neonatal-onset multisystem inflammatory disease (NOMID)/chronic infantile neurologic, cutaneous, and arthritis (CINCA) syndrome.[130] Infants with CAPS may present with a congenital urticarial rash that is characterized by sparse dermal neutrophils, and with lymphocytes and eosinophils (ie, nonspecific features compatible with an urticarial process). However, perieccrine neutrophils were recently documented.[131] Nuclear dust and necrobiotic collagen[132] may be present; edema is usually absent. Diagnosis can be confirmed through identification of a mutation of the cold-induced autoinflammatory syndrome-1 gene (CIAS-1), and the condition responds to interleukin-1 receptor antagonist therapy.[131] In contrast, another hereditary periodic fever syndrome, tumor necrosis factor receptor–associated periodic syndrome (TRAPS, OMIM 142680), is characterized by a nonspecific dermal perivascular and interstitial lymphocytic and monocytic infiltrate (without neutrophils).[133,134]

EOSINOPHILIC DERMATITIS
Flame Figures

Flames figures result from the deposition of eosinophil granules on dermal collagen fibers, imparting a flame-like profile. Although classically associated with eosinophilic cellulitis (Wells syndrome), the differential diagnosis for flame figures includes a wide variety of disorders that may exhibit prominent dermal eosinophils, including arthropod bite reaction; scabies and other parasitic infestations or infections; drug reactions; eosinophilic folliculitis[135]; eosinophilic ulcer of the oral mucosa; leukocytoclastic vasculitis,[136] including urticarial vasculitis[137]; Churg Strauss syndrome; cutaneous mastocytosis[138]; interstitial granulomatous dermatitis; dermatitis herpetiformis[139]; bullous pemphigoid; dermatitis cruris pustulosa et atrophicans[140]; and eosinophilic annular erythema (see later discussion).[141] Although most of these disorders seem to exhibit flame figures only occasionally, a review of case reports of bullous lesions containing flame figures (often classified as bullous Wells syndrome) suggests an association with Churg-Strauss syndrome.[142–144]

Dermal Hypersensitivity Reactions

Dermal hypersensitivity reaction (DHR) is not a single clinical diagnosis per se, but rather is a histologic diagnosis rendered in pathology reports for findings that are far more widely recognized by practicing dermatologists and dermatopathologists compared with its relatively scant documentation in the medical literature. Weedon[145] characterized DHR as "… the most controversial concept in dermatopathology, because of its inconsistent usage, its variable clinicopathologic

correlations, its enigmatic nature, and the emotive climate that accompanies the use of the term." Thus, terminology and definitions of DHR may vary; equivalent terms include urticarial hypersensitivity reaction,[146] cutaneous hypersensitivity reaction, and cutaneous hypersensitivity response. Published experience to date suggests that DHR is a relatively commonly encountered pattern characterized by sparse to moderately dense superficial and mid/deep perivascular lymphocytes with scattered eosinophils, and minimal if any epidermal alteration (usually mild spongiosis and/or excoriation).[47,147] Thus, compared with other forms of eosinophilic dermatitis, the inflammatory infiltrate in DHR is generally sparse and predominantly lymphocytic, not eosinophilic. Flame figures are not a typical feature. Sparse neutrophils are a variable finding. When encountered in initial sections, a low threshold for obtaining deeper sections is advised, because focal diagnostic features such as folliculitis may be demonstrated.

Clinically, many patients with DHR present with a generalized papular pruritic eruption centered on the trunk and proximal extremities, and many prove to have drug reactions or arthropod bite reactions. Rare examples have been associated with systemic malignancy, and idiopathic cases may receive one of several designations, including itchy red bump disease,[148] red itchy bump syndrome,[149] papular dermatitis,[150] subacute prurigo, prurigo simplex subacuta,[151] prurigo simplex,[152] or even DHR itself (as one example of histopathologic features defining a clinical entity for lack of a clear-cut diagnosis). Other patients with DHR present with patches or plaques that may be classified as urticarial dermatitis.[147] Many of these patients seem to have an urticarial variant of spongiotic dermatitis (eg, nummular dermatitis) (Maxwell A. Fung, MD, personal observation, 2012). Ultimately, a wide range of disorders may be considered in the differential diagnosis of the DHR reaction pattern.[153]

Treatment of patients with idiopathic DHR is challenging, because topical steroids and antihistamines generally fail to induce remission. Reports of efficacy have been attributed to phototherapy,[154] low-dose prednisone,[155] and mycophenolate mofetil.[156]

Eosinophilic Annular Erythema

Eosinophilic annular erythema is a rare disorder characterized by annular or figurate urticarial plaques and dermal eosinophilic infiltrates that arise on the trunk and extremities of children or adults. Vacuolar interface changes and increased interstitial mucin deposition have been described.[157] Flame figures were not a feature in the original cases but have recently been documented, suggesting this idiopathic disorder may fall within the spectrum of Wells syndrome (eosinophilic cellulitis).[141,157]

SUMMARY

The complex and fascinating spectrum of inflammatory skin disease, and the comprehension of it, is ever-expanding and evolving. The continued recognition of novel histologic reaction patterns and new variants of established disorders should be assumed. Although ancillary biomarker testing promises to enhance the ability to accurately diagnose and manage patients, the willingness and ability of a dermatopathologist to engage in clinical-pathologic correlation will remain critical to optimizing the accuracy of histologic interpretation.

REFERENCES

1. Smoller BR. Update on dermatopathology. In: Thiers BH, editor. Dermatologic clinics; No. 17. Philadelphia: Saunders; 1999.
2. Rajaratnam R, Smith AG, Biswas A, et al. The value of skin biopsy in inflammatory dermatoses. Am J Dermatopathol 2009;31(4):350–3.
3. Cerroni L, Argenyi Z, Cerio R, et al. Influence of evaluation of clinical pictures on the histopathologic diagnosis of inflammatory skin disorders. J Am Acad Dermatol 2010;63(4):647–52.
4. Karai LJ, Bergfeld WF. Recent advances in T-cell regulation relevant to inflammatory dermatopathology. J Cutan Pathol 2009;36(7):721–8.
5. Onoufriadis A, Simpson MA, Pink AE, et al. Mutations in IL36RN/IL1F5 are associated with the severe episodic inflammatory skin disease known as generalized pustular psoriasis. Am J Hum Genet 2011;89(3):432–7.
6. Callen JP, Bernardi DM, Clark RA, et al. Adult-onset recalcitrant eczema: a marker of noncutaneous lymphoma or leukemia. J Am Acad Dermatol 2000;43(2 Pt 1):207–10.
7. Reddy K, Bhawan J. Histologic mimickers of mycosis fungoides: a review. J Cutan Pathol 2007;34(7):519–25.
8. Martinez-Moran C, Sanz-Munoz C, Morales-Callaghan AM, et al. Lymphomatoid contact dermatitis. Contact Derm 2009;60(1):53–5.
9. Houck HE, Wirth FA, Kauffman CL. Lymphomatoid contact dermatitis caused by nickel. Am J Contact Dermat 1997;8(3):175–6.
10. Mendese G, Beckford A, Demierre MF. Lymphomatoid contact dermatitis to baby wipes. Arch Dermatol 2010;146(8):934–5.
11. Ezzedine K, Rafii N, Heenen M. Lymphomatoid contact dermatitis to an exotic wood: a very harmful toilet seat. Contact Derm 2007;57(2):128–30.
12. Fung MA. 'Epidermotropism' vs. 'exocytosis' of lymphocytes 101: definition of terms. J Cutan Pathol 2010;37(5):525–9.
13. Murphy MJ. Mycosis fungoides and related lesions. In: Murphy MJ, editor. Molecular diagnostics in dermatology and dermatopathology. New York: Humana Press Springer; 2011. p. 211.
14. Thurber SE, Zhang B, Kim YH, et al. T-cell clonality analysis in biopsy specimens from two different skin sites shows high specificity in the diagnosis of patients with suggested mycosis fungoides. J Am Acad Dermatol 2007;57(5):782–90.
15. Dabiri S, Morales A, Ma L, et al. The frequency of dual TCR-PCR clonality in granulomatous disorders. J Cutan Pathol 2011;38(9):704–9.
16. Boer A, Ackerman A. Prurigo pigmentosa (Nagashima's disease): textbook and atlas of a distinctive inflammatory disease of the skin. New York: Ardor Scribendi; 2004.
17. Erbagci Z. Prurigo pigmentosa in association with Helicobacter pylori infection in a Caucasian Turkish woman. Acta Derm Venereol 2002;82(4):302–3.
18. Missall TA, Pruden S, Nelson C, et al. Identification of Helicobacter pylori in Skin Biopsy of Prurigo Pigmentosa. Am J Dermatopathol 2012;34(4):446–8.
19. Uwaifo GI, Muzzammil A, Shoukri K, et al. Diabetes but not psoriasis. Lancet 1999;354(9177):480.
20. Abdallah MA, Ghozzi MY, Monib HA, et al. Necrolytic acral erythema: a cutaneous sign of hepatitis C virus infection. J Am Acad Dermatol 2005; 53(2):247–51.
21. El-Darouti MA, Mashaly HM, El-Nabarawy E, et al. Leukocytoclastic vasculitis and necrolytic acral erythema in patients with hepatitis C infection: do viral load and viral genotype play a role? J Am Acad Dermatol 2010;63(2):259–65.
22. Nofal AA, Nofal E, Attwa E, et al. Necrolytic acral erythema: a variant of necrolytic migratory erythema or a distinct entity? Int J Dermatol 2005;44(11):916–21.
23. Woldow A, Manton JS, Campanelli C, et al. The necrolytic erythemas: a continuous spectrum? Cutis 2011;88(4):185–8.
24. Maverakis E, Fung MA, Lynch PJ, et al. Acrodermatitis enteropathica and an overview of zinc metabolism. J Am Acad Dermatol 2007;56(1): 116–24.
25. Abdallah MA, Hull C, Horn TD. Necrolytic acral erythema: a patient from the United States successfully treated with oral zinc. Arch Dermatol 2005;141(1):85–7.
26. Kapoor R, Johnson RA. Necrolytic acral erythema. N Engl J Med 2011;364(15):1479–80.
27. Kao GF, Sulica VI. Focal acantholytic dyskeratosis occurring in pityriasis rubra pilaris. Am J Dermatopathol 1989;11(2):172–6.
28. Magro CM, Crowson AN. The clinical and histomorphological features of pityriasis rubra pilaris. A

comparative analysis with psoriasis. J Cutan Pathol 1997;24(7):416–24.

29. Ko CJ, Milstone LM, Choi J, et al. Pityriasis rubra pilaris: the clinical context of acantholysis and other histologic features. Int J Dermatol 2011;50(12):1480–5.

30. Sebastian A, Koff AB, Goldberg LJ. PRP with subcorneal acantholysis: case report and review. J Cutan Pathol 2010;37(1):99–101.

31. Hojyo-Tomoka MT, Vega-Memije ME, Cortes-Franco R, et al. Diagnosis and treatment of actinic prurigo. Dermatol Ther 2003;16(1):40–4.

32. Lane PR, Murphy F, Hogan DJ, et al. Histopathology of actinic prurigo. Am J Dermatopathol 1993;15(4): 326–31.

33. LeBoit PE. Interface dermatitis. How specific are its histopathologic features? Arch Dermatol 1993; 129(10):1324–8.

34. Maize JC Jr, Resneck JS Jr, Shapiro PE, et al. Ducking stray "magic bullets": a Melan-A alert. Am J Dermatopathol 2003;25(2):162–5.

35. Beltraminelli H, Shabrawi-Caelen LE, Kerl H, et al. Melan-a-positive "pseudomelanocytic nests": a pitfall in the histopathologic and immunohistochemical diagnosis of pigmented lesions on sun-damaged skin. Am J Dermatopathol 2009;31(3):305–8.

36. Abbas O, Bhawan J. Cutaneous perineural inflammation: a review. J Cutan Pathol 2010;37(12):1200–11.

37. Pincus LB, LeBoit PE, Goddard DS, et al. Marked papillary dermal edema–an unreliable discriminator between polymorphous light eruption and lupus erythematosus or dermatomyositis. J Cutan Pathol 2010;37(4):416–25.

38. Weaver J, Bergfeld WF. Quantitative analysis of eosinophils in acute graft-versus-host disease compared with drug hypersensitivity reactions. Am J Dermatopathol 2010;32(1):31–4.

39. Sharon VR, Konia TH, Barr KL, et al. Assessment of the 'no eosinophils' rule: are eosinophils truly absent in pityriasis lichenoides, connective tissue disease, and graft-vs.-host disease? J Cutan Pathol 2012; 39(4):413–8.

40. Gleason BC, Zembowicz A, Granter SR. Non-bullous neutrophilic dermatosis: an uncommon dermatologic manifestation in patients with lupus erythematosus. J Cutan Pathol 2006;33(11):721–5.

41. Brinster NK, Nunley J, Pariser R, et al. Nonbullous neutrophilic lupus erythematosus: a newly recognized variant of cutaneous lupus erythematosus. J Am Acad Dermatol 2012;66(1):92–7.

42. Barr KL, Konia TH, Fung MA. Lupus erythematosus-like imiquimod reaction: a diagnostic pitfall. J Cutan Pathol 2011;38(4):346–50.

43. Chan MP, Zimarowski MJ. Lupus erythematosus-like reaction in imiquimod-treated skin: a report of 2 cases. Am J Dermatopathol 2011;33(5):523–7.

44. Wenzel J, Tuting T. An IFN-associated cytotoxic cellular immune response against viral, self-, or tumor antigens is a common pathogenetic feature in "interface dermatitis". J Invest Dermatol 2008; 128(10):2392–402.

45. Burnett TJ, English JC 3rd, Ferris LK. Development of subacute cutaneous lupus erythematosus associated with the use of imiquimod to treat actinic keratoses. J Drugs Dermatol 2010;9(8):1022–4.

46. Gul U, Gonul M, Cakmak SK, et al. A case of generalized discoid lupus erythematosus: successful treatment with imiquimod cream 5%. Adv Ther 2006;23(5):787–92.

47. Fung MA. The clinical and histopathologic spectrum of "dermal hypersensitivity reactions," a nonspecific histologic diagnosis that is not very useful in clinical practice, and the concept of a "dermal hypersensitivity reaction pattern". J Am Acad Dermatol 2002;47(6):898–907.

48. Rottenberg S, von Tscharner C, Roosje PJ. Thymoma-associated exfoliative dermatitis in cats. Vet Pathol 2004;41(4):429–33.

49. Florizoone K. Thymoma-associated exfoliative dermatitis in a rabbit. Vet Dermatol 2005;16(4):281–4.

50. Tepper LC, Spiegel IB, Davis GJ. Diagnosis of erythema multiforme associated with thymoma in a dog and treated with thymectomy. J Am Anim Hosp Assoc 2011;47(2):e19–25.

51. Wadhera A, Maverakis E, Mitsiades N, et al. Thymoma-associated multiorgan autoimmunity: a graft-versus-host-like disease. J Am Acad Dermatol 2007;57(4):683–9.

52. Holder J, North J, Bourke J, et al. Thymoma-associated cutaneous graft-versus-host-like reaction. Clin Exp Dermatol 1997;22(6):287–90.

53. Sleijfer S, Kaptein A, Versteegh MI, et al. Full-blown graft-versus-host disease presenting with skin manifestations, jaundice and diarrhoea: an unusual paraneoplastic phenomenon of a thymoma. Eur J Gastroenterol Hepatol 2003;15(5):565–9.

54. Offerhaus GJ, Schipper ME, Lazenby AJ, et al. Graft-versus-host-like disease complicating thymoma: lack of AIRE expression as a cause of non-hereditary autoimmunity? Immunol Lett 2007; 114(1):31–7.

55. Maverakis E, Goodarzi H, Wehrli LN, et al. The etiology of paraneoplastic autoimmunity. Clin Rev Allergy Immunol 2012;42(2):135–44.

56. Spies J, Foucar K, Thompson CT, et al. The histopathology of cutaneous lesions of Kikuchi's disease (necrotizing lymphadenitis): a report of five cases. Am J Surg Pathol 1999;23(9):1040–7.

57. Atwater AR, Longley BJ, Aughenbaugh WD. Kikuchi's disease: case report and systematic review of cutaneous and histopathologic presentations. J Am Acad Dermatol 2008;59(1):130–6.

58. Kim JH, Kim YB, In SI, et al. The cutaneous lesions of Kikuchi's disease: a comprehensive analysis of 16 cases based on the clinicopathologic,

immunohistochemical, and immunofluorescence studies with an emphasis on the differential diagnosis. Hum Pathol 2010;41(9):1245–54.

59. Paradela S, Lorenzo J, Martinez-Gomez W, et al. Interface dermatitis in skin lesions of Kikuchi-Fujimoto's disease: a histopathological marker of evolution into systemic lupus erythematosus? Lupus 2008;17(12):1127–35.

60. Pilichowska ME, Pinkus JL, Pinkus GS. Histiocytic necrotizing lymphadenitis (Kikuchi-Fujimoto disease): lesional cells exhibit an immature dendritic cell phenotype. Am J Clin Pathol 2009;131(2):174–82.

61. Walsh NM, Green PJ, Burlingame RW, et al. Cocaine-related retiform purpura: evidence to incriminate the adulterant, levamisole. J Cutan Pathol 2010;37(12):1212–9.

62. Waller JM, Feramisco JD, Alberta-Wszolek L, et al. Cocaine-associated retiform purpura and neutropenia: is levamisole the culprit? J Am Acad Dermatol 2010;63(3):530–5.

63. Jacob RS, Silva CY, Powers JG, et al. Levamisole-Induced Vasculopathy: a Report of 2 Cases and a Novel Histopathologic Finding. Am J Dermatopathol 2012;34(2):208–13.

64. Chung C, Tumeh PC, Birnbaum R, et al. Characteristic purpura of the ears, vasculitis, and neutropenia–a potential public health epidemic associated with levamisole-adulterated cocaine. J Am Acad Dermatol 2011;65(4):722–5.

65. Graf J, Lynch K, Yeh CL, et al. Purpura, cutaneous necrosis, and antineutrophil cytoplasmic antibodies associated with levamisole-adulterated cocaine. Arthritis Rheum 2011;63(12):3998–4001.

66. Wiesner O, Russell KA, Lee AS, et al. Antineutrophil cytoplasmic antibodies reacting with human neutrophil elastase as a diagnostic marker for cocaine-induced midline destructive lesions but not autoimmune vasculitis. Arthritis Rheum 2004;50(9):2954–65.

67. Rongioletti F, Ghio L, Ginevri F, et al. Purpura of the ears: a distinctive vasculopathy with circulating autoantibodies complicating long-term treatment with levamisole in children. Br J Dermatol 1999;140(5):948–51.

68. Saleh Z, Mutasim DF. Macular lymphocytic arteritis: a unique benign cutaneous arteritis, mediated by lymphocytes and appearing as macules. J Cutan Pathol 2009;36(12):1269–74.

69. Lee JS, Kossard S, McGrath MA. Lymphocytic thrombophilic arteritis: a newly described medium-sized vessel arteritis of the skin. Arch Dermatol 2008;144(9):1175–82.

70. Kossard S, Lee JS, McGrath MA. Macular lymphocytic arteritis. J Cutan Pathol 2010;37(10):1114–5.

71. Al-Daraji W, Gregory AN, Carlson JA. "Macular arteritis": a latent form of cutaneous polyarteritis nodosa? Am J Dermatopathol 2008;30(2):145–9.

72. Munehiro A, Yoneda K, Koura A, et al. Macular lymphocytic arteritis in a patient with rheumatoid arthritis. Eur J Dermatol 2012;22(3):427–8.

73. Nikkels AF, Delvenne P, Herfs M, et al. Occult herpes simplex virus colonization of bullous dermatitides. Am J Clin Dermatol 2008;9(3):163–8.

74. Kosann MK, Fogelman JP, Stern RL. Kaposi's varicelliform eruption in a patient with Grover's disease. J Am Acad Dermatol 2003;49(5):914–5.

75. Lynch PJ, Moyal-Barracco M, Bogliatto F, et al. 2006 ISSVD classification of vulvar dermatoses: pathologic subsets and their clinical correlates. J Reprod Med 2007;52(1):3–9.

76. Roh MR, Choi YJ, Lee KG. Papular acantholytic dyskeratosis of the vulva. J Dermatol 2009;36(7):427–9.

77. Chorzelski TP, Kudejko J, Jablonska S. Is papular acantholytic dyskeratosis of the vulva a new entity? Am J Dermatopathol 1984;6(6):557–60.

78. Saenz AM, Cirocco A, Avendano M, et al. Papular acantholytic dyskeratosis of the vulva. Pediatr Dermatol 2005;22(3):237–9.

79. Frew JW, Murrell DF. Paraneoplastic pemphigus (paraneoplastic autoimmune multiorgan syndrome): clinical presentations and pathogenesis. Dermatol Clin 2011;29(3):419–25.

80. Anhalt GJ, Kim SC, Stanley JR, et al. Paraneoplastic pemphigus. An autoimmune mucocutaneous disease associated with neoplasia. N Engl J Med 1990;323(25):1729–35.

81. Nguyen VT, Ndoye A, Bassler KD, et al. Classification, clinical manifestations, and immunopathological mechanisms of the epithelial variant of paraneoplastic autoimmune multiorgan syndrome: a reappraisal of paraneoplastic pemphigus. Arch Dermatol 2001;137(2):193–206.

82. Czernik A, Camilleri M, Pittelkow MR, et al. Paraneoplastic autoimmune multiorgan syndrome: 20 years after. Int J Dermatol 2011;50(8):905–14.

83. Bouloc A, Joly P, Saint-Leger E, et al. Paraneoplastic pemphigus with circulating antibodies directed exclusively against the pemphigus vulgaris antigen desmoglein 3. J Am Acad Dermatol 2000;43(4):714–7.

84. Cummins DL, Mimouni D, Tzu J, et al. Lichenoid paraneoplastic pemphigus in the absence of detectable antibodies. J Am Acad Dermatol 2007;56(1):153–9.

85. Park GT, Lee JH, Yun SJ, et al. Paraneoplastic pemphigus without an underlying neoplasm. Br J Dermatol 2007;156(3):563–6.

86. Borradori L, Lombardi T, Samson J, et al. Anti-CD20 monoclonal antibody (rituximab) for refractory erosive stomatitis secondary to CD20(+) follicular lymphoma-associated paraneoplastic pemphigus. Arch Dermatol 2001;137(3):269–72.

87. Marzano AV, Grammatica A, Cozzani E, et al. Paraneoplastic pemphigus. A report of two cases associated with chronic B-cell lymphocytic leukaemia. Br J Dermatol 2001;145(1):127–31.

88. Barnadas MA, Curell R, Alomar A, et al. Paraneoplastic pemphigus with negative direct immunofluorescence in epidermis or mucosa but positive findings in adnexal structures. J Cutan Pathol 2009;36(1):34–8.

89. Fung MA, Sato N, Tida T, et al. Isolation and characterization of granuloma initiation factor. Am J Pathol 1992;141(6):1445–51.

90. Ball NJ, Kho GT, Martinka M. The histologic spectrum of cutaneous sarcoidosis: a study of twenty-eight cases. J Cutan Pathol 2004;31(2):160–8.

91. Gordon EA, Schmidt AN, Boyd AS. Palisaded neutrophilic and granulomatous dermatitis: a presenting sign of sarcoidosis? J Am Acad Dermatol 2011;65(3):664–5.

92. Resnik KS. The findings do not conform precisely: fibrosing sarcoidal expressions of panniculitis as example. Am J Dermatopathol 2004;26(2):156–61.

93. Siegfried EC, Prose NS, Friedman NJ, et al. Cutaneous granulomas in children with combined immunodeficiency. J Am Acad Dermatol 1991; 25(5 Pt 1):761–6.

94. Murakawa GJ, McCalmot T, Frieden IJ. Chronic plaques in a patient with ataxia telangiectasia. Cutaneous granulomatous lesions in a patient with AT. Arch Dermatol 1998;134(9):1145–8.

95. Murphy MJ. Necrotizing palisaded granulomatous dermatitis as a manifestation of familial hemophagocytic lymphohistiocytosis. J Cutan Pathol 2010; 37(8):907–10.

96. Emanuel PO, Phelps RG. Metastatic Crohn's disease: a histopathologic study of 12 cases. J Cutan Pathol 2008;35(5):457–61.

97. Chu P, Connolly MK, LeBoit PE. The histopathologic spectrum of palisaded neutrophilic and granulomatous dermatitis in patients with collagen vascular disease. Arch Dermatol 1994;130(10): 1278–83.

98. Sangueza OP, Caudell MD, Mengesha YM, et al. Palisaded neutrophilic granulomatous dermatitis in rheumatoid arthritis. J Am Acad Dermatol 2002;47(2):251–7.

99. Peroni A, Colato C, Schena D, et al. Interstitial granulomatous dermatitis: a distinct entity with characteristic histological and clinical pattern. Br J Dermatol 2012;166(4):775–83.

100. Magro CM, Crowson AN, Schapiro BL. The interstitial granulomatous drug reaction: a distinctive clinical and pathological entity. J Cutan Pathol 1998; 25(2):72–8.

101. Magro CM, Cruz-Inigo AE, Votava H, et al. Drug-associated reversible granulomatous T cell dyscrasia: a distinct subset of the interstitial granulomatous drug reaction. J Cutan Pathol 2010;37(Suppl 1):96–111.

102. Kaplan J, Burgin S, Sepehr A. Granulomatous pigmented purpura: report of a case and review of the literature. J Cutan Pathol 2011;38(12):984–9.

103. Wong WR, Kuo TT, Chen MJ, et al. Granulomatous variant of chronic pigmented purpuric dermatosis: report of two cases. Br J Dermatol 2001;145(1): 162–4.

104. Lin WL, Kuo TT, Shih PY, et al. Granulomatous variant of chronic pigmented purpuric dermatoses: report of four new cases and an association with hyperlipidaemia. Clin Exp Dermatol 2007;32(5): 513–5.

105. Lee SH, Kwon JE, Lee KG, et al. Granulomatous variant of chronic pigmented purpuric dermatosis associated with hyperlipidaemia. J Eur Acad Dermatol Venereol 2010;24(10):1243–5.

106. Sweet RD. An acute febrile neutrophilic dermatosis. Br J Dermatol 1964;76:349–56.

107. Su W, Liu H. Diagnostic criteria for Sweet syndrome. Cutis 1996;37:167–74.

108. von den Driesch P. Sweet's syndrome (acute febrile neutrophilic dermatosis). J Am Acad Dermatol 1994;31(4):535–56 [quiz: 557–60].

109. Apalla Z, Kanatli L, Sotiriou E, et al. Histiocytoid Sweet syndrome. Clin Exp Dermatol 2011;36(5): 562–3.

110. Malone JC, Slone SP, Wills-Frank LA, et al. Vascular inflammation (vasculitis) in sweet syndrome: a clinicopathologic study of 28 biopsy specimens from 21 patients. Arch Dermatol 2002;138(3): 345–9.

111. Cohen PR. Skin lesions of Sweet syndrome and its dorsal hand variant contain vasculitis: an oxymoron or an epiphenomenon? Arch Dermatol 2002; 138(3):400–3.

112. Cooper PH, Frierson HF, Greer KE. Subcutaneous neutrophilic infiltrates in acute febrile neutrophilic dermatosis. Arch Dermatol 1983;119(7):610–1.

113. Strutton G, Weedon D, Robertson I. Pustular vasculitis of the hands. J Am Acad Dermatol 1995; 32(2 Pt 1):192–8.

114. Galaria NA, Junkins-Hopkins JM, Kligman D, et al. Neutrophilic dermatosis of the dorsal hands: pustular vasculitis revisited. J Am Acad Dermatol 2000;43(5 Pt 1):870–4.

115. DiCaudo DJ, Connolly SM. Neutrophilic dermatosis (pustular vasculitis) of the dorsal hands: a report of 7 cases and review of the literature. Arch Dermatol 2002;138(3):361–5.

116. Weenig RH, Bruce AJ, McEvoy MT, et al. Neutrophilic dermatosis of the hands: four new cases and review of the literature. Int J Dermatol 2004; 43(2):95–102.

117. Callen JP. Neutrophilic dermatoses. Dermatol Clin 2002;20(3):409–19.

118. Walling HW, Snipes CJ, Gerami P, et al. The relationship between neutrophilic dermatosis of the dorsal hands and sweet syndrome: report of 9 cases and comparison to atypical pyoderma gangrenosum. Arch Dermatol 2006;142(1):57–63.

119. Jordaan HF. Acute febrile neutrophilic dermatosis. A histopathological study of 37 patients and a review of the literature. Am J Dermatopathol 1989;11(2):99–111.

120. Callen JP. Pyoderma gangrenosum. Lancet 1998; 351(9102):581–5.

121. Takahama H, Kanbe T. Neutrophilic dermatosis of the dorsal hands: a case showing HLA B54, the marker of Sweet's syndrome. Int J Dermatol 2010; 49(9):1079–80.

122. Requena L, Kutzner H, Palmedo G, et al. Histiocytoid Sweet syndrome: a dermal infiltration of immature neutrophilic granulocytes. Arch Dermatol 2005;141(7):834–42.

123. Camarillo D, McCalmont TH, Frieden IJ, et al. Two pediatric cases of nonbullous histiocytoid neutrophilic dermatitis presenting as a cutaneous manifestation of lupus erythematosus. Arch Dermatol 2008;144(11):1495–8.

124. Murase JE, Wu JJ, Theate I, et al. Bortezomib-induced histiocytoid Sweet syndrome. J Am Acad Dermatol 2009;60(3):496–7.

125. Wu AJ, Rodgers T, Fullen DR. Drug-associated histiocytoid Sweet's syndrome: a true neutrophilic maturation arrest variant. J Cutan Pathol 2008; 35(2):220–4.

126. Spencer B, Nanavati A, Greene J, et al. Dapsone-responsive histiocytoid Sweet's syndrome associated with Crohn's disease. J Am Acad Dermatol 2008;59(2 Suppl 1):S58–60.

127. Chow S, Pasternak S, Green P, et al. Histiocytoid neutrophilic dermatoses and panniculitides: variations on a theme. Am J Dermatopathol 2007; 29(4):334–41.

128. Gerami P, Guitart J. Panniculitis with histiocytoid/immature neutrophils is not limited to histiocytoid panniculitic Sweet syndrome. Am J Dermatopathol 2007;29(6):596.

129. Heymann WR. Histiocytoid Sweet syndrome. J Am Acad Dermatol 2009;61(4):693–4.

130. Goldbach-Mansky R. Current status of understanding the pathogenesis and management of patients with NOMID/CINCA. Curr Rheumatol Rep 2011;13(2):123–31.

131. Kolivras A, Theunis A, Ferster A, et al. Cryopyrin-associated periodic syndrome: an autoinflammatory disease manifested as neutrophilic urticarial dermatosis with additional perieccrine involvement. J Cutan Pathol 2011;38(2):202–8.

132. Kieffer C, Cribier B, Lipsker D. Neutrophilic urticarial dermatosis: a variant of neutrophilic urticaria strongly associated with systemic disease. Report of 9 new cases and review of the literature. Medicine (Baltimore) 2009;88(1):23–31.

133. Toro JR, Aksentijevich I, Hull K, et al. Tumor necrosis factor receptor-associated periodic syndrome: a novel syndrome with cutaneous manifestations. Arch Dermatol 2000;136(12):1487–94.

134. Schmaltz R, Vogt T, Reichrath J. Skin manifestations in tumor necrosis factor receptor-associated periodic syndrome (TRAPS). Dermatoendocrinol 2010;2(1):26–9.

135. Magro CM, Crowson AN. Necrotizing eosinophilic folliculitis as a manifestation of the atopic diathesis. Int J Dermatol 2000;39(9):672–7.

136. Ackerman A, Boer A, Bennin B, et al. Histologic diagnosis of inflammatory skin diseases. 3rd edition. New York: Ardor Scribendi; 2005.

137. McKee P, Calonje E, Granter SR. Pathology of the skin with clinical correlations. 3rd edition. Philadelphia: Elsevier Mosby; 2005.

138. Hunt SJ, Santa Cruz DJ. Eosinophilic cellulitis: histologic features in a cutaneous mastocytoma. Dermatologica 1991;182(2):132–4.

139. Rose C, Brocker EB, Krahl D. Dermatitis herpetiformis with flame figures mimicking an arthropod bite. Am J Dermatopathol 2003;25(3):277–8 [author reply: 278].

140. Bens G, Franck F, Diatto G, et al. Dermatitis cruris pustulosa et atrophicans—a frequent but poorly understood tropical skin condition—a case report from Burkina Faso. Int J Dermatol 2008;47(5):473–5.

141. Rongioletti F, Fausti V, Kempf W, et al. Eosinophilic annular erythema: an expression of the clinical and pathological polymorphism of Wells syndrome. J Am Acad Dermatol 2011;65(4):e135–7.

142. Schuttelaar ML, Jonkman MF. Bullous eosinophilic cellulitis (Wells' syndrome) associated with Churg-Strauss syndrome. J Eur Acad Dermatol Venereol 2003;17(1):91–3.

143. Fujimoto N, Wakabayashi M, Kato T, et al. Wells syndrome associated with Churg-Strauss syndrome. Clin Exp Dermatol 2011;36(1):46–8.

144. Lee SH, Roh MR, Jee H, et al. Wells' syndrome associated with Churg-Strauss syndrome. Ann Dermatol 2011;23(4):497–500.

145. Weedon D. Weedon's skin pathology. 3rd edition. Philadelphia: Churchill Livingstone Elsevier; 2010.

146. LeBoit PE. The last refuge of scoundrels. Am J Dermatopathol 2004;26(6):516–7.

147. Kossard S, Hamann I, Wilkinson B. Defining urticarial dermatitis: a subset of dermal hypersensitivity reaction pattern. Arch Dermatol 2006;142(1):29–34.

148. Ackerman A. Histologic diagnosis of inflammatory skin diseases: a method by pattern analysis. Philadelphia: Lea & Febiger; 1978.

149. RIBS. RxDerm archives 2012. Available at: http://dermatology.cdlib.org/rxderm-archives/itchy-red-bump-disease. Accessed January 19, 2012.

150. Sherertz EF, Jorizzo JL, White WL, et al. Papular dermatitis in adults: subacute prurigo, American style? J Am Acad Dermatol 1991;24(5 Pt 1): 697–702.

151. Uehara M, Ofuji S. Primary eruption of prurigo simplex subacuta. Dermatologica 1976;153(1): 49–56.

152. James WD, Berger TG, Elston DM. Andrews' diseases of the skin: Clinical dermatology. Philadelphia: Saunders Elsevier; 2006.

153. Tharp MD. Top-accessed article: defining urticarial dermatitis. Arch Dermatol 2011;147(12):1436.

154. Clark AR, Jorizzo JL, Fleischer AB. Papular dermatitis (subacute prurigo, "itchy red bump" disease): pilot study of phototherapy. J Am Acad Dermatol 1998;38(6 Pt 1):929–33.

155. Rietschel RL. A clinician's view of urticarial dermatitis. Arch Dermatol 2006;142(7):932 [author reply: 932–3].

156. Flugman SL. Long-term control of papular dermatitis ("dermal hypersensitivity reaction") with mycophenolate mofetil. Arch Dermatol 2006;142(11):1512–3.

157. Howes R, Girgis L, Kossard S. Eosinophilic annular erythema: a subset of Wells' syndrome or a distinct entity? Australas J Dermatol 2008;49(3):159–63.

158. Helm TN, Grover R, Beutner E. Neoplasia-induced autoimmunity encompasses a spectrum of changes. J Am Acad Dermatol 2008;58(4):713.

What's New in the Histologic Evaluation of Alopecia and Hair-Related Disorders?

Dirk M. Elston, MD

KEYWORDS

- Dermatopathology • Biopsy • Alopecia • Histology

KEY POINTS

- In most cases, an alopecia diagnosis can be reached with either vertical or transverse sections.
- The HoVert[1] technique for sectioning alopecia specimens is an ingenious method that provides vertical and transverse views of portions of a single scalp biopsy specimen.
- The Tyler technique has additional advantages.
- Large tufts of hair protruding from a common infundibulum ("six-packs" or "doll's hair") can be a clue to the quiescent phase of neutrophilic forms of alopecia, especially folliculitis decalvans and acne keloidalis nuchae.

ALOPECIA

Several recent articles have contributed to knowledge of alopecia and have refined the diagnostic criteria. Some have focused on practical questions of how to section biopsy specimens to optimize the diagnostic yield. The first portion of this article focuses on advances in the histologic evaluation of alopecia.

How to Section the Specimen When Only a Single Punch Biopsy is Received

In most cases, a diagnosis can be reached with either vertical or transverse sections. Vertical sections are superior for the diagnosis of scarring alopecia and comparable with transverse sections for alopecia areata.[2,3] Transverse sections have advantages in the diagnosis of other forms of non-scarring alopecia. Combining the two maximizes the diagnostic yield. When only a single specimen is received, various techniques have been proposed to provide vertical and transverse sections from a single specimen.

The HoVert[1] technique for sectioning alopecia specimens is an ingenious method that provides vertical and transverse views of portions of a single scalp biopsy specimen. The HoVert technique entails transecting the 4-mm punch scalp biopsy transversely, 1 mm below the epidermal surface, to create an epidermal disk and a lower portion. The epidermal disk is then bisected to provide vertical sections of the upper half of the specimen. On the slide, the lower portion of the specimen is viewed in transverse (horizontal) section, whereas the sections from the upper half are seen in vertical section to provide a higher diagnostic yield for such conditions as lichen planopilaris (LPP) that preferentially affect the follicular infundibulum and can be missed with transverse sectioning.

The Tyler technique[4] is an alternate method in which the specimen is first bisected vertically, and then one-half of the cylinder is sectioned transversely (**Fig. 1**). All sections are embedded together in a single cassette. The two resulting transverse half-moons are embedded side by side to create the impression of a single complete transverse section with an adjacent complete vertical section. An advantage of this technique is that it produces a full-vertical section (from the stratum corneum to the subcutaneous fat) rather than vertical sections

Ackerman Academy of Dermatopathology, 145 East 32nd Street, 10th Floor, New York, NY 10016, USA
E-mail address: delston@ameripath.com

Dermatol Clin 30 (2012) 685–694
http://dx.doi.org/10.1016/j.det.2012.06.010
0733-8635/12/$ – see front matter Published by Elsevier Inc.

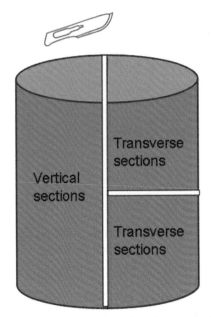

Fig. 1. Tyler technique for obtaining vertical and transverse sections from a single punch specimen.

that show only the upper half of the follicle. Another advantage is the ability to view all levels of the dermis in transverse sections, because serial sections show progressively higher transverse sections in one half-moon and progressively lower levels in the other half-moon (**Fig. 2**). The Tyler technique may be advantageous when a single specimen is received and the differential diagnosis includes such conditions as lupus erythematosus, central centrifugal cicatricial alopecia, or alopecia areata, where key histologic features are typically below the bisected level of HoVert specimens. However, it should be noted that because all portions of the specimen can ultimately be represented in serial sections with either technique, it may largely be a matter of individual preference. Both techniques have significant advantages over purely vertical or purely horizontal sectioning.

Tufting as a Clue to Neutrophil-Mediated Scarring Alopecia

Large tufts of hair protruding from a common infundibulum ("six-packs" or "doll's hair") can be a clue to the quiescent phase of neutrophilic forms of alopecia, especially folliculitis decalvans and acne keloidalis nuchae (**Fig. 3**). Lymphocyte-mediated forms tend to produce smaller clusters of hairs.[5] Large tufts can also be seen after burns and as physiologic tufting, especially in the occipital scalp, so the finding of six-packs must be interpreted in the context of the clinical presentation.[6]

Lymphoma Presenting as Alopecia

Alopecia in mycosis fungoides and Sézary syndrome

Alopecia can be an important manifestation of mycosis fungoides and Sézary syndrome. A retrospective study of 1550 patients noted 38 patients with patchy, total-scalp, or universal alopecia. Thirteen (34%) of the 38 had patchy alopecia clinically identical to alopecia areata.[7] Although alopecia areata is characterized by peribulbar lymphoid infiltrates, lymphocytes or eosinophils in fibrous tract remnants, pigment in fibrous tract remnants, catagen hairs, pigment casts, and dilated follicular infundibulae, mycosis fungoides is more likely to demonstrate epidermotropism of large angulated lymphocytes throughout the follicular epithelium, basilar tagging, and halos surrounding lymphocytes. Follicular mucinosis may be present. The histologic changes in Sézary syndrome are far more variable and can be nonspecific. The syndrome is best confirmed by the combination of clinical erythroderma and circulating Sézary cells.

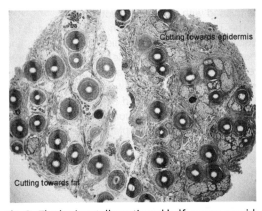

Fig. 2. The horizontally sectioned half-moons provide successive levels toward either the epidermis or subcutaneous tissue (hematoxylin-eosin, original magnification ×100).

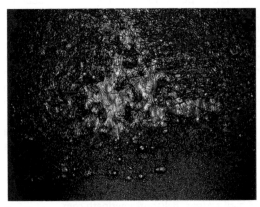

Fig. 3. Acne keloidalis nuchae demonstrating large follicular tufts ("six-packs").

Scarring alopecia in B-cell lymphoma

Primary cutaneous follicle center cell lymphoma of the scalp has recently been reported presenting as scarring alopecia.[8] There is overlap at scanning magnification with lupus erythematosus presenting with prominent germinal centers. Careful attention should be paid to the symmetry and regularity of the lymphoid nodules, symmetry of the surrounding mantle zone, and presence or absence of tangible body macrophages. Both demonstrate follicles composed mostly of CD20+ centrocytes, but the lymphomas often demonstrate disruption of the CD21+ network of dendritic cells within the lymphoid follicles and wandering of BCL-6+ follicle center cells beyond the confines of the follicle.

Subtle Clues to the Diagnosis of Trichotillomania

Histologic features of trichotillomania (trichotillosis) include empty anagen follicles, multiple catagen hairs, pigment casts in the follicular channel, and trichomalacia. Of these, the most specific finding is trichomalacia, which can produce striking findings, such as the "hamburger bun sign." This involves a vertically oriented split in the hair shaft, containing proteinaceous material and erythrocytes, morphologically reminiscent of a hamburger in a bun (**Fig. 4**).[9] Degeneration of the hair fiber can take other forms, such as the "hot dog" sign (**Fig. 5**).

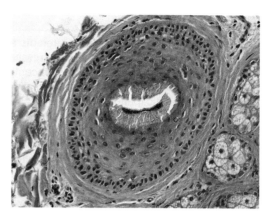

Fig. 5. Hot dog sign in trichotillomania (hematoxylin-eosin, original magnification, ×400). (*Courtesy of* Michael Ioffreda, MD.)

Subtle Clues to the Diagnosis of Alopecia Areata

Helpful diagnostic signs in alopecia areata include the presence of peribulbar lymphoid infiltrates, follicular miniaturization, dystrophic follicles, catagen hairs, pigment incontinence in fibrous tract remnants, lymphocytes or eosinophils in fibrous tract remnants, and pigment casts within follicular channels. Several of these features overlap with other entities, and careful attention must be paid to the entire constellation of findings and the clinical presentation. Yellow dots have been noted on dermoscopy, which correspond histologically with dilated follicular infundibula, and this finding can help to distinguish alopecia areata from trichotillomania, telogen effluvium, and pattern alopecia. The finding has been likened to a Swiss cheese appearance.[10]

Reflectance Confocal Microscopy

Reflectance confocal microscopy was evaluated in seven white patients with LPP or discoid lupus erythematosus involving the scalp. Discoid lupus erythematosus and LPP demonstrated spongiosis, exocytosis, interface dermatitis, periadnexal infiltration of inflammatory cells, dilated dermal vessels, and melanophages. In LPP, bright rims around the adnexal epithelium and dermal papillae were obscured by inflammatory cell infiltrates along a large front, whereas this is a focal finding in discoid lupus erythematosus. During therapeutic follow-up, marked reduction or absence of inflammatory cells at the level of the epidermis, upper dermis, and adnexal structures was considered evidence of complete remission. The authors concluded that reflectance confocal microscopy demonstrated promise in diagnosis and evaluation of therapeutic response.[11]

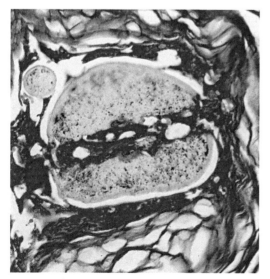

Fig. 4. Hamburger sign in trichotillomania (hematoxylin-eosin, original magnification, ×400). (*Courtesy of* Leonard Sperling, MD, and Michael Royer, MD.)

Overlap Alopecia

Flares of LPP are commonplace after attempts at scar revision or hair transplantation. Progressive scarring alopecia secondary to LPP was recently described in the setting of follicular unit transplantation for androgenetic (pattern) alopecia, emphasizing the need to be alert for the presence of scarring alopecia superimposed on a background of pattern alopecia.[12] LPP has also been reported after trauma from breakdancing. The resulting apical alopecia mimicked pattern alopecia.[13]

Ethnic Variation in Alopecia

A study of scarring alopecia in Indian patients revealed 18 (49%) of 37 patients with a diagnosis of lupus erythematosus, 15 (41%) of 37 with a diagnosis of LPP, one patient with folliculitis, and three with alopecia areata. Important differentiating features for lupus erythematosus included epidermal atrophy, papillary dermal fibrosis, mucin, peribulbar inflammation, and haphazard spacing of scars, compared with LPP, which typically demonstrated a normal epidermis, peri-infundibular infiltrate, and regular spacing of scars. Twelve cases demonstrated total absence of follicles but could be classified based on the connective tissue changes, emphasizing the importance of dermal changes and elastic tissue stains in the diagnosis of alopecia (see later). Not surprisingly, patients described as "pseudopelade" clinically were most likely to show LPP on histologic examination.[14]

In another recent histologic study of alopecia areata in Indian patients, the diagnosis was made on vertical sections in all 20 cases. The anagen/nonanagen ratio was 1:1.62. Miniaturization of follicles was noted in five (25%) cases. Peribulbar inflammation was noted in all the cases with a dominance of lymphocytes, and pigment casts were present in five cases. These findings suggest that clinicians had biopsied early lesions of alopecia areata.[15]

According to a recent study, central hair loss in African American women does not seem to be associated with relaxer or hot comb use; a history of seborrheic dermatitis; or reaction to a hair care product, bacterial infection, or male-pattern hair loss in fathers of subjects.[16] Future studies need to address the influence of recall bias. I myself have had patients flatly deny ever having straightened their hair, only to have a family member remind them that they practiced straightening for years.

Langerhans Cells in LPP and Traction Alopecia

A study comparing the Langerhans cell concentration in LPP with traction alopecia was performed using double immunostaining with CD1a and CD3. The 16 biopsy specimens evaluated included nine biopsies of LPP and seven biopsies of traction alopecia. The mean ratio of the concentration of Langerhans cells to T lymphocytes was 1.28 for LPP and 0.59 for traction alopecia, suggesting the inflammation in LPP may be influenced by Langerhans cells and suggesting that traction alopecia is not immune-mediated. It should be noted that isolated cases of traction alopecia demonstrated ratios similar to those seen in LPP, limiting the diagnostic utility in individual cases. It may be that these cases represented cicatricial marginal alopecia, rather than traction alopecia.[17]

Elastic Tissue Patterns in Alopecia

Characteristic patterns of elastic tissue loss can be helpful in the diagnosis of scarring alopecia. The biopsy must be taken from a mature area of alopecia and does not require the presence of inflammation. Normal fibrous tract remnants are surrounded by a thick elastic tissue sheath (Fig. 6). LPP and folliculitis decalvans demonstrate loss of the elastic sheath in the late stage when the infiltrate is no longer identifiable (Fig. 7). In vertical sections, LPP and folliculitis decalvans demonstrate superficial wedge-shaped scars centered about the infundibulum (Fig. 8), whereas end-stage lesions of chronic cutaneous lupus erythematosus usually demonstrate loss of elastic tissue throughout the entire dermis. Idiopathic pseudopelade (ie, those cases that do not represent LPP) demonstrates broad hyalinized fibrous tract remnants with preservation and duplication of the elastic sheath and thick interstitial elastic fibers (Fig. 9).[18] Although an elastic van Gieson stain is most commonly used to demonstrate the characteristic patterns, an alternative is to view hematoxylin-eosin stained sections under a fluorescent microscope, taking advantage of the

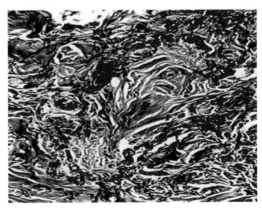

Fig. 6. Elastic tissue stain demonstrating the normal elastic tissue sheath (elastic van Gieson, original magnification ×200).

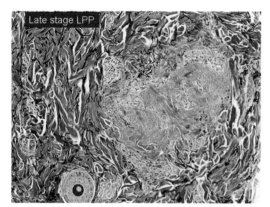

Fig. 7. Lichen planopilaris demonstrates loss of the elastic sheath (transverse section, elastic van Gieson, original magnification ×200).

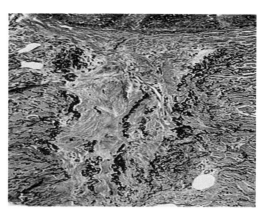

Fig. 9. Idiopathic pseudopelade demonstrates broad hyalinized fibrous tract remnants with preservation and duplication of the elastic sheath (elastic van Gieson, original magnification ×100).

autofluorescence of the eosinophilic elastic fibers (**Fig. 10**).[19] This compares favorably with elastic van Gieson stained sections (**Fig. 11**). It should be emphasized that elastic staining provides prognostic and diagnostic information, because scarring at the level of the germinative epithelium (bulge area) correlates with permanent hair loss.

Selenium

Selenium excess and selenium deficiency have been associated with alopecia, mostly through a mechanism of telogen effluvium. In a mouse model of alopecia and poliosis associated with excessive and deficient selenium, biopsy from the alopecic patches showed increased telogen hair follicles and epidermal atrophy. There was an accompanying decrease in antiapoptotic Bcl-2 and an increase in proapoptotic Bax in the group with excessive selenium.[20]

Telepathology

A study of a World Wide Web–based process for histopathologic consultations found that melanocytic lesions, inflammatory dermatoses, and squamous lesions comprised 82% of the specimens, but the technology was also useful for cases of alopecia. Improved turnaround time was one of the major advantages of World Wide Web–based consultation.[21]

Anti–Tumor Necrosis Factor-α Therapy

Anti–tumor necrosis factor-α therapy can produce nonscarring patterns of alopecia, and

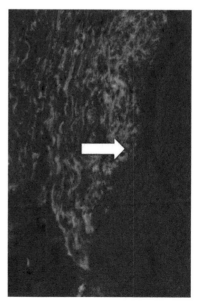

Fig. 10. Loss of elastic tissue visible in sections viewed under a fluorescent microscope. The *arrow* indicates the border of the scar (traumatic alopecia, vertical section, hematoxylin-eosin, original magnification ×100).

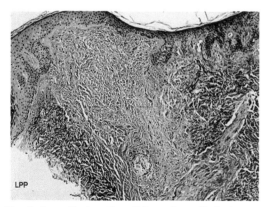

Fig. 8. In vertical section, lichen planopilaris demonstrates wedge-shaped loss of elastic tissue (elastic van Gieson, original magnification ×100).

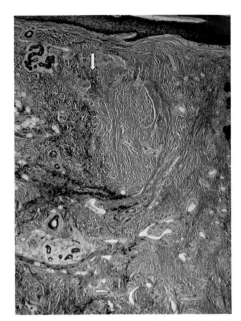

Fig. 11. Loss of elastic tissue visible in elastic tissue stained sections. The *arrow* indicates the border of the scar (elastic van Gieson, original magnification ×40).

dermatopathologists must remain alert to this possibility. All scalp biopsies in a recent study of this phenomenon revealed psoriasiform epidermal features (acanthosis and confluent parakeratosis with neutrophils and frank pustules) and alopecia areata–like dermal changes (markedly increased catagen/telogen, miniaturized hairs, and peribulbar lymphocytic inflammation). The presence of numerous plasma cells and eosinophils can be an important clue to the diagnosis.[22]

Progenitor Cells Populations and Cellular Proliferation in Pattern Alopecia

A recent study suggests that men with androgenetic alopecia retain hair follicle stem cells but lack CD200-rich and CD34-positive hair follicle progenitor cells. These progenitor cells localize to the stem cell–rich bulge area but are larger and more proliferative than the KRT15 (hi) stem cells. These findings suggest a defect in conversion of hair follicle stem cells to progenitor cells.[23]

A study of biopsies from the frontal (bald) area and occipital (hair-bearing) area of 15 male patients with androgenetic alopecia compared with specimens from the frontal area of five age-matched control subjects demonstrated a low proliferation rate in the bald area of patients and a perifollicular inflammatory infiltrate with antiapoptotic Bcl-2 expression in dermal lymphocytes.[24]

L-Threonate, an ascorbate metabolite, seems promising as a treatment for androgen-driven balding, based on its ability to suppress dihydrotestosterone-induced dickkopf-1 expression in human hair dermal papilla cells.[25] This finding has to be validated by clinical studies, but suggests that stem cells represent a promising target for the nonsurgical treatment of alopecia.

Loose Anagen Hair Syndrome

An ultrastructural study of the abnormal inner root sheath of the hair follicle in the loose anagen hair syndrome found intercellular edema in the prekeratinized Huxley cell zone and dyskeratosis of Henle and cuticle cells within the inner root sheath. On light microscopy, the keratinized Henle cell layer showed tortuous and irregular swellings. Irregular keratinization of the inner root sheath cuticle cells and swelling of Huxley cells were also noted.[26] These changes predispose to the rumpled silk stocking appearance of the inner root sheath remnants at the base of easily extracted anagen hairs (**Fig. 12**).

OTHER HAIR-RELATED DISORDERS

There have been significant recent advances in the understanding of hair-related disorders that do not result in alopecia. This section focuses on new findings in these hair-related disorders.

Viral-Associated Trichodysplasia Spinulosa

Viral-associated trichodysplasia spinulosa presents as a folliculocentric papular disorder in the setting of immunosuppression, mostly secondary to solid organ transplantation or hematopoietic malignancies. Clinically, the lesions are concentrated in the central portion of the face. Variable degrees of hair loss are present, especially affecting

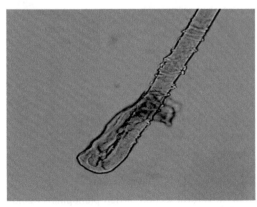

Fig. 12. Rumpled silk stocking appearance of the inner root sheath remnants in loose anagen syndrome.

facial hair. Histologically, the affected follicles are dilated by an expansion of dystrophic inner root sheath with enlarged trichohyaline cytoplasmic granules and central keratotic and parakeratotic debris (**Fig. 13**). It is caused by a polyomavirus, and may respond to oral valganciclovir.[27,28]

Subtle Signs of Fox-Fordyce Disease

Fox-Fordyce disease may demonstrate infundibular plugging, acanthosis, focal parakeratosis, focal spongiosis near the entry point of the apocrine duct, and a nonspecific and variable infiltrate. Newly recognized clues to the diagnosis of Fox-Fordyce disease include perifollicular foamy histiocytes and prominent dilation of apocrine coils. The foamy histiocytes have been referred to as "perifollicular xanthomatosis" and "perifollicular muciphages" (**Fig. 14**).[29,30] These are important clues, because the histologic changes may otherwise be subtle, and the spongiotic focus at the entrance of the apocrine duct is not commonly seen.

Pseudolymphomatous Folliculitis

Pseudolymphomatous folliculitis occurs in men and women, with a mean age of about 38. The lesions present as dome-shaped or sessile nodules on the face suggestive of cutaneous lymphoid hyperplasia or lymphoma. Most present with solitary lesions measuring less than 1.5 cm, although multiple nodules can occur.[31] Rapid regression has been noted after incisional biopsy and excision is usually curative, although recurrence has been reported.[32] Histopathologically, the lesions demonstrate dense lymphocytic infiltrates extending from the dermis to the subcutis simulating a cutaneous lymphoma. Atypical lymphocytes may be prominent, but hair follicles are enlarged and deformed with their outlines blurred by lymphocytic infiltrates.[33] This is in contrast to the distinct absence of epithelial reaction in most biopsies of

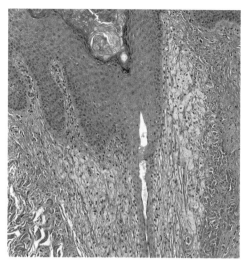

Fig. 14. Fox-Fordyce disease can be quite subtle in histologic sections, but the presence of a few perifollicular foamy histiocytes can suggest the diagnosis (hematoxylin-eosin, original magnification ×100). (*Courtesy of* Adolpho Bormate, MD, Philip LeBoit, MD, and Timothy McCalmont, MD.)

lymphoma. Most authors have found that the infiltrate is predominantly composed of B cells, but some authors have reported T-cell predominance in their series. A common finding is an increased number of perifollicular Langerhans histiocytes that express anti–S-100 protein and CD1a. These Langerhans cells may occur in aggregates.

Because true lymphoma can also be folliculotropic, careful attention should be paid to cytology and epithelial and vascular reaction. Pseudolymphomatous folliculitis demonstrates hair follicle hyperplasia, and the dense infiltrate is predominantly composed of small well-differentiated lymphocytes, lymphoplasmacytoid cells, plasma cells, and epithelioid histiocytes that form small aggregates or granulomas. Features worrisome for lymphoma include eccrine/apocrine duct hyperplasia (syringolymphoid hyperplasia); muscle infiltration; smudging of lymphocytes; single file infiltration; and the presence of large atypical cells, although scattered large atypical CD30[+] cells can be identified in some cases of pseudolymphoma. Usually, pseudolymphomatous folliculitis demonstrates a polyclonal pattern of kappa and lambda light-chain expression, although a subset of patients may demonstrate clonality. This group does not differ clinically from patients with polyclonality. Helpful diagnostic features to distinguish clonal pseudolymphomatous folliculitis from lymphoma are the presence of reactive pilosebaceous units and the presence of abundant CD1a-positive and S-100 protein–positive histiocytes or dendritic Langerhans cells.[34]

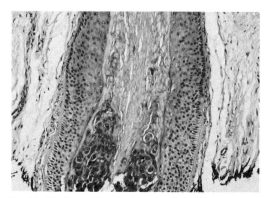

Fig. 13. Viral-associated trichodysplasia (hematoxylin-eosin, original magnification ×200).

Genetic Syndromes

The ichthyosis follicularis, alopecia, and photophobia syndrome

The ichthyosis follicularis, alopecia, and photo-phobia syndrome (OMIM 308205) is a rare X-linked genodermatosis characterized by follicular kera-totic papules, total or subtotal alopecia, and photophobia. Although prior reports focused on the presence of follicular plugging and hypoplastic pilosebaceous structures, a recent study using vertical and transverse sectioning techniques showed miniaturized anagen hair follicles with characteristic follicular plugs in vertical sections and abortive sebaceous glands in hair follicles seen in transverse sections. The total number of hair follicles was not significantly decreased.[35]

Vitamin D–resistant rickets with alopecia

1,25-Dihydroxyvitamin D_3 mediates its actions by binding to the vitamin D receptor. Mutations in the vitamin D receptor cause hereditary vitamin D–resistant rickets. A recent report of two unre-lated young female patients with severe early onset rickets, hypocalcemia, and hypophosphate-mia noted partial alopecia with unusual patterns of scant residual hair. Both patients harbored the same unique nonsense mutation resulting in a premature stop codon (R50X) in the vitamin D receptor gene.[36]

Fibrodysplasia ossificans progressiva

Fibrodysplasia ossificans progressiva is charac-terized by progressive ossification of soft tissues. According to a recent French study, scalp nodules that may be associated with alopecia may be found in roughly 40% of patients and usually represent the first manifestation of the disease. Patients also have characteristic skeletal malfor-mations involving the great toes, and less commonly the fingers, and vertebrae.[37] The histo-pathologic changes of the scalp biopsies demon-strated a range of findings, and the authors noted significant overlap with histopathologic features of cranial fasciitis. Findings included proliferation of short spindle cells negative or weakly positive for desmin, and negative for CD34 and S100. The proliferation involved the deep subcutaneous tissue and also focally the superficial muscle tissue. The spindle cells were either randomly arranged with a surrounding myx-oid stroma or formed short fascicles embedded in a collagenous stroma. Numerous small vessels were noted in the surrounding tissue. The accom-panying inflammatory infiltrate consisted mainly of T lymphocytes. A few scattered mast cells were present. Dermatopathologists should be familiar with these findings, to avoid misdiagnosis as cranial fasciitis.

Pseudocyst of the Scalp

Alopecic and aseptic nodules of the scalp, also known as pseudocyst of the scalp, is a recently described entity first reported in Japan. The nodules have a predilection for the occiput, and the associated alopecia is nonscarring. The condi-tion seems to overlap with dissecting cellulitis of the scalp. Histopathologically, the lesions were characterized by deep granulomata in half of the 14 patients reported and nonspecific inflammation in the other half. The lesions often respond to doxycycline.[38]

SUMMARY

The diagnosis of alopecia and other hair-related disorders can be challenging. An appreciation of the newest diagnostic techniques and newly described entities can help provide the best care for patients. Advances in the understanding of disease mechanisms can help in treating hair disorders that proved refractory in the past. I applaud all of the investigators who contributed to the work summarized in this article.

REFERENCES

1. Nguyen JV, Hudacek K, Whitten JA, et al. The HoVert technique: a novel method for the sectioning of alopecia biopsies. J Cutan Pathol 2011;38(5): 401–6.
2. Elston DM, Ferringer T, Dalton S, et al. A comparison of vertical versus transverse sections in the evalua-tion of alopecia biopsy specimens. J Am Acad Der-matol 2005;53(2):267–72.
3. Peckham SJ, Sloan SB, Elston DM. Histologic features of alopecia areata other than peribulbar lymphocytic infiltrates. J Am Acad Dermatol 2011; 65(3):615–20.
4. Elston DM. The Tyler technique for alopecia biop-sies. J Cutan Pathol 2012;39(2):306.
5. Pincus LB, Price VH, McCalmont TH. The amount counts: distinguishing neutrophil-mediated and lymphocyte-mediated cicatricial alopecia by compound follicles. J Cutan Pathol 2011;38(1):1–4.
6. Elston DM. Tufted folliculitis. J Cutan Pathol 2011; 38(7):595–6.
7. Bi MY, Curry JL, Christiano AM, et al. The spectrum of hair loss in patients with mycosis fungoides and Sézary syndrome. J Am Acad Dermatol 2011; 64(1):53–63.
8. Kluk J, Charles-Holmes R, Carr RA. Primary cuta-neous follicle centre cell lymphoma of the scalp

presenting with scarring alopecia. Br J Dermatol 2011;165(1):205–7.

9. Royer MC, Sperling LC. Splitting hairs: the 'hamburger sign' in trichotillomania. J Cutan Pathol 2006;33(Suppl 2):63–4.

10. Müller CS, El Shabrawi-Caelen L. 'Follicular Swiss cheese' pattern: another histopathologic clue to alopecia areata. J Cutan Pathol 2011;38(2):185–9.

11. Agozzino M, Tosti A, Barbieri L, et al. Confocal microscopic features of scarring alopecia: preliminary report. Br J Dermatol 2011;165(3):534–40.

12. Crisóstomo MR, Crisóstomo MC, Crisóstomo MG, et al. Hair loss due to lichen planopilaris after hair transplantation: a report of two cases and a literature review. An Bras Dermatol 2011;86(2): 359–61.

13. Monselise A, Chan LJ, Shapiro J. Break dancing: a new risk factor for scarring hair loss. J Cutan Med Surg 2011;15(3):177–9.

14. Inchara YK, Tirumalae R, Kavdia R, et al. Histopathology of scarring alopecia in Indian patients. Am J Dermatopathol 2011;33(5):461–7.

15. Chaitra V, Rajalakshmi T, Kavdia R. Histopathologic profile of alopecia areata in Indian patients. Int J Trichology 2010;2(1):14–7.

16. Olsen EA, Callender V, McMichael A, et al. Central hair loss in African American women: incidence and potential risk factors. J Am Acad Dermatol 2011;64(2):245–52.

17. Hutchens KA, Balfour EM, Smoller BR. Comparison between Langerhans cell concentration in lichen planopilaris and traction alopecia with possible immunologic implications. Am J Dermatopathol 2011;33(3):277–80.

18. Elston DM, McCollough ML, Warschaw KE, et al. Elastic tissue in scars and alopecia. J Cutan Pathol 2000;27:147–52.

19. Elston DM. Medical pearl: fluorescence microscopy of hematoxylin-eosin-stained sections. J Am Acad Dermatol 2002;47:777–9.

20. Hwang SW, Lee HJ, Suh KS, et al. Changes in murine hair with dietary selenium excess or deficiency. Exp Dermatol 2011;20(4):367–9.

21. Zembowicz A, Ahmad A, Lyle SR. A comprehensive analysis of a web-based dermatopathology second opinion consultation practice. Arch Pathol Lab Med 2011;135(3):379–83.

22. Doyle LA, Sperling LC, Baksh S, et al. Psoriatic alopecia/alopecia areata-like reactions secondary to anti-tumor necrosis factor-α therapy: a novel cause of noncicatricial alopecia. Am J Dermatopathol 2011;33(2):161–6.

23. Garza LA, Yang CC, Zhao T, et al. Bald scalp in men with androgenetic alopecia retains hair follicle stem cells but lacks CD200-rich and CD34-positive hair follicle progenitor cells. J Clin Invest 2011;121(2): 613–22.

24. El-Domyati M, Attia S, Saleh F, et al. Evaluation of apoptosis regulatory markers in androgenetic alopecia. J Cosmet Dermatol 2010;9(4):267–75.

25. Kwack MH, Ahn JS, Kim MK, et al. Preventable effect of L-threonate, an ascorbate metabolite, on androgen-driven balding via repression of dihydrotestosterone-induced dickkopf-1 expression in human hair dermal papilla cells. BMB Rep 2010; 43(10):688–92.

26. Mirmirani P, Uno H, Price VH. Abnormal inner root sheath of the hair follicle in the loose anagen hair syndrome: an ultrastructural study. J Am Acad Dermatol 2011;64(1):129–34.

27. Matthews MR, Wang RC, Reddick RL, et al. Viral-associated trichodysplasia spinulosa: a case with electron microscopic and molecular detection of the trichodysplasia spinulosa-associated human polyomavirus. J Cutan Pathol 2011;38(5):420–31.

28. Benoit T, Bacelieri R, Morrell DS, et al. Viral-associated trichodysplasia of immunosuppression: report of a pediatric patient with response to oral valganciclovir. Arch Dermatol 2010;146(8):871–4.

29. Macarenco RS, Garces SJC. Dilation of apocrine glands. A forgotten but helpful histopathological clue to the diagnosis of axillary Fox-Fordyce disease. Am J Dermatopathol 2009;31(4):393–7.

30. Bormate AB Jr, Leboit PE, McCalmont TH. Perifollicular xanthomatosis as the hallmark of axillary Fox-Fordyce disease: an evaluation of histopathologic features of 7 cases. Arch Dermatol 2008;144(8):1020–4.

31. Nakamura M, Kabashima K, Tokura Y. Pseudolymphomatous folliculitis presenting with multiple nodules. Eur J Dermatol 2009;19(3):263–4.

32. Kwon EJ, Kristjansson AK, Meyerson HJ, et al. A case of recurrent pseudolymphomatous folliculitis: a mimic of cutaneous lymphoma. J Am Acad Dermatol 2009;60(6):994–1000.

33. Petersson F. Pseudolymphomatous folliculitis with marked lymphocytic folliculo- and focal epidermotropism: expanding the morphologic spectrum. Am J Dermatopathol 2011;33(3):323–5.

34. Kazakov DV, Belousova IE, Kacerovska D, et al. Hyperplasia of hair follicles and other adnexal structures in cutaneous lymphoproliferative disorders: a study of 53 cases, including so-called pseudolymphomatous folliculitis and overt lymphomas. Am J Surg Pathol 2008;32(10):1468–78.

35. Kamo M, Ohyama M, Kosaki K, et al. Ichthyosis follicularis, alopecia, and photophobia syndrome: a case report and a pathological insight into pilosebaceous anomaly. Am J Dermatopathol 2011;33(4): 403–6.

36. Forghani N, Lum C, Krishnan S, et al. Two new unrelated cases of hereditary 1,25-dihydroxyvitamin D-resistant rickets with alopecia resulting from the same novel nonsense mutation in the vitamin D receptor gene. J Pediatr Endocrinol Metab 2010;23(8):843–50.

37. Piram M, Le Merrer M, Bughin V, et al. Scalp nodules as a presenting sign of fibrodysplasia ossificans progressiv a: a register-based study. J Am Acad Dermatol 2011;64(1):97–101.

38. Abdennader S, Vignon-Pennamen MD, Hatchuel J, et al. Alopecic and aseptic nodules of the scalp (pseudocyst of the scalp): a prospective clinicopathological study of 15 cases. Dermatology 2011;222(1):31–5.

Emerging Adverse Cutaneous Drug Reactions

Joshua W. Hagen[a], Cynthia M. Magro[b],
A. Neil Crowson[c,d,e,f,]*

KEYWORDS

- Monoclonal antibody therapy • Cutaneous drug reaction • Infliximab • Etanercept • Adalimumab
- Rituximab

KEY POINTS

- More than 2 decades have passed since the Food and Drug Administration approval of muromonab-CD3 (Orthoclone OKT3) ushered in the era of monoclonal antibody therapy for the treatment of human disease.[1]
- Despite having relatively favorable safety profiles overall, these drugs are not without potential side effects, some of which are occasionally severe enough to prompt discontinuation of the drug.[2]
- The market for tumor necrosis factor α (TNFα) inhibitors is currently occupied by 4 monoclonal antibodies (adalimumab, infliximab, certolizumab pegol, and golimumab) directed against the TNFα protein, and 1 TNF-receptor fusion protein (etanercept).

INTRODUCTION

The past several decades have seen the advent and rapidly expanding use of biological agents in the treatment of chronic disease states ranging from organ transplant rejection to rheumatoid arthritis and lymphoproliferative disorders. As increasingly large pools of patients have been enrolled in treatment protocols using these agents, physicians have become acquainted with both desired and adverse events associated with their use. Dermatologists frequently encounter patients affected by cutaneous drug reactions associated with the use of biological agents, and should therefore be familiar with the full range of side effects that have been reported in the literature. This review discusses these adverse cutaneous effects, their underlying mechanisms, and efforts to predict and minimize their occurrence.

ADVERSE REACTIONS TO MONOCLONAL ANTIBODIES

More than 2 decades have passed since Food and Drug Administration (FDA) approval of muromonab-CD3 (Orthoclone OKT3) ushered in the era of monoclonal antibody therapy for the treatment of human disease.[1] With the introduction of infliximab (Remicade), etanercept (Enbrel), and adalimumab (Humira) to inhibit activity of tumor necrosis factor α (TNFα), physicians augmented their armamentarium in the battle against autoimmune diseases such as rheumatoid arthritis (RA), Crohn disease, and psoriasis. Monoclonal antibodies directed against vascular endothelial cell growth factor (VEGF) (bevacizumab), ErbB2 (trastuzumab), and CD20 (rituximab) have joined the anti-TNFα agents as the most extensively prescribed drugs in this class, which together account for some of the

[a] Tri-Institutional MD-PhD Program, Weill Medical College of Cornell University, New York, NY 10065, USA;
[b] Department of Pathology and Laboratory Medicine, Weill Medical College of Cornell University, New York, NY 10065, USA; [c] Department of Dermatology, University of Oklahoma, Oklahoma, OK, USA; [d] Department of Pathology, University of Oklahoma, Tulsa, OK, USA; [e] Department of Surgery, University of Oklahoma, Tulsa, OK, USA; [f] St John Medical Center and Regional Medical Laboratory, Tulsa, OK, USA
* Corresponding author. Regional Medical Laboratory, 4142 South Mingo Road, Tulsa, OK 74146.
E-mail address: ncrowson@sjmc.org

Dermatol Clin 30 (2012) 695–730
http://dx.doi.org/10.1016/j.det.2012.06.016
0733-8635/12/$ – see front matter © 2012 Elsevier Inc. All rights reserved.

top-selling biotechnology drugs. To date more than 20 monoclonal antibody therapies have been approved for use by the FDA.

Despite having relatively favorable safety profiles overall, these drugs are not without potential side effects, some of which are occasionally severe enough to prompt discontinuation of the drug.[2] Although adverse reactions affecting the skin are usually tolerated sufficiently to allow continued use, they can be distressing to the patients, who will often seek the attention of their physician(s). As a consequence it is important that rheumatologists and dermatologists who might encounter these adverse reactions in their clinical practice be familiar with the incidence and, when known, the pathogenesis of these reaction processes. In many cases, the adverse reactions fall under the rubric of a "class effect" and can therefore be expected from any of the agents using the same mechanism of action, whereas in other cases there appear to be reaction patterns that are specific to individual agents that are rare or unreported with remaining members of the class. This article reviews the reaction patterns observed across the broad range of biologics in use currently, while discussing possible underlying mechanisms and efforts to minimize their occurrence.

TNFα Inhibitors

The market for TNFα inhibitors is currently occupied by 4 monoclonal antibodies (adalimumab, infliximab, certolizumab pegol, golimumab) directed against the TNFα protein, and 1 TNF-receptor fusion protein (etanercept). These medications are used to treat a broad range of autoimmune conditions including psoriasis, RA, Crohn disease, ankylosing spondylitis, and various off-label conditions.

Injection-site and infusion reactions

The most common dermatologic complaint associated with the use of monoclonal antibodies is the injection-site reaction defined by edema, erythema, pruritus, and/or pain. The incidence of injection-site reactions ranges from 3% to 49%, and appears to be a function of both the specific anti-TNFα agent used and the underlying disease process.[3–10] These studies indicate that RA patients, especially those treated with etanercept, are at significantly increased risk of developing injection-site reactions in comparison to patients with psoriasis or Crohn disease. While patients typically experience a decrease in frequency and severity of injection site reactions over the course of treatment, worsening reactions with continued administration are reported.[3,6,11,12] Histologically, infiltrates of CD8+ T cells characterize the primary and recurrent

reactions, consistent with a type IV delayed hypersensitivity reaction.[11]

Infusion reactions include pruritus, urticaria, chills/fevers, anaphylaxis, and vital-sign alterations that occur, by definition, within 2 to 24 hours following infusion of the drug. Rates of infusion reactions with TNFα inhibitors range from 3% to 24%, depending on the trial and the disease under treatment.[13–16] Pretreatment with corticosteroids in an effort to reduce infusion reactions appears to have little value, and may even have the paradoxic effect of increasing rates of infusions reactions.[17–21] Instead, regular administration without prolonged interdose intervals seems to be the most effective means of preventing antibody formation leading to infusion reactions.[22,23]

Infections

Numerous case reports have surfaced that suggest an association between infections and the use of TNFα inhibitors.[15,24,25] Both systemic and cutaneous infections have been observed,[26] suggesting that immunosuppression related to anti-TNFα therapies renders patients more susceptible to infectious pathogens. However, RA patients, one of the major patient demographics receiving TNFα inhibitors, exhibit higher infection rates compared with the general population, which may account for some of the observed infectious complications.[27] That said, comparison between RA patients using anti-TNFα antibodies and those prescribed other disease-modifying antirheumatic drugs (DMARDs) revealed an adjusted relative risk of 4.28 (95% confidence interval, 1.06–17.17).[28] Lee and colleagues[24] reported 13 patients (of 150 in total) who developed cutaneous infections while on infliximab, adalimumab, or etanercept, which included pityriasis versicolor, tinea corporis, impetiginized eczema, herpes simplex, and Staphylococcus aureus.

Fungal, bacterial, and viral infections have all been reported at higher rates in patients using anti-TNFα agents, but none severe enough to require hospitalization.[25] A study of 500 patients using infliximab described 48 patients with infectious events including cases of abscesses, upper respiratory tract infections, pneumonia, cellulitis, shingles, chicken pox, genital herpes, and candidal onychomycosis.[15] As regards viral infections, a prospective cohort study comparing monoclonal anti-TNFα antibodies, etanercept, and DMARDs indicated a statistically significant increased risk for herpes zoster specific to the monoclonal agents, although the investigators considered that the risk fell below the level of clinical significance.[29] Psoriasis patients treated with etanercept also experienced an increased incidence of viral warts.[30,31] An important side effect directly linked with TNFα blockade therapy is the development of reactivated pulmonary tuberculosis, hence a relative contraindication to the use of the drug is a positive purified protein derivative test.

Inflammatory reactions of the skin

A broad range of inflammatory reactions of the skin has been reported in patients with TNFα blockade. Infliximab-induced acne is reported (**Fig. 1**)[32,33] New-onset dermatitis herpetiformis, alopecia areata, pityriasis rosea, and dermatitis sicca (anhidrosis) have been reported with use of various TNFα inhibitors, typically within the first year of initiating treatment.[24] Leukocytoclastic vasculitis, lichenoid drug reactions, perniosis-like eruptions, superficial granuloma annulare, and acute folliculitis following infliximab therapy were reported in patients treated for Crohn disease or RA.[34] Eczema, including dyshidrotic, nummular, contact, papular, and unspecified types, has also been associated with the use of infliximab and etanercept (**Fig. 2**).[24,25,35] Lichenoid reactions have been noted with the entire range of TNF-blocking agents (**Fig. 3**).[25,36–39]

Several case reports suggest a relationship between the development of palisading neutrophilic and granulomatous dermatitis and TNFα-inhibitor therapy (**Fig. 4**).[40–42] It has been proposed that TNFα inhibition initiates a leukocytoclastic vasculitis, possibly through interference with self-tolerance mechanisms or immune complex formation, which is followed by a granulomatous inflammatory process. Some investigators have postulated a granulomatous koebnerization in those cases associated with underling RA. Among the granulomatous infiltrates associated with TNFα therapy are rheumatoid nodules,[43–45] interstitial granulomatous dermatitis,[46] granuloma annulare,[47] and sarcoid-like granulomas.[48–52]

There have been 5 reported cases of erythema multiforme–like reactions to TNFα inhibitors, after which the offending medication was stopped and the patients' lesions resolved with topical and oral steroids.[36,53,54] The authors have encountered an adalimumab-triggered lymphocytic interface dermatitis mimicking erythema multiforme histologically in a patient with a drug-induced lupus-like symptom complex associated with a positive lupus band test (**Fig. 5**); this histology mimics acute lupus erythematosus. One case of an eosinophilic cellulitis–like reaction following etanercept[55] and one associated with adalimumab[56] have also been reported.

Cutaneous neoplasms

Immunosuppressed patients experience an increased incidence of cutaneous neoplasms including melanoma, nonmelanoma skin cancer (NMSC), and cutaneous lymphoproliferative disorders.[57–61] It has been postulated that the immunomodulatory effects of TNFα inhibition might effect an increase in rates of skin cancers among patients requiring long-term therapy. TNFα was initially identified as a potent proapoptotic signal for tumor cells.[62,63] Animal studies in rats have indicated that anti-TNFα antibodies interfere with antitumor immune surveillance in response to implanted tumor cells that are otherwise robustly attacked in untreated animals.[64] Similar results were obtained with the use of TNF knockout mice.[65]

These findings suggest that antitumor surveillance mechanisms in humans might also be impaired by the chronic administration of anti-TNFα agents. The challenge in addressing the question of iatrogenic neoplasms resulting from anti-TNFα therapy remains the documented predisposition for malignancies associated with the underlying diseases.[66,67] Sporadic case reports have laid claim to an association between TNFα inhibitors and the

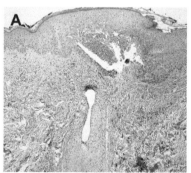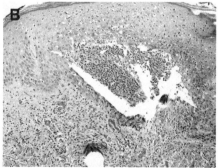

Fig. 1. (*A, B*) A patient taking adalimumab (Humira) for psoriasis developed new pustules on the trunk and extremities. The skin biopsy shows a neutrophilic folliculitis with localization of the pustule to involve the ostium and superficial isthmic part of the hair follicle. There is an element of acantholysis.

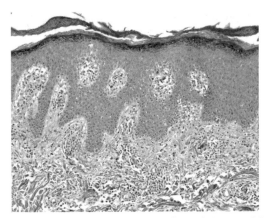

Fig. 2. A 55-year-old man taking infliximab (Remicade) for Crohn disease developed eczematous plaques in a widespread distribution. The clinical impression included eczema versus parapsoriasis. Biopsies showed a psoriasiform dermatitis.

development of NMSCs and cutaneous lymphoproliferative disorders.[66,68–70] Animal studies, however, have not borne out the association between de novo neoplasms and loss of TNFα,[71,72] suggesting that the associations observed clinically may arise from susceptibilities independent of anti-TNFα therapy, and that the induced loss of immune surveillance creates a permissive environment that coincides with the inherently proneoplastic nature of the diseases being treated.

Infliximab has been associated with acute development of keratoacanthoma and squamous cell carcinoma (SCC),[73] and rapid onset of SCCs has been noted following use of etanercept.[74–76] The question of whether this implies promotion of underlying precancerous lesions or de novo carcinogenesis was brought into focus by a report describing basal cell carcinoma (BCC) and SCC in psoriasis patients with extensive prior exposure to

light therapy who later began anti-TNFα therapy.[77] A large national cohort study of RA patients showed an elevated risk for development of NMSC that was most closely associated with use of prednisone or TNFα inhibitors alone or with concomitant methotrexate.[66] As is often the case, however, reports have surfaced that argue against such associations. A meta-analysis of randomized controlled trials using TNFα inhibitors in psoriasis patients (N = 6810) did not confirm an increased risk of malignancy.[78] Lebwohl and colleagues[79] also reported no evidence for increased risk of cutaneous SCC in patients receiving etanercept for up to 5 years. Aside from BCC and SCC, a single case of Merkel cell carcinoma has been reported in the context of adalimumab, methotrexate, and prednisone administration for RA.[70]

In addition to the reports of NMSCs, there have been occasional reported cases of associated melanoma. In 2 patients with a remote history of surgically excised melanoma there was a late recurrence (6 and 9 years after excision) of eruptive locoregional metastases following the initiation of etanercept and adalimumab, respectively.[80] Late recurrence of melanoma, however, is part of the natural history of melanoma, and whether this phenomenon can be attributed to TNFα inhibition in such cases is questionable. Although melanomas have been reported in patients with RA and Crohn disease receiving TNFα inhibitors,[81,82] strong evidence for a causal association is lacking.

Other forms of melanocytic proliferation influenced by anti-TNFα therapy include cutaneous nevi associated with infliximab therapy in the setting of Crohn disease[83] and eruptive melanocytic nevi associated with use of infliximab and etanercept in Crohn disease and psoriasis, respectively.[84] Balato and colleagues[85] extended

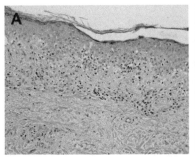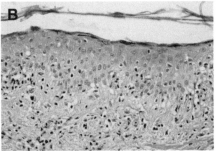

Fig. 3. A 65-year-old man was on etanercept (Enbrel) for 3 months and developed a patchy papulosquamous erythematous rash involving the trunk and lower legs. A skin biopsy showed an interface dermatitis. Features unlike lichen planus are the epidermal attenuation, lack of an increased granular cell layer, and only slight hyperkeratosis (A). There is basilar vacuolar change with a few lymphocytes present along the dermal-epidermal junction (B).

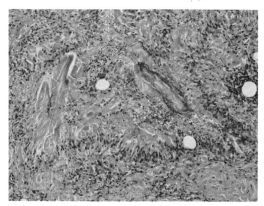

Fig. 4. A 46-year-old woman with a 30-year history of rheumatoid arthritis developed an asymptomatic erythematous eruption on the posterior bilateral lower extremities of 1 month's duration. She was taking multiple medications including adalimumab (Humira) every other week for 2 years, methotrexate 10 mg weekly for 4 months, and long-term prednisone. The skin biopsy shows a palisading neutrophilic and granulomatous dermatitis. The adalimumab was discontinued after 2 months, and the eruption cleared completely.

the hypothesis that the proinflammatory cytokine milieu of psoriasis might establish relative inhibition of melanogenesis and melanocyte growth in light of the reduced incidence of pigmented lesions in these patients. If true, it is possible that initiation of TNFα inhibitors releases this inhibitory state and restores a native level of melanogenesis and melanocyte proliferation that is, by comparison, hyperactive.

Lymphoproliferative disorders are also among the list of cutaneous neoplasms reported in patients using TNFα inhibitors. Among these are

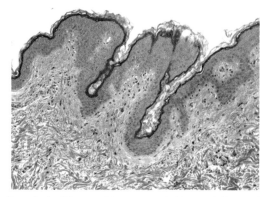

Fig. 5. A 35-year-old woman taking adalimumab (Humira) developed a widespread macular rash that was photoaccentuated. A biopsy showed a cell-poor interface dermatitis in the setting of a positive lupus band test from sun-protected skin.

reports of cutaneous γδ T-cell lymphoma in an RA patient using etanercept,[86] mycosis fungoides (MF) in 2 patients using etanercept and infliximab,[87] CD30+ T-cell lymphoma following cyclosporin and infliximab,[88] MF-associated follicular mucinosis after 7 months of adalimumab,[89] CD8+ cutaneous T-cell lymphoma with infliximab,[90] Sezary syndrome associated with infliximab and etanercept,[69,91] and cutaneous anaplastic large cell lymphoma following infliximab.[69] Because of their inherent rarity and the small number of case reports available, the association between TNFα inhibitors and cutaneous T-cell lymphoma is tenuous. No large-scale trials have addressed this question.

Although additional investigation is required to establish a concrete link between cutaneous malignancies and the use of TNFα inhibitors, many of the alternative treatments for the intended patient population (eg, psoriasis patients) have well-established risks of malignancy with long-term use (eg, photochemotherapy, methotrexate, mycophenolate mofetil).[92]

Other cutaneous reactions

Not infrequently, patients develop autoantibodies during their course of TNFα blockade. Following 6 months of treatment with etanercept or infliximab, 11% and 34% of patients, respectively, developed antinuclear antibodies. Anti–double-stranded DNA antibodies were found in 15% of patients taking etanercept and in 9% of patients using infliximab.[93,94] Perhaps it is not surprising, then, that there are reports of patients developing systemic lupus erythematosus while on etanercept, sometimes with cutaneous involvement.[95–100] There have been similar reports of new-onset cutaneous lupus with the use of infliximab[101–103] and adalimumab.[104–106] Meta-analysis of several hundred reported cases of autoimmune diseases associated with TNFα inhibitors revealed that cutaneous vasculitis, lupus-like syndromes, systemic lupus erythematosus, and interstitial lung disease were the most common.[107,108] Dermatomyositis has also been reported in association with TNFα inhibition.[109]

The anti-TNFα agents appear to have a negative impact on the control of psoriasis in some patients. Case reports of worsening or new-onset psoriasis are not infrequent in the TNF-inhibitor literature.[110–115] A retrospective analysis of 12 years' experience at the Mayo Clinic showed 56 patients with either new-onset psoriasis or exacerbation of underlying psoriasis who were treated with infliximab, adalimumab, or etanercept for Crohn disease or RA.[116] New-onset psoriatic palmoplantar pustulosis has also been noted in 2 patients treated with infliximab for RA.[117] Certolizumab for Crohn disease has been associated with development of psoriatic lesions.[118] Cytokine imbalance with increased levels of interferon-α (IFN-α) has been proposed as a possible pathogenetic mechanism.[119]

Interleukin-2 Inhibitors

To date there are 3 biological agents designed to target interleukin (IL)-2 signaling. Basiliximab (Simulect) is a chimeric mouse-human monoclonal antibody directed against the IL-2 receptor α subunit (CD25), used to prolong renal allograft survival. Daclizumab (Zenapax) is a humanized monoclonal antibody that targets the same α subunit of IL-2 receptor. Denileukin diftitox (Ontak) is an engineered protein, used in some cases of T-cell and B-cell lymphoma and advanced melanoma, which combines IL-2 with diphtheria toxin, thereby killing cells bearing IL-2 receptors that bind and internalize the toxin. Reports of cutaneous reactions to administration of these agents are sparse in the literature, perhaps reflecting a relatively benign profile as regards skin biology, but it is conceivable that basiliximab played a role in the pathogenesis of nephrogenic fibrosing dermopathy in 2 liver transplant patients.[120]

A small dose-escalation study using denileukin diftitox reported a 14% incidence of generalized maculopapular/vesicular rashes and a single case of mild vascular leak syndrome.[121] Capillary leak syndrome presenting with facial erythema and edema has been previously reported with denileukin diftitox,[122] and presents in a manner similar to that seen with IL-2 immunotherapy for cancer.[123,124] Pretreatment with corticosteroids appears to be effective in reducing the frequency of this complication.[125,126] There has also been a report of a fatal rash consistent with toxic epidermal necrolysis occurring in a patient with follicular large-cell lymphoma receiving denileukin diftitox.[127]

CD20 Inhibitors

Currently there are 3 FDA-approved monoclonal antibodies directed against the B-cell antigen CD20: rituximab (Rituxan), ibritumomab tiuxetan (Zevalan), and tositumomab (Bexxar). Of this class, rituximab has been most often reported to have significant adverse cutaneous reactions, although the remaining 2 agents have been available for a shorter period and have a less extensive history to mine for potential reactions.

Infusion reactions

Urticaria appears to be a common side effect in patients receiving rituximab, with incidence ranging from 3% to 14% in clinical trials.[128–132] Severe infusion reactions have also been noted.[133,134]

Infections

While systemic infectious complications have been reported in association with the use of rituximab, specific mention of cutaneous infections has been largely absent.[128,135] Of the handful of cutaneous infections reported in patients treated for non-Hodgkin lymphoma, herpes simplex and herpes zoster constituted the majority.[136,137]

Cutaneous malignancies

Associated malignancies with rituximab included reports of 6 BCCs, 2 SCCs, and 2 melanomas in a group of 1039 patients undergoing treatment for RA.[138] Merkel cell carcinoma has also been reported in a patient using rituximab.[139]

Other adverse cutaneous reactions

Although it appears to be a rare occurrence, there is a report of a patient experiencing Stevens-Johnson syndrome characterized by grade 1 mucositis after treatment with rituximab, which persisted for over a year until the patient's death.[140] Although there have yet to be any reports in humans of toxic epidermal necrolysis (TEN) with rituximab alone, reactions consistent with this classification have been observed in rhesus macaques following administration.[141] There have been postmarketing reports of erythema multiforme, Stevens-Johnson syndrome, TEN, bullous dermatitis, and exfoliative dermatitis in patients receiving the combined regimen of radiolabeled ibritumomab with rituximab (ie, the Zevalin therapeutic regimen).[142]

CD30 Antagonists

Brentuximab is a chimeric monoclonal antagonist of the CD30 molecule and is used in CD30+ lymphoproliferative lesions. A patient with CD30+ anaplastic large-cell lymphoma developed an eczematous eruption while on brentuximab (Fig. 6).

VEGF Inhibitors

Bevacizumab (Avastin) and ranibizumab (Lucentis) comprise the family of monoclonal antibodies currently approved to target VEGF in the treatment of various cancers, macular degeneration, and diabetic retinopathy. The bulk of reported reactions have been for the parent drug bevacizumab while the affinity-matured Fab fragment, ranibizumab, has comparatively few reports of adverse cutaneous effects to date. Among the dermatologic complaints in patients using bevacizumab, general rash is the most commonly

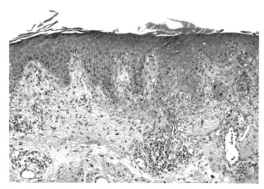

Fig. 6. A 67-year-old man with CD30-positive cutaneous anaplastic large cell lymphoma was treated with the anti-CD30 monoclonal chimeric antibody brentuximab (Adcetris), only to develop an eczematous eruption on the forearms, trunk, and thighs. Biopsy showed a heavy perivascular mononuclear cell infiltrate. No CD30-positive cells were identified in the infiltrate. (*Courtesy of* Dr Renee Grau, Oklahoma City, OK.)

reported.[143–146] More specific classification of skin reactions includes reports of papulopustular eruptions,[147] perforating dermatosis,[148] and cutaneous lupus erythematosus.[149] There has also been a report of impaired wound healing and skin-flap necrosis in a patient taking paclitaxel and bevacizumab after undergoing mastectomy for locally advanced breast cancer.[150] An episode of acute generalized exanthematous pustulosis was reported in association with ranibizumab following intravitreal administration.[151]

Epidermal Growth Factor Receptor Inhibitors

Monoclonal antibodies currently FDA approved for clinical use in targeting the epidermal growth factor receptor (EGFR) include cetuximab (Erbitux) and panitumumab (Vectibix). Both are indicated for metastatic colorectal cancer, and cetuximab is additionally approved for treatment of recurrent or metastatic SCC of the head and neck. The majority of the cutaneous reactions reported have been associated with cetuximab. The most common of these are eruptions of acneiform and rosaceiform lesions that serve as surrogate markers of tumor response.[152–157] One report demonstrated the presence of coagulase-positive *Staphylococcus* infection in association with a papulopustular drug eruption.[158] There have also been reports of eyelash trichomegaly,[159,160] xeroderma pigmentosum,[161] Grover disease,[162] ecthymatous skin eruption,[163] cicatricial ectropion,[164] paronychia,[165] and severe radiation dermatitis/TEN-like reactions.[166–168] Panitumumab has also been associated with similar acneiform, papulopustular eruptions, but few

reactions apart from this have been reported.[169] Dose-escalation studies with cetuximab suggested that severity of skin reactions did not follow a dose-sensitive distribution.[170] While both antibodies target the same effector molecule, there have been reports of differences in the patterns of toxicity seen for each agent when administered sequentially, suggesting possible non–class effect cutaneous toxicities.[171]

Efalizumab (Raptiva)

Efalizumab targets the CD11a antigen involved in cellular adhesion and costimulatory signaling between leukocytes. Compared with several of the monoclonal agents discussed previously, efalizumab has low reported rates of infusion reactions.[12,172–174] Its administration has been associated with increased incidence (in the range of ~3%) of herpes infections.[175,176] CD11a is one of the variable α-chain components of the leukocyte function–associated antigen (LFA)-1, which plays an important role in antibody-dependent cellular cytotoxicity directed against herpes-infected cells.[177] Cell-culture studies have shown that monoclonal antibodies directed against CD11a, but not CD11b or CD11c, inhibit the early phase of the IFN-α response normally generated by exposure to herpes virus, suggesting a potential mechanism behind the increased incidence of herpetic lesions in patients using efalizumab.[178] Along similar lines, there has been a report of disseminated eruptive giant molluscum contagiosum in a psoriasis patient using efalizumab.[179] A small increase (~1%) in the rate of impetigo and cellulitis has also been observed.[172]

Efalizumab has been reported to increase the rate of acne compared with placebo (4% vs 1%) in a large double-blind study comprising 1928 patients.[180] In addition to the adverse effects reported in larger studies, there have been specific reports of efalizumab-induced subacute cutaneous lupus erythematosus,[181] DRESS (Drug Reaction with Eosinophilia and Systemic Symptoms) syndrome,[182,183] dermatitis/lichen simplex chronicus,[184] exacerbation of pityriasis rubra pilaris,[185] eruptive seborrheic keratoses,[186] eruptive dermatofibromas,[187] and guttate psoriasis.[188]

Efalizumab is approved for the treatment of psoriasis, so it has been a point of special interest among clinicians and researchers that subsets of patients using the agent develop de novo psoriatic lesions or experience worsening of preexisting psoriasis (ie, rebound psoriasis). Numerous placebo-controlled trials with large patient populations have reported psoriasis-related adverse events in 2.2% to 13.6% of patients, which frequently exceeds the rates reported for placebo (ranging from 0.8% to 11.2%).[175,176,180] A unique type of inflammatory reaction has also been reported with the use of efalizumab in psoriasis patients resulting in the formation of eruptive papules composed of CD11b[+], CD11c[+], and inducible nitric oxide synthase–positive myeloid leukocytes with minimal CD3[+] cells.[189] It was proposed that these lesions arise from the expression of alternative β2 integrins that alter trafficking of circulating leukocytes to the skin.

Alefacept (Amevive)

Alefacept is an immunoglobulin G (IgG)1–LFA-3 fusion protein used in the treatment of chronic plaque psoriasis. It compares favorably with the anti-TNFα agents with regard to infusion reactions, with rates reported up to 8% higher than with placebo.[190,191] Marketing studies of 1869 patients associated alefacept with NMSCs, including BCCs (n = 20) and SCCs (n = 26), in addition to a small number of melanomas (n =3).[191] A smaller study with 201 patients reported 3 patients with BCC and 1 with SCC.[192] Schmidt and colleagues[193] reported the development of transformed MF after treatment with alefacept. Similar to several of the anti-TNFα agents, there have been reports of associated eruptive benign melanocytic nevi.[84]

Trastuzumab (Herceptin)

Trastuzumab is a humanized monoclonal antibody that targets the HER2/neu receptor, the product of a gene (ERBB2) commonly overexpressed in a subset of aggressive breast cancers. As with many of the monoclonal therapies, infusion reactions are not uncommon.[133] Although it is often used in concert with radiation therapy in the treatment of breast cancer, it does not appear that trastuzumab contributes significantly to rates of dermatitis beyond levels associated with radiation therapy alone.[194] Several reports have surfaced regarding photosensitivity in combination with the taxane class of chemotherapeutics,[195,196] although photosensitivity has been observed with taxanes in isolation.[197,198] Tufted folliculitis of the scalp with scaling and pruritus was also reported in a patient following the transition from doxorubicin and cyclophosphamide to trastuzumab.[199]

Alemtuzumab (Campath)

Mature T and B lymphocytes express CD52, a glycosylphosphatidylinositol-anchored antigen that serves as the target of the monoclonal antibody, alemtuzumab, in the treatment of lymphoproliferative disorders. Various reports have implicated alemtuzumab in disseminated molluscum contagiosum,[200] generalized herpes simplex,[201] varicella zoster,[202,203] sarcoidosis,[204] and acute CD30[+] transformation of cutaneous T-cell lymphoma in a manner reminiscent of Richter syndrome.[205,206]

Natalizumab (Tysabri)

Natalizumab is a humanized antibody directed against α4-integrin, an important cellular adhesion molecule target in the treatment of multiple sclerosis and Crohn disease. While there have been reports of generalized drug eruptions[207] and severe cutaneous candidal infection[208] in patients using natalizumab, perhaps the most striking adverse cutaneous effect involves the controversy surrounding accelerated evolution of nevi into melanoma.[209–213] Studies performed more than a decade ago implicated α4-integrin expression at the primary tumor site as an important inhibitor for dyshesive growth. At the same time, however, once metastatic cells are present in the blood, α4-integrin expression appeared to aid in transendothelial migration at specific tissues.[214,215] Future studies will likely clarify the potential risks posed by natalizumab therapy with regard to development and progression of melanoma. The authors have encountered a patient with multiple sclerosis who developed urticarial plaques while taking natalizumab, with a dermal hypersensitivity morphology on biopsy (**Fig. 7**).

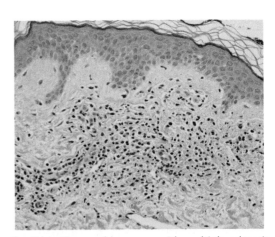

Fig. 7. A 48-year-old woman with multiple sclerosis was started on natalizumab (Tysabri) and within 1 week developed a fixed urticarial rash involving the back, chest, and left thigh. Skin biopsy showed a superficial to mid dermal interstitial and perivascular lymphocytic and histiocytic infiltrate with accompanying eosinophils, compatible with a dermal hypersensitivity reaction.

ADVERSE CUTANEOUS REACTIONS TO INTRAVENOUS IMMUNOGLOBULIN THERAPY

Because of its favorable safety profile, intravenous immunoglobulin (IVIG) therapy for a wide range of neurologic, dermatologic, and rheumatologic conditions has gained in popularity over recent years. As reviewed here, there has been an association between the use of IVIG and eruptions of eczematous lesions, most frequently affecting the palms and soles, which are usually self-limited and resolve after withdrawing IVIG treatment; some have required topical or systemic corticosteroids. In the vast majority of cases, treatments are well tolerated by patients, with minor adverse effects including headache, chills, myalgias, arthralgias, and nausea, but relatively few significant adverse effects.[216,217] The frequency of localized and generalized cutaneous adverse effects associated with IVIG varies between 0.4% and 6%.[218–220] As early as 1997 reports began to emerge that suggested an association between eczema and IVIG therapy.[221] The current literature contains more than 60 cases of IVIG-associated eczematous reactions.[221–243] Patients' ages ranged from 7 years to the mid 70s, with the majority falling in the fifth through seventh decades of life. More than half of the patients presented with a picture of dyshidrotic eczema/pompholyx, which typically presented during the first infusion of IVIG, often within 5 to 10 days. Pompholyx is a relatively rare manifestation within the broader classification of eczema and can be seen following a variety of stimuli, including allergic and irritant contact reactions and dermatophytids. Among a series of 120 patients with pompholyx, IVIG was identified as the likely etiologic agent in only 1.[232] Outside the context of IVIG use, pompholyx does not exhibit an unbalanced gender distribution[244] while the majority of the patients experiencing this reaction in association with IVIG were males, perhaps signifying a male predominance for the underlying conditions being treated with IVIG, such as multifocal motor neuropathy,[240] chronic inflammatory demyelinating polyneuropathy,[239] and Guillain-Barré syndrome.[228,229,233]

IVIG is composed of pooled IgG from the plasma of more than 1000 blood donors that is subsequently processed to remove infectious agents, with variable allowances for the level of immunoglobulin A content, sucrose, glucose, and preservatives. No single IVIG preparation is associated with the development of eczematous reactions, implying that formulation alone was not responsible, but there have been cases whereby switching between different manufacturers resulted in improvement.[222] Whether this represents desensitization with subsequent infusions or a true variability in the reactivity of various IVIG products is unclear, as is the mechanism underlying IVIG-associated eczematous reactions as a whole.

There are 2 separate reports of IVIG reactions associated with hypocomplementemia of C4 with accompanying low levels of CH50[222] or CH100.[238] In the case reported by Sarmiento and colleagues,[238] a 39-year-old man receiving IVIG for progressive myopathy developed a widely distributed erythrodermic eczematous reaction and pompholyx with new-onset hypocomplementemia of C4 with low CH100, the levels of which normalized alongside resolution of the skin reaction. It was hypothesized that low complement levels might represent the formation of immune complexes containing fixed complement that triggered the observed skin reaction. Elevated IgG complement-fixing immune complexes have been observed in children with atopic eczema.[245] Hypocomplementemia of C4 has led some investigators to suggest that complement-fixing immune complexes may play a role in the pathogenesis. It has been noted in cell-culture studies that IgG has the capacity to regulate the CD1 expression profile of dendritic cells. High IgG levels promote the expression of CD1d with low levels of CD1a, CD1b, and CD1c. IVIG treatment reverses this pattern of expression.[246] Eczematous skin harbors elevated numbers of CD1a-positive Langerhans cells when compared with normal skin.[247] Whether IVIG treatment influences the numbers of CD1a-expressing dendritic cells in the skin or the levels of CD1a expression in patients who develop the eczematous reaction has yet to be determined, although this remains an interesting question in light of the differential self-antigen versus foreign-antigen-presenting capabilities of the different isoforms.[248–252]

CUTANEOUS DRUG REACTIONS ASSOCIATED WITH CHRONIC HYDROXYUREA THERAPY

Hydroxyurea or hydroxycarbamide is an antineoplastic agent that interferes with DNA synthesis by way of ribonucleotide reductase inhibition, and is used in the treatment of myeloproliferative disorders, including chronic myelogenous leukemia (CML), essential thrombocythemia, and polycythemia vera. It has been used as a treatment for recalcitrant psoriasis[253–255] and as a means to reduce the frequency of painful attacks in patients with sickle-cell disease.[256,257] Well-known systemic and metabolic side effects include leukopenia and thrombocytopenia, but there are also less well-known cutaneous sequelae of long-term hydroxyurea use.

Pseudodermatomyositis with Chronic Hydroxyurea Therapy

For many years it was recognized that patients undergoing long-term hydroxyurea therapy were subject to a host of skin reactions including xerosis, pigmentary change, ulcer formation, alopecia, palmar/plantar keratoderma, tissue atrophy, and chromonychia.[258–261] Many of these reactions are common to the antineoplastic agents as a family. The first reports of hydroxyurea-induced erythematosquamous lesions involving the dorsa of metacarpophalangeal and interphalangeal joints came in 1975 with a description of 3 patients treated for CML who developed lesions 3 to 4 years after initiation of therapy.[258] Following this initial report, Burns and colleagues[262] reported a 31-year-old male patient with similar lesions that developed after 7 years of therapy. In 1984, Sigal and colleagues[261] published a report describing 3 additional patients presenting with band-like erythema on the dorsum of the fingers and toes in a morphology that was highly reminiscent of dermatomyositis. There have since been widespread reports of what has since been referred to as pseudodermatomyositis lesions after chronic hydroxyurea therapy,[263–278] typified by the erythematous, linear, scaly plaques often on the dorsal aspect of the interphalangeal and metacarpophalangeal joints. Lesions can also develop outside the classic joint distribution and may include scaly, poikilodermatous plaques or violaceous papules on the feet, elbows, palms, and face. Facial involvement can also result in edema (**Fig. 8**A, B). Atrophic change with the development of telangiectasias is common, similar to that seen in dermatomyositis proper.[270] In many such cases there were concomitant ulcers, most commonly affecting the legs and feet.[279–285]

Skin biopsies show perivascular mononuclear cell infiltrates with vacuolar degeneration of basal keratinocytes and accumulation of colloid bodies in the papillary dermis (**Fig. 8**C). Reaction patterns such as these are nonspecific and support a differential diagnosis that includes dermatomyositis, poikiloderma, lichenoid reactions, and graft-versus-host disease. There is no accompanying muscle involvement in hydroxyurea-associated dermatomyositis-like reactions. Prolonged presence of lesions has been suggested to lead to an atrophied, cigarette paper–like appearance that can be characterized by signs of accelerated physiologic photoaging of the skin, seen histologically as severe dermal elastosis.[286] The mechanism that underlies the dermatomyositis-like lesions that develop with chronic hydroxyurea is still uncertain, but similar reactions have been observed for a variety of medications including several statins,[287–289] penicillamine,[290] bacillus Calmette-Guérin vaccination,[291]

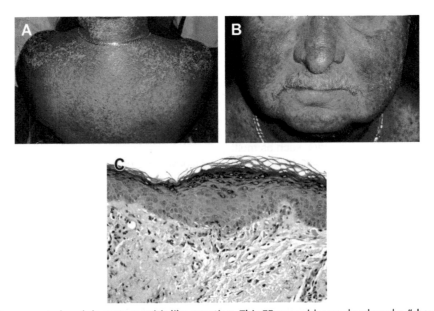

Fig. 8. Hydroxyurea-induced dermatomyositis-like eruption. This 55-year-old man developed a "shawl sign" (A) with superimposed scale and marked facial edema (B) while on hydroxyurea. Skin biopsy showed a cell-poor interface dermatitis with postinflammatory pigment incontinence and vascular density reduction of the superficial vascular plexus, mimicking dermatomyositis (C). (*Courtesy of* Dr George Monks, Tulsa, OK.)

the 5-fluorouracil derivative tegafur,[292] cyclophosphamide, and etoposide.[293] It is interesting that psoriasis patients who are treated with lower doses of hydroxyurea experience mucocutaneous reactions, pigmentation of nails and skin, and occasionally xerosis and alopecia, but do not appear to develop dermatomyositis-like reactions with the same frequency as do those patients with myeloproliferative disorders.[283,294] This finding suggests that perhaps dose and underlying disease state influence the pathogenesis.

Nonmelanoma Skin Cancers and Hydroxyurea

As far back as the early 1980s it was recognized that hydroxyurea had the potential to enhance tumorigenesis in the skin of mice when administered before exposure to the carcinogen N-methyl-N-nitrosourea.[295] There have been many observations of the propensity for patients using hydroxyurea to develop accelerated photoaging and actinic damage of the skin. Disdier and colleagues[296] were the first to report an association between the rapid development of SCC and the use of hydroxyurea in a CML patient. Patients tend to develop NMSC in sun-exposed and non–sun-exposed areas after a 2- to 13-year latency period,[271,297–308] while precursor epithelial dysplasia has also been observed to improve after discontinuation of hydroxyurea therapy.[309] There has been a report of Merkel cell carcinoma arising in a patient using hydroxyurea.[310] Most reported SCC cases arose in patients with Fitzpatrick skin types I and II, primarily in sun-exposed areas. For these lesions, ultraviolet (UV) irradiation and mutagenesis is likely to have played a role, but the temporal association and the well-documented latency period suggest that hydroxyurea participates in the process. By interfering with DNA synthesis, hydroxyurea inhibits DNA damage repair mechanisms that would normally be triggered by UV-induced DNA damage.[311] Hydroxyurea is also converted into free radical nitroxide within cells, which can inflict oxidative damage on cellular proteins and lipids as well as disrupt normal biosynthetic and signaling pathways that control growth and proliferation.[312] Random mutations in p53 as a primary initiating event is postulated in sporadic SCC, and normal UV-exposed skin harbors pockets of cells carrying p53 mutations[313] that expand with further exposure.[314] Chronic oxidative stress provided by hydroxyurea-derived nitroxides is also a source of tumor promotion that, in concert with UVB irradiation, tips the balance toward rapid development and progression of precancerous lesions. Skin biopsy specimens from hydroxyurea-induced pseudodermatomyositis patients have demonstrated aberrant p53 expression patterns, coinciding in at least one patient with the development of NMSCs that prompted cessation of therapy and eventual death due to myelodysplasia.[309,315]

Ulcer Formation Following Hydroxyurea Administration

Some patients who presented with pseudodermatomyositis lesions following long-term (ie, more than 5 years) use of hydroxyurea developed painful, fibrous, recalcitrant ulcers of the leg, often accompanied by surrounding atrophy,[281,316–327] characteristically localized to the malleolar or perimalleolar regions. Ulcers can also arise independently of the dermatomyositis-like reactions. In one large series, it was reported that the first occurrence was associated with multiple ulcers in 70% of the patients.[327] Although ulcers on the leg typify the distribution pattern of this reaction, there have been cases reported with the feet and genitalia predominantly involved.[328,329] Biopsied ulcers typically manifest epidermal atrophy and dermal fibrosis in the absence of an underlying vascular injury such as a leukocytoclastic vasculitis or diabetic microangiopathy (**Fig. 9A–C**).[327] Thrombotic microangiopathy may be seen (**Fig. 10**).

In one large series of patients with chronic myeloproliferative disease who developed leg ulcers, the mean duration of the ulcers was 10 months, despite attentive wound care. Cessation of hydroxyurea was necessary to achieve resolution of the ulcers, which typically resolved within 3 months of discontinuation.[327] There is a variety of treatment protocols aimed at speeding the resolution of hydroxyurea-induced ulcers, which include prostaglandin E_1/pentoxifylline combinations,[330] granulocyte-macrophage colony-stimulating factor,[331] Apligraf,[332] topical fibroblast growth factor,[333] or use of a protease-modulating matrix.[334]

The antimetabolic properties of hydroxyurea are likely to blame for the pathogenesis of the associated ulcers. Slowing of keratinocyte turnover and growth impedes wound repair at the level of the basal keratinocyte layer, which is damaged secondary to either hydroxyurea dermopathy or concomitant microtrauma, as is common on the legs.[316,319,320,335] Velez and colleagues[336] has suggested that macroerythrocytosis (a common laboratory finding associated with the use of hydroxyurea that arises from inhibition of DNA synthesis) may contribute to the development of ulceration. Indeed, there is generally an increase of roughly 12% in size of red blood cells

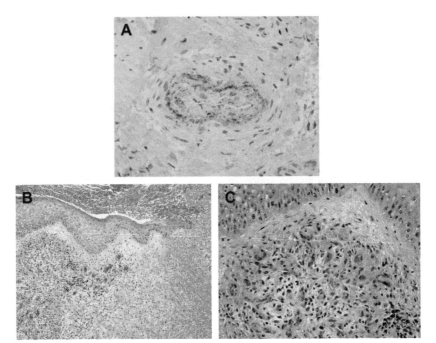

Fig. 9. (*A, B*) A 71-year-old woman with a long-standing history of polycythemia vera on hydroxyurea developed 6-cm ulcers on the lower extremity. A skin biopsy showed an ulcer associated with glomeruloid neovascularization, indicating an ischemic-based etiology. The glomeruloid foci manifest luminal and mural fibrin deposition, defining the presence of a pauci-inflammatory necrotizing thrombotic diathesis. There is prominent deposition of C5b-9 within vessels (*C*).

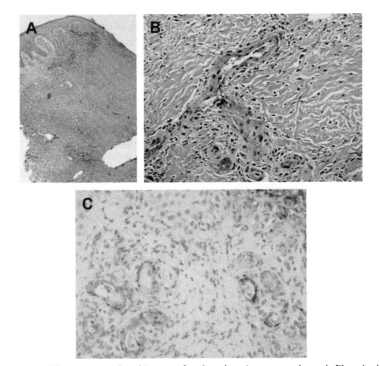

Fig. 10. (*A, B*) A 54-year-old woman with a history of polycythemia vera and myelofibrosis developed painful ankle ulcers on hydroxyurea and interferon. Biopsies showed epidermal and dermal necrosis associated with compensatory glomeruloid neovascularization with occlusive luminal thrombi accompanied by ectatic vessels, defining a pattern that is atrophie blanche/livedoid vasculopathy-like but with evidence of an underlying procoagulant state with vascular thrombosis. The C5b-9 assay shows extensive deposition in the blood vessels in the zones of glomeruloid neovascularization (*C*). Based on the extreme degree of C5b-9 deposition, the patient received eculizumab (Soliris), with an excellent clinical response.

associated with a corresponding decrease in deformability,[337] which could theoretically lead to reduced microvascular perfusion and parallel the ulceration seen with arterial insufficiency. Ulcer patients who were transitioned from hydroxyurea to pipobroman saw a subsequent decrease in the mean corpuscular volume from 121 μm^3 to 100 μm^3 over the course of a month with subsequent ulcer resolution.[327] Wirth and colleagues[338] explored a possible role of hydroxyurea-resistant thrombocytosis in ulcer formation in a 54-year-old woman with CML who showed improvement following anagrelide treatment to normalize platelet counts. The interpretation of this finding is clouded, however, by the paucity of data relating thrombocytosis and ulcer formation, along with the distinct possibility that the ulcers were due to the preceding, year-long course of hydroxyurea and the fact that healing coincided with discontinuation of hydroxyurea 5 months prior.[339]

ADVERSE CUTANEOUS REACTIONS TO OTHER CHEMOTHERAPY DRUGS

Other chemotherapeutic agents to exhibit cutaneous toxicities, especially with prolonged use, are reviewed elsewhere.[340-342]

Sunitinib (Sutent)

Sunitinib is a multitargeted tyrosine kinase inhibitor that is used to treat renal cell carcinoma and imatinib-resistant gastrointestinal stromal tumors (GISTs). The mechanism of action is one of inhibition of various tyrosine kinases, including VEGF receptor, platelet-derived growth factor receptor, and CD117. Mucocutaneous reactions include stomatitis and an acneiform folliculitis with acrosyringeal accentuation (**Fig. 11**); the authors have also

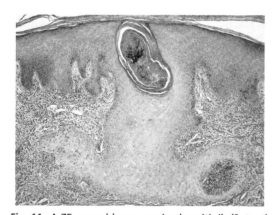

Fig. 11. A 75-year-old man received sunitinib (Sutent) for colon cancer. He developed an acneiform eruption that showed a neutrophilic pustular reaction of hair follicles and acrosyringia on biopsy.

observed a photodistributed eruption mimicking subacute cutaneous lupus erythematosus.

RETIFORM PURPURA IN ASSOCIATION WITH LEVAMISOLE-ADULTERATED COCAINE

The past several years have seen numerous reports of a distinct vasculitis-like syndrome with retiform purpura (**Fig. 12A**), frequently involving the earlobes and face in association with the use of levamisole-adulterated cocaine.[343-348] Levamisole is an anthelmintic with a well-documented capacity to induce vasculitic and thrombotic damage. Leukopenia, neutropenia, antiphospholipid antibodies, and antineutrophil cytoplasmic antibodies (ANCAs) have been reported in these patients alongside microvascular thrombosis and occasional small-vessel vasculitis (**Fig. 12B, D**).

More than 70% of cocaine shipments seized on entry into the United States have been found to contain levamisole,[349] and 194 of 249 (78%) cocaine-positive urine toxicology studies at a 500-bed Denver hospital tested positive for levamisole using gas chromatography–mass spectrometry.[350]

The earliest reports of vasculitis associated with use of cocaine described involvement of small vessels of the cerebral circulation.[351-355] In vitro studies suggest that cocaine use facilitates the migration of monocytes across the blood-brain barrier and, as a result, may contribute to the development of vasculitis.[356] Generalized cutaneous vasculitic lesions of the skin and Henoch-Schönlein purpura with necrotizing vasculitis have been reported following cocaine use,[346,357] as has upper extremity large-vessel vasculitis diagnosed by angiography.[358] There has been a single report of Stevens-Johnson syndrome related to the use of cocaine[359] in a patient who had used cocaine on a daily basis for an extended period and reported the lesions only after procuring cocaine from a new source, suggesting that these lesions represented the effect of an adulterant not present in the previous supply. A similar presentation with scrotal gangrene requiring debridement was reported in a 22-year-old man 3 hours after smoking crack cocaine.[360] An association between smoking of crack cocaine and Churg-Strauss vasculitis has been suggested in one case report, with eosinophilic angiitis seen on skin and muscle biopsies.[361] Necrotizing granulomatous vasculitis associated with nasal destruction has also been reported in a chronic cocaine user,[362] although most cases involving loss of nasal tissue do not show granulomatous infiltrates. Though considered controversial, there has been a suggestion that some patients with Buerger disease may actually represent the sequelae of recreational cocaine use

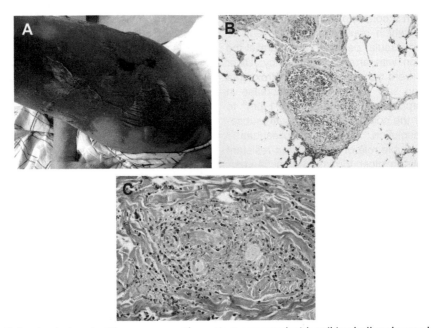

Fig. 12. (*A, B*) Cocaine-induced retiform purpura. The patient presented with striking bullous hemorrhagic infarction of the upper and lower extremities. There is epidermal and dermal necrosis extending to the dermal subcutaneous interface. (*C*) The histopathology of cocaine-induced retiform purpura is varied. Likely at the inception of the vasculopathy is endothelial cell apoptosis with denudement and concomitant vascular thrombosis, resulting in a pauci-inflammatory thrombogenic vasculopathy, well exemplified by this photomicrograph. The chronicity of the process is revealed by the organizing luminal thrombi with neovascularization. The thrombotic diathesis involves both the venous and arterial systems.

because of the significant overlap of the clinico-pathologic presentations.[363]

The term cocaine-induced pseudovasculitis has been floated in the literature to reflect the observation that cocaine use in some patients produces symptoms mimicking Wegener granulomatosis (WG) without producing the histopathologic findings of a true vasculitis.[364–366] Differentiation between a true vasculitis (such as WG) and the pseudovasculitis associated with cocaine use is important, because it spares the patient unnecessary treatment with high-dose corticosteroids and immunosuppressants. The use of ANCA positivity to differentiate vasculitis versus pseudovasculitis has been flagged as a potential pitfall, as there are situations whereby proteinase-3 (PR3)-ANCA (or cytoplasmic ANCA [C-ANCA]) is positive in individuals using cocaine.[367–369] Whereas the PR3-ANCA may not reliably differentiate cocaine-induced lesions from WG, human neutrophil elastase ANCA (HNE-ANCA) has been proposed as a more discriminating assay, as it is positive following cocaine abuse.

Levamisole was introduced in 1966 as an anthelmintic agent before the recognition that it possessed antitumor properties useful in the adjunctive treatment of colon cancer, melanoma,

and cancers of the head and neck. It was apparent early on that it could induce agranulocytosis,[370] and could stimulate circulating immune complexes leading to vasculitis,[371,372] typically a mixed leukocytoclastic vasculitis with microvascular thrombosis or microvascular thrombosis alone (**Fig. 12**C, D).[373] Levamisole acts as a hapten, which can trigger the immune response.[373,374] Children who were treated for nephrotic syndrome with levamisole occasionally went on to develop a vasculitic picture that was accompanied by circulating antinuclear, antiphospholipid, and anti-cytoplasmic autoantibodies that persisted long after the resolution of the skin lesions.[373] Because of the high incidence of adverse effects, the drug was withdrawn from the market by the FDA in 2000, but remains in use primarily as a deworming agent in veterinary medicine. Beginning in 2005, levamisole surfaced as a cutting agent in cocaine samples within the United States, possibly because of its stimulant-enhancing properties and similar appearance to cocaine.

Beginning in 2010 a handful of reports emerged describing patients, frequently female, who presented with distinctive retiform purpuric lesions of varying severity often localized to the ears, cheeks, nose, and extremities (see

Table 1 for a summary of reported cases) in the setting of current or recent cocaine use. The similarity of the lesions to the morphology and distribution reported previously for levamisole,[373] taken together with Drug Enforcement Agency reports of the rise of levamisole contamination in street cocaine, led to the recognition that these reactions were likely due to the presence of this cutting agent. Biopsies from the majority of patients reported in Table 1 showed microvascular thrombosis, leukocytoclastic vasculitis, or a mixture of both.[375–380] Neutropenia was a common finding in the majority of patients, although there were several patients with normal absolute neutrophil counts at presentation. Consistent with prior reports of autoantibody formation following levamisole exposure, 88% of the cases reviewed in Table 1 were perinuclear-ANCA or C-ANCA positive, often PR3-ANCA, myeloperoxidase-ANCA, and HNE-ANCA subtypes. Anticardiolipin antibody was positive in 13 patients (52%), and 20% of patients had positive antinuclear antibody (ANA) tests. Several patients were also found to have elevated erythrocyte sedimentation rate, C-reactive protein, D-dimer, and partial thromboplastin time. One patient exhibited low protein C and protein S levels.[378,379] Patients often presented with a history of spontaneously resolving lesions that would recur whenever they used cocaine, whereas others had persistent lesions that responded to treatment with steroids or antibiotics (see Table 1). In one patient whose lesions failed to resolve spontaneously or with steroids, surgical debridement was necessary, followed by multiple reconstructive procedures.[380] Although neutropenia was severe in some patients after their exposure to levamisole, most rebounded spontaneously to normal neutrophil counts after sustained abstinence from adulterated cocaine or following filgrastim (G-CSF) therapy.[379–385]

CUTANEOUS DRUG REACTIONS WITH INTERFERON THERAPY

IFN proteins are host-derived defenses released in response to viral, bacterial, and parasitic pathogens, and also provide a host response to tumor cells. IFN-α is a type I IFN produced by leukocytes, which has also become very useful in synthetic forms as a treatment for a variety of human diseases. IFN-α2a has been approved for treatment of hairy-cell leukemia,[386,387] AIDS-related Kaposi sarcoma,[388,389] Behçet disease,[390,391] and CML.[392,393] IFN-α2b is approved for use in hepatitis B and C,[394,395] melanoma,[396,397] condyloma acuminata,[398] and Kaposi sarcoma.

Injection-Site Reactions

As with many of the biological agents, hypersensitivity and injection-site reactions have occasionally been associated with IFN-α although they are infrequently reported in the literature. Maurtua and colleagues[399] reported a patient who developed injection-site erythema and induration after starting a second round of IFN-α2b, in whom skin biopsy showed a sparse perivascular mixed inflammatory infiltrate with activated CD8[+], HLA-DR[+] T cells on flow cytometry, consistent with a delayed type hypersensitivity reaction, as has also been reported for recombinant IFN-α2c.[400] Broad sensitivity to the class has been noted in a patient who developed an urticarial skin reaction following 2 different formulations of pegylated IFN, but treatment was continued and the symptoms were adequately managed with topical steroids and antihistamines.[401]

In addition to the hypersensitivity reactions reported, there have been several reports of necrotizing cutaneous lesions at the site of IFN-α injections[402,403] associated with a necrotizing vasculitis. The mechanism underlying this reaction pattern is unclear, and may be due to the high concentration of the drug present at the site of the injection or preservatives present in the preparation. Variation in the injection site is recommended to avoid this potential complication.

Psoriasis with Interferon-α Therapy

One of the more commonly observed cutaneous reactions with IFN-α is the de novo development of psoriatic lesions[404–410] or exacerbation of pre-existing psoriasis.[411–420] It is well established that IFN-α plays an important role in activating the immune response against infectious agents, and mounting evidence from these reports indicates that it also has the potential to trigger or accelerate the aberrant immune-system activity underlying psoriasis. Plasmacytoid dendritic cells (PDCs) are the natural factories for IFN-α production; trophic to the skin of psoriasis patients, they become activated and produce large quantities of IFN-α that promote disease activity. Inhibition of IFN-α production by the PDCs prevents the development of psoriasis.[421] T cells derived from psoriasis patients have increased sensitivity and prolonged responses to IFN-α.[422] Boyman and colleagues[423] showed that transient expression of IFN-α was implicated in the proliferation of T cells during development of early-stage psoriasis but was not found at elevated levels once the disease was fully established in plaque stage.[424]

Table 1
Reported cases of cocaine-associated retiform purpura and vasculitis

Authors[Ref.]	Age/Sex	Distribution	Neutropenia	Autoantibodies	Treatment and Outcome
Chung et al[380]	46, F	b/l ears, cheeks, upper and lower extremities	No	MPO- and PR3-ANCA+, anticardiolipin IgM+	Steroids (improved)
	57, F	b/l ears and cheeks	Yes	MPO- and PR3-ANCA+, anticardiolipin IgM+	IV antibiotics and filgrastim (improved)
	46, F	b/l ears, neck, trunk, extremities	Yes	P-ANCA+, C-ANCA+, anticardiolipin IgM+	Methylprednisone (improved)
	22, F	b/l ears, cheeks, nose, buttocks, thighs	Yes	P-ANCA+, anticardiolipin IgM+	Methylprednisone (improved)
	37, M	b/l ears	No	P-ANCA+, elevated CRP, ESR, D-dimer; +ANA	Supportive
	50, M	b/l ears, trunk, extremities	No	P-ANCA+, elevated CRP, ESR, D-dimer, PTT; +ANA	Antibiotics (rapidly improved)
Farhat et al[374]	43, F	b/l lower extremities	N/A	P-ANCA+	Pain control
	41, F	b/l thighs, buttocks, trunk, upper extremities, nose	N/A	P-ANCA+, anticardiolipin IgM+	N/A
Buchanan et al[381]	N/A, M	b/l ears	Yes	N/A	Supportive
Walsh et al[375]	39, F	Legs and trunk	N/A	HNE-ANCA+, P-ANCA+, C-ANCA+, +ANA	N/A
	49, F	Legs and trunk	Yes	HNE-ANCA+, P-ANCA+, C-ANCA+, +ANA, elevated ESR	N/A
Waller et al[376]	38, F	Ear, cheeks, right breast, b/l upper and lower extremities	Yes	PR3-ANCA+, lupus anticoagulant+	N/A
	43, F	b/l lower extremity and ear, b/l arms and thighs	Yes	MPO-ANCA+, elevated PTT, anti-dsDNA+, lupus anticoagulant+, anticardiolipin IgM+	N/A
Lung et al[382]	44, F	b/l lower extremities, abdomen, face	Yes	N/A	N/A

Study	Age, Sex	Location		Laboratory findings	Treatment (outcome)
Ullrich et al[383]	45, M	Extremities and ears	Yes	P-ANCA+, MPO- and PR3-ANCA+, anticardiolipin IgM+, +ANA	Prednisone (with some improvement)
	49, F	Trunk and extremities	Yes	C-ANCA+, PR3-ANCA+	Conservative
	27, F	Lower extremities	Yes	P-ANCA+, MPO- and PR3-ANCA+	Prednisone (improved)
	29, F	Left foot and b/l ears	No	P-ANCA+, MPO- and PR3-ANCA+, anticardiolipin IgM+	Prednisone (improved)
	55, F	Face, trunk and extremities	No	P-ANCA+, MPO- and PR3-ANCA+, anticardiolipin IgM+, thyroglobulin and thyroid peroxidase antibody+	Steroids and cyclophosphamide (improved)
Fthenakis and Klein[377]	48, F	Face, abdomen, legs	No	+ANA, mildly reduced protein C and protein S	Spontaneous remission with relapse
Bradford et al[378]	57, F	b/l cheeks and earlobes	Yes	P-ANCA+, anticardiolipin IgM+	Filgrastim and spontaneous skin resolution
	22, F	Face, ears, legs, thighs, buttocks	Yes	P-ANCA+, anticardiolipin IgM+, serine IgM+	Steroids (resolved)
Muirhead and Eide[379]	54, F	Face, ears, breasts, extremities	Yes	P-ANCA+, C-ANCA+	Steroids (unresolved) and debridement
Han et al[384]	52, F	Arms, legs, nose, cheeks, ears	Yes	P-ANCA+, PR3-ANCA+, anticardiolipin IgM+	Steroids, dalteparin (improved)
Geller et al[385]	50, F	b/l arms, breasts, upper back, ears	Yes	Anticardiolipin IgM+, P-ANCA+, elevated CRP	N/A

Abbreviations: +, positive; ANA, antinuclear antibody; ANCA, antineutrophil cytoplasmic antibody; b/l, bilateral; C-ANCA, cytoplasmic ANCA; P-ANCA, perinuclear ANCA; CRP, C-reactive protein; dsDNA, double-stranded DNA; ESR, erythrocyte sedimentation rate; F, female; HNE, human neutrophil elastase; IgM, immunoglobulin M; IV, intravenous; M, male; MPO, myeloperoxidase; N/A, no data available; PR3, proteinase 3; PTT, partial thromboplastin time.

When psoriatic lesions develop in patients treated with IFN-α, there is a variety of therapeutic options including acitretin, a second-generation retinoid used frequently in patients with chronic psoriasis that has been used successfully to treat IFN-α–triggered psoriasis,[418] and UV light, effective in exacerbations of psoriasis in this setting.[425]

Cutaneous Sarcoidosis in Patients Using Interferon-α

Beginning in the mid to late 1990s, there were scattered reports of patients using IFN-α for hepatitis C and CML who later developed papules, macules, and subcutaneous nodules consistent with features of sarcoidosis, confirmed by skin biopsies.[426,427] Over the next decade, a substantial number of similar cases were reported for patients using IFN-α to treat a wide range of diseases including melanoma, RA, CML, and hepatitis C.[428–456] Lesions developed in patients receiving both pegylated and nonpegylated forms of IFN-α. In many cases, there was both systemic and cutaneous disease.

Sarcoidosis patients suffer sarcoidal granulomata that present as nodules in various organs such as lungs, lymph nodes, and skin; in the skin these manifest as macules, papules, and plaques distributed singly or in groups. As these granulomas are generally believed to be a host response to microbial pathogens or foreign material, it is not surprising that patients treated with IFN-α who go on to develop sarcoidosis will express lesions in skin that has been injected with facial fillers,[440,444] or at sites of tattoos[431,434,435,446,457] or prior trauma with introduced foreign material.[443]

Despite speculation that these observations of cutaneous sarcoidosis are related more to the underlying disease than to the use of IFN-α,[458] human genetics studies suggested otherwise. In a cohort of Japanese patients with sarcoidosis, investigators found overrepresentation of an IFN-α allele that is associated with higher levels of expression, suggesting that IFN-α itself is a likely culprit in the pathogenesis.[459] High levels of IFN-α have been shown to induce the expression of STAT1,[460] which has also been hypothesized as a key pathogenetic factor in the development of sarcoidosis.[461]

Sarcoidal granulomata contain epithelioid histiocytes and encircling $CD4^+$ T lymphocytes of the T-helper cells type 1 (Th1) subset, which secrete IL-2 and IFN-γ.[462] Phenotypic analysis of the T lymphocytes in patients with chronic sarcoidosis reveals a population of lymphocytes that are $CD4^+$, $CD28^-$, whereas normal lymphocyte populations are $CD28^+$.[463] In one patient with IFN-α–induced sarcoidosis, T-cell subtype analysis showed a dramatic diminution of CD28, which corresponds with a subtype of sarcoidosis that is generally characterized as having greater proinflammatory and tissue-damaging behavior.[447]

For patients who develop cutaneous (or systemic) sarcoidosis during their course of IFN-α treatment, withdrawal of the offending medication is considered an effective means of alleviating symptoms; the anti-TNFα monoclonal antibody infliximab has been proved to be therapeutically effective.[464] The success of this approach follows from the observation that activated Th1 cells secrete cytokines that activate macrophage production of TNFα, which further promotes the granulomatous response.[465]

Other Cutaneous Reactions Observed with Interferon-α

Other cutaneous reactions that have been reported, in more limited numbers, include development of oral aphthae, genital ulceration, erythema nodosum, and a positive pathergy test consistent with a picture of Behçet disease in a subset of CML patients using IFN-α.[466–468] Ironically, IFN-α is frequently used to manage Behçet disease.[390,391] In one study, 7 of 29 CML patients (24%) who were using IFN-α were found to have a positive pathergy test while none of the CML patients without IFN-α treatment (n = 15) reacted to the needle stick.[468] It was proposed that the development of pathergy, much like in Behçet disease, is due to IFN-α–mediated alterations in neutrophil activity in a malignant clone of cells.

Dalekos and colleagues[469] reported on 3 hepatitis patients who developed lichen planus (LP) while using IFN-α, with lesions developing 3 to 6 months after the initiation of treatment. Cessation of therapy was not required because of the mild nature of the lesions, which resolved promptly after therapy was completed. The investigators reported the presence of ANAs in these patients before the initiation of therapy, and suggested that the development of LP lesions might represent an autoimmune diathesis augmented by IFN-α. Hepatitis C virus (HCV) infection alone is considered an etiologic factor in the development of LP,[470] suggesting that the drug may not be a cause of the eruption in this setting. Reports of oral LP lesions worsening after initiation of pegylated IFN and ribavirin[471] suggest a possible facilitative role.

Although typical injection-site reactions were noted earlier, a series by Arrue and colleagues[472] described a distinct lupus-like reaction to IFN-α or IFN-β at injection sites in patients undergoing treatment for melanoma or multiple sclerosis. Skin biopsies showed dermal mucin deposition with dense periadnexal and interface lymphocytic dermatitis. The lupus-like lesions were self-resolving over a period of several weeks to months, but would occasionally develop anew at subsequent injection sites.

Atopic eczema-like lesions are among the less frequent cutaneous reactions induced by IFN-α.[473–475] In a case series of 20 patients using IFN-α and ribavirin to treat HCV infection, eczematoid lesions occurred on the extremities 2 to 4 months following the initiation of treatment; biopsies showing perivascular mononuclear cell infiltrates and skin testing for allergy to the treatment regimen were found to be nonpredictive of relapse.[475] The immunomodulatory role of IFN, as opposed to a specific allergic mechanism, is suggested.[473] Some investigators have considered the expression of eczema as a rationale for discontinuation of treatment, but others recommend use of topical corticosteroids and emollients to permit continued IFN therapy for the underlying disease.[476,477]

An unusual transient eczematous eruption surrounding melanocytic nevi, known as the Meyerson phenomenon, has been noted in several patients treated with IFN-α and ribavirin,[478,479] including one patient with dysplastic nevus syndrome.[480] The pigmented nevi with this halo pattern do not undergo regressive change as seen in classic halo nevi.

Lingual hyperpigmentation has been reported in a handful of cases to date in chronic HCV patients using pegylated IFN-α and ribavirin.[481–485] A similar case series reported hyperpigmented patches on the upper arms and thighs, including over injection sites, with biopsies showing increased focal epidermal keratinocyte pigmentation, perivascular lymphocytic infiltrate in the superficial dermis, numerous pigmented macrophages, and lack of hemosiderin deposition.[486] The mechanism for this rarely encountered hyperpigmentation is not entirely understood, although there is speculation that upregulation of melanocyte stimulating hormone receptors and increased production of the corresponding ligand are potentially involved.[483] Patients with darker skin appear to develop these hyperpigmented lesions with greater frequency, as do patients who use the pegylated form of IFN, presumably because of higher serum concentrations and a longer half-life.[482]

Combined IFN-α and ribavirin treatment has been associated with reversible[487–489] or irreversible[490] alopecia. Hair regrowth usually began within 3 months of completion of treatment and because the vast majority of the observed cases have been reversible, patients can usually continue treatment until virologic response has been achieved.

Two separate reports describe patients developing lesions of pyoderma gangrenosum during a course of IFN-α therapy.[420,491] In one of the patients in whom the lesions developed, TNF, IL-6, and soluble IL-2 receptor were elevated at the time when the lesion appeared, and subsequently fell to within normal limits at the time that the lesion healed following discontinuation of IFN-α and treatment with prednisone and cyclosporine A.[491] Sanders and colleagues[492] described 2 patients with ulcerating, erythematous plaques with granulomatous and suppurative dermatitis, which demonstrated histopathology remarkably similar to that seen in pyoderma gangrenosum, including intravascular thrombi.[493]

SUMMARY

With novel drugs coming to market as specific targeted therapies for neoplastic and autoinflammatory disease, the medical community is entering hitherto uncharted territory. Pathologists must be alert for perplexing reactions and symptom complexes with which they are unfamiliar, and be prepared to alert their colleagues in clinical medicine, the pharmaceutical industry, and regulatory agencies to these previously undescribed or ill-recognized adverse reactions.

REFERENCES

1. Smith SL. Ten years of Orthoclone OKT3 (muromonab-CD3): a review. J Transpl Coord 1996;6(3): 109–19 [quiz: 120–1].
2. Rahier JF, Buche S, Peyrin-Biroulet L, et al. Severe skin lesions cause patients with inflammatory bowel disease to discontinue anti-tumor necrosis factor therapy. Clin Gastroenterol Hepatol 2010;8(12):1048–55.
3. Moreland LW, Schiff MH, Baumgartner SW, et al. Etanercept therapy in rheumatoid arthritis. A randomized, controlled trial. Ann Intern Med 1999;130(6):478–86.
4. Tyring S, Gottleib A, Papp K, et al. Etanercept and clinical outcomes, fatigue, and depression in psoriasis: double-blind placebo-controlled randomised phase III trial. Lancet 2006;367(9504):29–35.
5. Papp KA, Tyring S, Lahfa M, et al. A global phase III randomized controlled trial of etanercept in psoriasis: safety, efficacy, and effect of dose reduction. Br J Dermatol 2005;152(6):1304–12.
6. Zeltser R, Valle L, Tanck C, et al. Clinical, histological, and immunophenotypic characteristics of injection site reactions associated with etanercept: a recombinant tumor necrosis factor alpha

receptor: Fc fusion protein. Arch Dermatol 2001; 137(7):893–9.

7. Mease PJ, Gladman DD, Ritchlin CT, et al. Adalimumab for the treatment of patients with moderately to severely active psoriatic arthritis: results of a double-blind, randomized, placebo-controlled trial. Arthritis Rheum 2005;52(10):3279–89.

8. Menter A, Tyring SK, Gordon K, et al. Adalimumab therapy for moderate to severe psoriasis: a randomized, controlled phase III trial. J Am Acad Dermatol 2008;58(1):106–15.

9. van de Putte LB, Atkins C, Malaise M, et al. Efficacy and safety of adalimumab as monotherapy in patients with rheumatoid arthritis for whom previous disease modifying antirheumatic drug treatment has failed. Ann Rheum Dis 2004;63(5):508–16.

10. Colombel JF, Sandborn WJ, Rutgeerts P, et al. Adalimumab for maintenance of clinical response and remission in patients with Crohn's disease: the CHARM trial. Gastroenterology 2007;132(1): 52–65.

11. Edwards KR, Mowad CM, Tyler WB. Worsening injection site reactions with continued use of etanercept. J Drugs Dermatol 2003;2(2):184–7.

12. Leonardi CL, Papp KA, Gordon KB, et al. Extended efalizumab therapy improves chronic plaque psoriasis: results from a randomized phase III trial. J Am Acad Dermatol 2005;52(3 Pt 1):425–33.

13. Maini RN, Breedveld FC, Kalden JR, et al. Sustained improvement over two years in physical function, structural damage, and signs and symptoms among patients with rheumatoid arthritis treated with infliximab and methotrexate. Arthritis Rheum 2004;50(4):1051–65.

14. Kapetanovic MC, Larsson L, Truedsson L, et al. Predictors of infusion reactions during infliximab treatment in patients with arthritis. Arthritis Res Ther 2006;8(4):R131.

15. Colombel JF, Loftus EV Jr, Tremaine WJ, et al. The safety profile of infliximab in patients with Crohn's disease: the Mayo clinic experience in 500 patients. Gastroenterology 2004;126(1):19–31.

16. Cohen RD, Tsang JF, Hanauer SB. Infliximab in Crohn's disease: first anniversary clinical experience. Am J Gastroenterol 2000;95(12):3469–77.

17. Wolbink GJ, Vis M, Lems W, et al. Development of antiinfliximab antibodies and relationship to clinical response in patients with rheumatoid arthritis. Arthritis Rheum 2006;54(3):711–5.

18. Cheifetz A, Mayer L. Monoclonal antibodies, immunogenicity, and associated infusion reactions. Mt Sinai J Med 2005;72(4):250–6.

19. Sany J, Kaiser MJ, Jorgensen C, et al. Study of the tolerance of infliximab infusions with or without betamethasone premedication in patients with active rheumatoid arthritis. Ann Rheum Dis 2005;64(11): 1647–9.

20. Wasserman MJ, Weber DA, Guthrie JA, et al. Infusion-related reactions to infliximab in patients with rheumatoid arthritis in a clinical practice setting: relationship to dose, antihistamine pretreatment, and infusion number. J Rheumatol 2004;31(10): 1912–7.

21. Jacobstein DA, Markowitz JE, Kirschner BS, et al. Premedication and infusion reactions with infliximab: results from a pediatric inflammatory bowel disease consortium. Inflamm Bowel Dis 2005; 11(5):442–6.

22. Farrell RJ, Alsahli M, Jeen YT, et al. Intravenous hydrocortisone premedication reduces antibodies to infliximab in Crohn's disease: a randomized controlled trial. Gastroenterology 2003;124(4): 917–24.

23. Kugathasan S, Levy MB, Saeian K, et al. Infliximab retreatment in adults and children with Crohn's disease: risk factors for the development of delayed severe systemic reaction. Am J Gastroenterol 2002; 97(6):1408–14.

24. Lee HH, Song IH, Friedrich M, et al. Cutaneous side-effects in patients with rheumatic diseases during application of tumour necrosis factor-alpha antagonists. Br J Dermatol 2007;156(3):486–91.

25. Flendrie M, Vissers WH, Creemers MC, et al. Dermatological conditions during TNF-alpha-blocking therapy in patients with rheumatoid arthritis: a prospective study. Arthritis Res Ther 2005;7(3): R666–76.

26. Bongartz T, Sutton AJ, Sweeting MJ, et al. Anti-TNF antibody therapy in rheumatoid arthritis and the risk of serious infections and malignancies: systematic review and meta-analysis of rare harmful effects in randomized controlled trials. JAMA 2006;295(19):2275–85.

27. Doran MF, Crowson CS, Pond GR, et al. Frequency of infection in patients with rheumatoid arthritis compared with controls: a population-based study. Arthritis Rheum 2002;46(9):2287–93.

28. Dixon WG, Watson K, Lunt M, et al. Rates of serious infection, including site-specific and bacterial intracellular infection, in rheumatoid arthritis patients receiving anti-tumor necrosis factor therapy: results from the British Society for Rheumatology Biologics Register. Arthritis Rheum 2006;54(8): 2368–76.

29. Strangfeld A, Listing J, Herzer P, et al. Risk of herpes zoster in patients with rheumatoid arthritis treated with anti-TNF-alpha agents. JAMA 2009; 301(7):737–44.

30. Paller AS, Siegfried EC, Eichenfield LF, et al. Long-term etanercept in pediatric patients with plaque psoriasis. J Am Acad Dermatol 2010; 63(5):762–8.

31. Paller AS, Siegfried EC, Langley RG, et al. Etanercept treatment for children and adolescents with

plaque psoriasis. N Engl J Med 2008;358(3): 241–51.

32. Sladden MJ, Clarke PJ, Mitchell B. Infliximab-induced acne: report of a third case. Br J Dermatol 2008;158(1):172.

33. Bassi E, Poli F, Charachon A, et al. Infliximab-induced acne: report of two cases. Br J Dermatol 2007;156(2):402–3.

34. Devos SA, Van Den Bossche N, De Vos M, et al. Adverse skin reactions to anti-TNF-alpha monoclonal antibody therapy. Dermatology 2003;206(4): 388–90.

35. Wang LC, Medenica MM, Shea CR, et al. Infliximab-induced eczematid-like purpura of Doucas and Kapetenakis. J Am Acad Dermatol 2003; 49(1):157–8.

36. Vergara G, Silvestre JF, Betlloch I, et al. Cutaneous drug eruption to infliximab: report of 4 cases with an interface dermatitis pattern. Arch Dermatol 2002;138(9):1258–9.

37. Battistella M, Rivet J, Bachelez H, et al. Lichen planus associated with etanercept. Br J Dermatol 2008;158(1):188–90.

38. Bovenschen HJ, Kop EN, Van De Kerkhof PC, et al. Etanercept-induced lichenoid reaction pattern in psoriasis. J Dermatolog Treat 2006; 17(6):381–3.

39. De Simone C, Caldarola G, D'Agostino M, et al. Lichenoid reaction induced by adalimumab. J Eur Acad Dermatol Venereol 2008;22(5):626–7.

40. Stephenson SR, Campbell SM, Drew GS, et al. Palisaded neutrophilic and granulomatous dermatitis presenting in a patient with rheumatoid arthritis on adalimumab. J Cutan Pathol 2011; 38(8):644–8.

41. Collaris EJ, van Marion AM, Frank J, et al. Cutaneous granulomas in rheumatoid arthritis. Int J Dermatol 2007;46(Suppl 3):33–5.

42. Bremner R, Simpson E, White CR, et al. Palisaded neutrophilic and granulomatous dermatitis: an unusual cutaneous manifestation of immune-mediated disorders. Semin Arthritis Rheum 2004;34(3):610–6.

43. Kekow J, Welte T, Kellner U, et al. Development of rheumatoid nodules during anti-tumor necrosis factor alpha therapy with etanercept. Arthritis Rheum 2002;46(3):843–4.

44. Cunnane G, Warnock M, Fye KH, et al. Accelerated nodulosis and vasculitis following etanercept therapy for rheumatoid arthritis. Arthritis Rheum 2002;47(4):445–9.

45. Scrivo R, Spadaro A, Iagnocco A, et al. Appearance of rheumatoid nodules following anti-tumor necrosis factor alpha treatment with adalimumab for rheumatoid arthritis. Clin Exp Rheumatol 2007; 25(1):117.

46. Deng A, Harvey V, Sina B, et al. Interstitial granulomatous dermatitis associated with the use of tumor necrosis factor alpha inhibitors. Arch Dermatol 2006;142(2):198–202.

47. Voulgari PV, Markatseli TE, Exarchou SA, et al. Granuloma annulare induced by anti-tumour necrosis factor therapy. Ann Rheum Dis 2008; 67(4):567–70.

48. Kudrin A, Chilvers ER, Ginawi A, et al. Sarcoid-like granulomatous disease following etanercept treatment for RA. J Rheumatol 2007;34(3):648–9.

49. Ishiguro T, Takayanagi N, Kurashima K, et al. Development of sarcoidosis during etanercept therapy. Intern Med 2008;47(11):1021–5.

50. Peno-Green L, Lluberas G, Kingsley T, et al. Lung injury linked to etanercept therapy. Chest 2002; 122(5):1858–60.

51. Verschueren K, Van Essche E, Verschueren P, et al. Development of sarcoidosis in etanercept-treated rheumatoid arthritis patients. Clin Rheumatol 2007;26(11):1969–71.

52. Hashkes PJ, Shajrawi I. Sarcoid-related uveitis occurring during etanercept therapy. Clin Exp Rheumatol 2003;21(5):645–6.

53. Beuthien W, Mellinghoff HU, von Kempis J. Skin reaction to adalimumab. Arthritis Rheum 2004; 50(5):1690–2.

54. Soliotis F, Glover M, Jawad AS. Severe skin reaction after leflunomide and etanercept in a patient with rheumatoid arthritis. Ann Rheum Dis 2002; 61(9):850–1.

55. Winfield H, Lain E, Horn T, et al. Eosinophilic cellulitis-like reaction to subcutaneous etanercept injection. Arch Dermatol 2006;142(2):218–20.

56. Boura P, Sarantopoulos A, Lefaki I, et al. Eosinophilic cellulitis (Wells' syndrome) as a cutaneous reaction to the administration of adalimumab. Ann Rheum Dis 2006;65(6):839–40.

57. Adamson R, Obispo E, Dychter S, et al. High incidence and clinical course of aggressive skin cancer in heart transplant patients: a single-center study. Transplant Proc 1998;30(4):1124–6.

58. Lampros TD, Cobanoglu A, Parker F, et al. Squamous and basal cell carcinoma in heart transplant recipients. J Heart Lung Transplant 1998;17(6): 586–91.

59. Lesnoni La Parola I, Masini C, Nanni G, et al. Kaposi's sarcoma in renal-transplant recipients: experience at the Catholic University in Rome, 1988-1996. Dermatology 1997;194(3):229–33.

60. Ravat FE, Spittle MF. Russell-Jones: primary cutaneous T-cell lymphoma occurring after organ transplantation. J Am Acad Dermatol 2006;54(4): 668–75.

61. Randle HW. The historical link between solid-organ transplantation, immunosuppression, and skin cancer. Dermatol Surg 2004;30(4 Pt 2):595–7.

62. Pennica D, Nedwin GE, Hayflick JS, et al. Human tumour necrosis factor: precursor structure, expression

and homology to lymphotoxin. Nature 1984; 312(5996):724–9.

63. Lejeune FJ, Liénard D, Matter M, et al. Efficiency of recombinant human TNF in human cancer therapy. Cancer Immun 2006;6:6.

64. Larmonier N, Cathelin D, Larmonier C, et al. The inhibition of TNF-alpha anti-tumoral properties by blocking antibodies promotes tumor growth in a rat model. Exp Cell Res 2007;313(11):2345–55.

65. Baxevanis CN, Voutsas IF, Tsitsilonis OE, et al. Compromised anti-tumor responses in tumor necrosis factor-alpha knockout mice. Eur J Immunol 2000;30(7):1957–66.

66. Chakravarty EF, Michaud K, Wolfe F. Skin cancer, rheumatoid arthritis, and tumor necrosis factor inhibitors. J Rheumatol 2005;32(11):2130–5.

67. Margolis D, Bilker W, Hennessy S, et al. The risk of malignancy associated with psoriasis. Arch Dermatol 2001;137(6):778–83.

68. Patel RV, Clark LN, Lebwohl M, et al. Treatments for psoriasis and the risk of malignancy. J Am Acad Dermatol 2009;60(6):1001–17.

69. Adams AE, Zwicker J, Curiel C, et al. Aggressive cutaneous T-cell lymphomas after TNFalpha blockade. J Am Acad Dermatol 2004;51(4):660–2.

70. Krishna SM, Kim CN. Merkel cell carcinoma in a patient treated with adalimumab: case report. Cutis 2011;87(2):81–4.

71. Bernert H, Sekikawa K, Radcliffe RA, et al. TNFa and IL-10 deficiencies have contrasting effects on lung tumor susceptibility: gender-dependent modulation of IL-10 haploinsufficiency. Mol Carcinog 2003;38(3):117–23.

72. Scott KA, Moore RJ, Arnott CH, et al. An anti-tumor necrosis factor-alpha antibody inhibits the development of experimental skin tumors. Mol Cancer Ther 2003;2(5):445–51.

73. Esser AC, Abril A, Fayne S, et al. Acute development of multiple keratoacanthomas and squamous cell carcinomas after treatment with infliximab. J Am Acad Dermatol 2004;50(Suppl 5):S75–7.

74. Smith KJ, Skelton HG. Rapid onset of cutaneous squamous cell carcinoma in patients with rheumatoid arthritis after starting tumor necrosis factor alpha receptor IgG1-Fc fusion complex therapy. J Am Acad Dermatol 2001;45(6):953–6.

75. Ly L, Czarnecki D. The rapid onset of multiple squamous cell carcinomas during etanercept treatment for psoriasis. Br J Dermatol 2007;157(5):1076–8.

76. Fryrear RS 2nd, Wiggins AK, Sangueza O, et al. Rapid onset of cutaneous squamous cell carcinoma of the penis in a patient with psoriasis on etanercept therapy. J Am Acad Dermatol 2004;51(6):1026.

77. Sheppard J, Raza K, Buckley CD. Skin cancer in psoriatic arthritis treated with anti-TNF therapy. Rheumatology (Oxford) 2007;46(10):1622–3.

78. Dommasch ED, Abuabara K, Shin DB, et al. The risk of infection and malignancy with tumor necrosis factor antagonists in adults with psoriatic disease: a systematic review and meta-analysis of randomized controlled trials. J Am Acad Dermatol 2011;64(6):1035–50.

79. Lebwohl M, Blum R, Berkowitz E, et al. No evidence for increased risk of cutaneous squamous cell carcinoma in patients with rheumatoid arthritis receiving etanercept for up to 5 years. Arch Dermatol 2005;141(7):861–4.

80. Fulchiero GJ Jr, Salvaggio H, Drabick JJ, et al. Eruptive latent metastatic melanomas after initiation of antitumor necrosis factor therapies. J Am Acad Dermatol 2007;56(Suppl 5):S65–7.

81. Katoulis AC, Kanelleas A, Zambacos G, et al. Development of two primary malignant melanomas after treatment with adalimumab: a case report and review of the possible link between biological therapy with TNF-alpha antagonists and melanocytic proliferation. Dermatology 2010; 221(1):9–12.

82. Fogo AJ, Hunt JB, Clement M. Multiple cutaneous malignancies arising in a patient with Crohn disease treated with concomitant azathioprine and antitumour necrosis factor-alpha. Clin Exp Dermatol 2010;35(7):793–5.

83. Katsanos KH, Christodoulou DK, Zioga A, et al. Cutaneous nevi pigmentosus during infliximab therapy in a patient with Crohn's disease: fallacy or coincidence? Inflamm Bowel Dis 2003;9(4):279.

84. Bovenschen HJ, Tjioe M, Vermaat H, et al. Induction of eruptive benign melanocytic naevi by immune suppressive agents, including biologicals. Br J Dermatol 2006;154(5):880–4.

85. Balato N, Di Costanzo L, Balato A, et al. Psoriasis and melanocytic naevi: does the first confer a protective role against melanocyte progression to naevi? Br J Dermatol 2011;164(6):1262–70.

86. Koens L, Senff NJ, Vermeer MH, et al. Cutaneous gamma/delta T-cell lymphoma during treatment with etanercept for rheumatoid arthritis. Acta Derm Venereol 2009;89(6):653–4.

87. Lourari S, Prey S, Livideanu C, et al. Cutaneous T-cell lymphoma following treatment of rheumatoid arthritis with tumour necrosis factor-alpha blocking agents: two cases. J Eur Acad Dermatol Venereol 2009;23(8):967–8.

88. Mahé E, Descamps V, Grossin M, et al. CD30+ T-cell lymphoma in a patient with psoriasis treated with cyclosporin and infliximab. Br J Dermatol 2003;149(1):170–3.

89. Dalle S, Balme B, Berger F, et al. Mycosis fungoides-associated follicular mucinosis under adalimumab. Br J Dermatol 2005;153(1):207–8.

90. Berthelot C, Cather J, Jones D, et al. Atypical CD8+ cutaneous T-cell lymphoma after immunomodulatory

therapy. Clin Lymphoma Myeloma 2006;6(4): 329–32.

91. Dauendorffer JN, Rivet J, Allard A, et al. Sezary syndrome in a patient receiving infliximab for ankylosing spondylitis. Br J Dermatol 2007; 156(4):742–3.

92. Naldi L. Malignancy concerns with psoriasis treatments using phototherapy, methotrexate, cyclosporin, and biologics: facts and controversies. Clin Dermatol 2011;28(1):88–92.

93. Weinblatt ME, Kremer JM, Bankhurst AD, et al. A trial of etanercept, a recombinant tumor necrosis factor receptor: Fc fusion protein, in patients with rheumatoid arthritis receiving methotrexate. N Engl J Med 1999;340(4):253–9.

94. Lipsky PE, van der Heijde DM, St Clair EW, et al. Infliximab and methotrexate in the treatment of rheumatoid arthritis. Anti-Tumor Necrosis Factor Trial in Rheumatoid Arthritis with Concomitant Therapy Study Group. N Engl J Med 2000;343(22):1594–602.

95. Abourazzak FE, Guggenbuhl P, Perdriger A, et al. Cutaneous lupus induced by etanercept in rheumatoid arthritis. Rev Med Interne 2008;29(9):744–7 [in French].

96. Bleumink GS, ter borg EJ, Ramselaar CG, et al. Etanercept-induced subacute cutaneous lupus erythematosus. Rheumatology (Oxford) 2001; 40(11):1317–9.

97. Debandt M, Vittecoq O, Descamps V, et al. Anti-TNF-alpha-induced systemic lupus syndrome. Clin Rheumatol 2003;22(1):56–61.

98. Kang MJ, Lee YH, Lee J. Etanercept-induced systemic lupus erythematosus in a patient with rheumatoid arthritis. J Korean Med Sci 2006; 21(5):946–9.

99. Shakoor N, Michalska M, Harris CA, et al. Drug-induced systemic lupus erythematosus associated with etanercept therapy. Lancet 2002;359(9306): 579–80.

100. Williams VL, Cohen PR. TNF alpha antagonist-induced lupus-like syndrome: report and review of the literature with implications for treatment with alternative TNF alpha antagonists. Int J Dermatol 2011;50(5):619–25.

101. Schneider SW, Staender S, Schlüter B, et al. Infliximab-induced lupus erythematosus tumidus in a patient with rheumatoid arthritis. Arch Dermatol 2006;142(1):115–6.

102. Richez C, Dumoulin C, Schaeverbeke T. Infliximab induced chilblain lupus in a patient with rheumatoid arthritis. J Rheumatol 2005;32(4):760–1.

103. High WA, Muldrow ME, Fitzpatrick JE. Cutaneous lupus erythematosus induced by infliximab. J Am Acad Dermatol 2005;52(4):E5.

104. Vezzoli P, Violetti SA, Serini SM, et al. Cutaneous lupus erythematosus induced by adalimumab. J Dermatol 2011;38(3):283–4.

105. Levine D, Switlyk SA, Gottlieb A. Cutaneous lupus erythematosus and anti-TNF-alpha therapy: a case report with review of the literature. J Drugs Dermatol 2010;9(10):1283–7.

106. Sheth N, Greenblatt D, Patel S, et al. Adalimumab-induced cutaneous lupus. Clin Exp Dermatol 2007; 32(5):593–4.

107. Ramos-Casals M, Brito-Zerón P, Muñoz S, et al. Autoimmune diseases induced by TNF-targeted therapies: analysis of 233 cases. Medicine (Baltimore) 2007;86(4):242–51.

108. Ramos-Casals M, Brito-Zerón P, Soto MJ, et al. Autoimmune diseases induced by TNF-targeted therapies. Best Pract Res Clin Rheumatol 2008; 22(5):847–61.

109. Klein R, Rosenbach M, Kim EJ, et al. Tumor necrosis factor inhibitor-associated dermatomyositis. Arch Dermatol 2010;146(7):780–4.

110. Richetta A, Mattozzi C, Carlomagno V, et al. A case of infliximab-induced psoriasis. Dermatol Online J 2008;14(11):9.

111. Borrás-Blasco J, Gracia-Perez A, Nuñez-Cornejo C, et al. Exacerbation of psoriatic skin lesions in a patient with psoriatic arthritis receiving adalimumab. J Clin Pharm Ther 2008;33(3):321–5.

112. de Gannes GC, Ghoreishi M, Pope J, et al. Psoriasis and pustular dermatitis triggered by TNF-{alpha} inhibitors in patients with rheumatologic conditions. Arch Dermatol 2007;143(2):223–31.

113. Sari I, Akar S, Birlik M, et al. Anti-tumor necrosis factor-alpha-induced psoriasis. J Rheumatol 2006; 33(7):1411–4.

114. Severs GA, Lawlor TH, Purcell SM, et al. Cutaneous adverse reaction to infliximab: report of psoriasis developing in 3 patients. Cutis 2007;80(3):231–7.

115. Lebas D, Staumont-Sallé D, Solau-Gervais E, et al. Cutaneous manifestations during treatment with TNF-alpha blockers: 11 cases. Ann Dermatol Venereol 2007;134(4 Pt 1):337–42 [in French].

116. Shmidt E, Wetter DA, Ferguson SB, et al. Psoriasis and palmoplantar pustulosis associated with tumor necrosis factor-alpha inhibitors: the mayo clinic experience, 1998 to 2010. J Am Acad Dermatol 2011. [Epub ahead of print].

117. Roux CH, Brocq O, Leccia N, et al. New-onset psoriatic palmoplantaris pustulosis following infliximab therapy: a class effect? J Rheumatol 2007;34(2):434–7.

118. Klein RQ, Spivack J, Choate KA. Psoriatic skin lesions induced by certolizumab pegol. Arch Dermatol 2010;146(9):1055–6.

119. Seneschal J, Milpied B, Vergier B, et al. Cytokine imbalance with increased production of interferon-alpha in psoriasiform eruptions associated with antitumour necrosis factor-alpha treatments. Br J Dermatol 2009;161(5):1081–8.

120. Baron PW, Cantos K, Hillebrand DJ, et al. Nephrogenic fibrosing dermopathy after liver transplantation

successfully treated with plasmapheresis. Am J Dermatopathol 2003;25(3):204–9.

121. Martin A, Gutierrez E, Muglia J, et al. A multicenter dose-escalation trial with denileukin diftitox (ONTAK, DAB(389)IL-2) in patients with severe psoriasis. J Am Acad Dermatol 2001;45(6):871–81.

122. Railan D, Fivenson DP, Wittenberg G. Capillary leak syndrome in a patient treated with interleukin 2 fusion toxin for cutaneous T-cell lymphoma. J Am Acad Dermatol 2000;43(2 Pt 1):323–4.

123. Cicardi M, Gardinali M, Bisiani G, et al. The systemic capillary leak syndrome: appearance of interleukin-2-receptor-positive cells during attacks. Ann Intern Med 1990;113(6):475–7.

124. Lissoni P, Barni S, Cattaneo G, et al. Activation of the complement system during immunotherapy of cancer with interleukin-2: a possible explanation of the capillary leak syndrome. Int J Biol Markers 1990;5(4):195–7.

125. Rosenstein M, Ettinghausen SE, Rosenberg SA. Extravasation of intravascular fluid mediated by the systemic administration of recombinant interleukin 2. J Immunol 1986;137(5):1735–42.

126. Foss FM, Bacha P, Osann KE, et al. Biological correlates of acute hypersensitivity events with DAB(389)IL-2 (denileukin diftitox, ONTAK) in cutaneous T-cell lymphoma: decreased frequency and severity with steroid premedication. Clin Lymphoma 2001;1(4):298–302.

127. Polder K, Wang C, Duvic M, et al. Toxic epidermal necrolysis associated with denileukin diftitox (DAB389IL-2) administration in a patient with follicular large cell lymphoma. Leuk Lymphoma 2005; 46(12):1807–11.

128. Cohen SB, Emery P, Greenwald MW, et al. Rituximab for rheumatoid arthritis refractory to anti-tumor necrosis factor therapy: results of a multicenter, randomized, double-blind, placebo-controlled, phase III trial evaluating primary efficacy and safety at twenty-four weeks. Arthritis Rheum 2006;54(9):2793–806.

129. Errante D, Bernardi D, Bianco A, et al. Rituximab-related urticarial reaction in a patient treated for primary cutaneous B-cell lymphoma. Ann Oncol 2006;17(11):1720–1.

130. Rey J, Wickenhauser S, Ivanov V, et al. A case of rituximab-related urticarial reaction in cutaneous B-cell lymphoma. J Eur Acad Dermatol Venereol 2009;23(2):210.

131. Witzig TE, Vukov AM, Habermann TM, et al. Rituximab therapy for patients with newly diagnosed, advanced-stage, follicular grade I non-Hodgkin's lymphoma: a phase II trial in the North Central Cancer Treatment Group. J Clin Oncol 2005; 23(6):1103–8.

132. Piro LD, White CA, Grillo-López AJ, et al. Extended Rituximab (anti-CD20 monoclonal antibody) therapy for relapsed or refractory low-grade or follicular non-Hodgkin's lymphoma. Ann Oncol 1999;10(6): 655–61.

133. Dillman RO. Infusion reactions associated with the therapeutic use of monoclonal antibodies in the treatment of malignancy. Cancer Metastasis Rev 1999;18(4):465–71.

134. Callen JP. Complications and adverse reactions in the use of newer biologic agents. Semin Cutan Med Surg 2007;26(1):6–14.

135. Emery P, Fleischmann R, Filipowicz-Sosnowska A, et al. The efficacy and safety of rituximab in patients with active rheumatoid arthritis despite methotrexate treatment: results of a phase IIB randomized, double-blind, placebo-controlled, dose-ranging trial. Arthritis Rheum 2006;54(5):1390–400.

136. Yawn BP, Saddier P, Wollan PC, et al. A population-based study of the incidence and complication rates of herpes zoster before zoster vaccine introduction. Mayo Clin Proc 2007;82(11):1341–9.

137. Del Poeta G, Del Principe MI, Buccisano F, et al. Consolidation and maintenance immunotherapy with rituximab improve clinical outcome in patients with B-cell chronic lymphocytic leukemia. Cancer 2008;112(1):119–28.

138. Keystone E, Fleischmann R, Emery P, et al. Safety and efficacy of additional courses of rituximab in patients with active rheumatoid arthritis: an open-label extension analysis. Arthritis Rheum 2007; 56(12):3896–908.

139. Robak E, Biernat W, Krykowski E, et al. Merkel cell carcinoma in a patient with B-cell chronic lymphocytic leukemia treated with cladribine and rituximab. Leuk Lymphoma 2005;46(6):909–14.

140. Lowndes S, Darby A, Mead G, et al. Stevens-Johnson syndrome after treatment with rituximab. Ann Oncol 2002;13(12):1948–50.

141. Allen KP, Funk AJ, Mandrell TD. Toxic epidermal necrolysis in two rhesus macaques (Macaca mulatta) after administration of rituximab. Comp Med 2005;55(4):377–81.

142. Biogen-Idec: Zevalin (ibritumomab tiuxetan) label update. 2005. Available at: http://www.accessdata. fda.gov/drugsatfda_docs/label/2005/125019_0092lbl. pdf. Accessed August, 2011.

143. Gotlib V, Khaled S, Lapko I, et al. Skin rash secondary to bevacizumab in a patient with advanced colorectal cancer and relation to response. Anticancer Drugs 2006;17(10):1227–9.

144. Ladas ID, Moschos MM, Papakostas TD, et al. Skin rash associated with intravitreal bevacizumab in a patient with macular choroidal neovascularization. Clin Ophthalmol 2009;3:129–31.

145. Saif MW, Longo WL, Israel G. Correlation between rash and a positive drug response associated with bevacizumab in a patient with advanced colorectal cancer. Clin Colorectal Cancer 2008;7(2):144–8.

146. Wozel G, Sticherling M, Schon MP. Cutaneous side effects of inhibition of VEGF signal transduction. J Dtsch Dermatol Ges 2010;8(4):243–9.

147. Amselem L, Diaz-Llopis M, Garcia-Delpech S, et al. Papulopustular eruption after intravitreal bevacizumab (Avastin). Acta Ophthalmol 2009;87(1):110–1.

148. Vano-Galvan S, Moreno C, Medina J, et al. Perforating dermatosis in a patient receiving bevacizumab. J Eur Acad Dermatol Venereol 2009;23(8): 972–4.

149. Vihinen P, Paija O, Kivisaari A, et al. Cutaneous lupus erythematosus after treatment with paclitaxel and bevacizumab for metastatic breast cancer: a case report. J Med Case Rep 2011;5:243.

150. Lazzati V, Zygoń J, Lohsiriwat V, et al. Impaired wound healing and bilateral mastectomy flap necrosis in a patient with locally advanced breast cancer after neoadjuvant Paclitaxel with bevacizumab. Aesthetic Plast Surg 2010;34(6):796–7.

151. Bosanquet DC, Davies WL, May K, et al. Acute generalised exanthematous pustulosis following intravitreal Ranibizumab. Int Wound J 2011;8(3): 317–9.

152. Bragg J, Pomeranz MK. Papulopustular drug eruption due to an epidermal growth factor receptor inhibitors, erlotinib and cetuximab. Dermatol Online J 2007;13(1):1.

153. Cholongitas E, Pipili C, Ioannidou D. Malassezia folliculitis presented as acneiform eruption after cetuximab administration. J Drugs Dermatol 2009; 8(3):274–5.

154. Cotena C, Gisondi P, Colato C, et al. Acneiform eruption induced by cetuximab. Acta Dermatovenerol Croat 2007;15(4):246–8.

155. Fernandez-Torres R, Martinez Gomez W, Cuevas Santos J, et al. Rosaceiform eruption induced by cetuximab. Eur J Dermatol 2010;20(3):392–3.

156. Gutzmer R, Werfel T, Mao R, et al. Successful treatment with oral isotretinoin of acneiform skin lesions associated with cetuximab therapy. Br J Dermatol 2005;153(4):849–51.

157. Walon L, Gilbeau C, Lachapelle JM. Acneiform eruptions induced by cetuximab. Ann Dermatol Venereol 2003;130(4):443–6 [in French].

158. Amitay-Laish I, David M, Stemmer SM. Staphylococcus coagulase-positive skin inflammation associated with epidermal growth factor receptor-targeted therapy: an early and a late phase of papulopustular eruptions. Oncologist 2010;15(9): 1002–8.

159. Kerob D, Dupuy A, Reygagne P, et al. Facial hypertrichosis induced by Cetuximab, an anti-EGFR monoclonal antibody. Arch Dermatol 2006; 142(12):1656–7.

160. Vano-Galvan S, Rios-Buceta L, Ma DL, et al. Cetuximab-induced hypertrichosis of the scalp and eyelashes. J Am Acad Dermatol 2010;62(3):531–3.

161. Rubió Casadevall J, Graña-Suarez B, Hernandez-Yague X, et al. Xeroderma pigmentosum: neck lymph node metastasis of a squamous cell carcinoma of the skin treated with cetuximab. Eur J Dermatol 2009;19(2):163–5.

162. Tscharner GG, Bühler S, Borner M, et al. Grover's disease induced by cetuximab. Dermatology 2006;213(1):37–9.

163. Navarini AA, Kamacharova I, Kerl K, et al. Ecthymatous skin eruption during therapy with cetuximab. Eur J Dermatol 2011;21(2):282–3.

164. Garibaldi DC, Adler RA. Cicatricial ectropion associated with treatment of metastatic colorectal cancer with cetuximab. Ophthal Plast Reconstr Surg 2007;23(1):62–3.

165. Eames T, Grabein B, Kroth J, et al. Microbiological analysis of epidermal growth factor receptor inhibitor therapy-associated paronychia. J Eur Acad Dermatol Venereol 2010;24(8):958–60.

166. Lee SS, Chu PY. Toxic epidermal necrolysis caused by cetuximab plus minocycline in head and neck cancer. Am J Otolaryngol 2010;31(4):288–90.

167. Billan S, Abdah-Bortnyak R, Kuten A. Severe desquamation with skin necrosis: a distinct pattern of skin toxicity secondary to head and neck irradiation with concomitant cetuximab. Isr Med Assoc J 2008;10(3):247.

168. Berger B, Belka C. Severe skin reaction secondary to concomitant radiotherapy plus cetuximab. Radiat Oncol 2008;3:5.

169. Korman JB, Ward DB, Maize JC Jr. Papulopustular eruption associated with panitumumab. Arch Dermatol 2010;146(8):926–7.

170. Ho C, Sangha R, Beckett L, et al. Escalating weekly doses of cetuximab and correlation with skin toxicity: a phase I study. Invest New Drugs 2011;29(4):680–7.

171. Lopez-Gómez M, Gómez-Raposo C, Sereno M, et al. Different patterns of toxicity after sequential administration of two anti-EGFR monoclonal antibodies. Clin Transl Oncol 2010;12(11):775–7.

172. Gordon KB, Papp KA, Hamilton TK, et al. Efalizumab for patients with moderate to severe plaque psoriasis: a randomized controlled trial. JAMA 2003;290(23):3073–80.

173. Menter A, Gordon K, Carey W, et al. Efficacy and safety observed during 24 weeks of efalizumab therapy in patients with moderate to severe plaque psoriasis. Arch Dermatol 2005;141(1):31–8.

174. Gottlieb AB, Gordon KB, Lebwohl MG, et al. Extended efalizumab therapy sustains efficacy without increasing toxicity in patients with moderate to severe chronic plaque psoriasis. J Drugs Dermatol 2004;3(6):614–24.

175. Papp KA, Bressinck R, Fretzin S, et al. Safety of efalizumab in adults with chronic moderate to severe plaque psoriasis: a phase IIIb, randomized, controlled trial. Int J Dermatol 2006;45(5):605–14.

176. Dubertret L, Sterry W, Bos JD, et al. Clinical experience acquired with the efalizumab (Raptiva) (CLEAR) trial in patients with moderate-to-severe plaque psoriasis: results from a phase III international randomized, placebo-controlled trial. Br J Dermatol 2006;155(1):170–81.

177. Kohl S, Loo LS, Schmalstieg FS, et al. The genetic deficiency of leukocyte surface glycoprotein Mac-1, LFA-1, p150,95 in humans is associated with defective antibody-dependent cellular cytotoxicity in vitro and defective protection against herpes simplex virus infection in vivo. J Immunol 1986;137(5):1688–94.

178. Cederblad B, Sandberg K, Alm GV. The leukocyte function-associated antigen-1 (LFA-1) is involved in the interferon-alpha response induced by herpes simplex virus in blood leukocytes. J Interferon Res 1993;13(3):203–8.

179. Weisenseel P, Kuznetsov AV, Flaig M, et al. Disseminated eruptive giant mollusca contagiosa in an adult psoriasis patient during efalizumab therapy. Dermatology 2008;217(1):85–6.

180. US-FDA. Raptiva (efalizumab): postmarket drug safety information for patients and providers. 2009. Available at: http://www.fda.gov/downloads/Drugs/DrugSafety/PostmarketDrugSafetyInformationfor PatientsandProviders/UCM143346.pdf. Accessed August, 2011.

181. Bentley DD, Graves JE, Smith DI, et al. Efalizumab-induced subacute cutaneous lupus erythematosus. J Am Acad Dermatol 2006;54(Suppl 5): S242–3.

182. de Groot M, de Rie MA, Bos JD. DRESS syndrome caused by efalizumab: comment. Clin Exp Dermatol 2009;34(3):413–4.

183. White JM, Smith CH, Robson A, et al. DRESS syndrome caused by efalizumab. Clin Exp Dermatol 2008;33(1):50–2.

184. de Groot M, de Rie MA, Bos JD. Dermatitis during efalizumab treatment in a patient with psoriasis vulgaris. Br J Dermatol 2005;153(4):843–4.

185. Klein A, Szeimies RM, Landthaler M, et al. Exacerbation of pityriasis rubra pilaris under efalizumab therapy. Dermatology 2007;215(1):72–5.

186. Vestergaard ME, Kossard S, Murrell DF. Seborrhoeic keratoses appearing in sites of previous psoriasis plaques during treatment with efalizumab. Clin Exp Dermatol 2009;34(8):e564–6.

187. Santos-Juanes J, Coto-Segura P, Mallo S, et al. Multiple eruptive dermatofibromas in a patient receiving efalizumab. Dermatology 2008;216(4):363.

188. Balato A, La Bella S, Gaudiello F, et al. Efalizumab-induced guttate psoriasis. Successful management and re-treatment. J Dermatolog Treat 2008; 19(3):182–4.

189. Lowes MA, Chamian F, Abello MV, et al. Eruptive papules during efalizumab (anti-CD11a) therapy of psoriasis vulgaris: a case series. BMC Dermatol 2007;7:2.

190. Lebwohl M, Christophers E, Langley R, et al. An international, randomized, double-blind, placebo-controlled phase 3 trial of intramuscular alefacept in patients with chronic plaque psoriasis. Arch Dermatol 2003;139(6):719–27.

191. US-FDA. Amevive (alefacept) package insert. 2005. Available at: http://www.accessdata.fda.gov/drugsatfda_docs/label/2005/125036s044lbl.pdf. Accessed August, 2011.

192. Perlmutter A, Cather J, Franks B, et al. Alefacept revisited: our 3-year clinical experience in 200 patients with chronic plaque psoriasis. J Am Acad Dermatol 2008;58(1):116–24.

193. Schmidt A, Robbins J, Zic J. Transformed mycosis fungoides developing after treatment with alefacept. J Am Acad Dermatol 2005;53(2):355–6.

194. Caussa L, Kirova YM, Gault N, et al. The acute skin and heart toxicity of a concurrent association of trastuzumab and locoregional breast radiotherapy including internal mammary chain: a single-institution study. Eur J Cancer 2011;47(1):65–73.

195. Akay BN, Unlu E, Buyukcelik A, et al. Photosensitive rash in association with porphyrin biosynthesis possibly induced by docetaxel and trastuzumab therapy in a patient with metastatic breast carcinoma. Jpn J Clin Oncol 2010;40(10):989–91.

196. Cohen AD, Mermershtain W, Geffen DB, et al. Cutaneous photosensitivity induced by paclitaxel and trastuzumab therapy associated with aberrations in the biosynthesis of porphyrins. J Dermatolog Treat 2005;16(1):19–21.

197. Ee HL, Yosipovitch G. Photo recall phenomenon: an adverse reaction to taxanes. Dermatology 2003;207(2):196–8.

198. Cohen PR. Photodistributed erythema multiforme: paclitaxel-related, photosensitive conditions in patients with cancer. J Drugs Dermatol 2009;8(1):61–4.

199. Rosman IS, Anadkat MJ. Tufted hair folliculitis in a woman treated with trastuzumab. Target Oncol 2010;5(4):295–6.

200. Pitini V, Arrigo C, Barresi G. Disseminated molluscum contagiosum in a patient with chronic lymphocytic leukaemia after alemtuzumab. Br J Haematol 2003;123(4):565.

201. Lundin J, Hagberg H, Repp R, et al. Phase 2 study of alemtuzumab (anti-CD52 monoclonal antibody) in patients with advanced mycosis fungoides/Sezary syndrome. Blood 2003;101(11):4267–72.

202. Venkatachalapathy S, Crowe J, Gray A. Atypical presentation of varicella zoster in a patient on alemtuzumab. Br J Haematol 2007;138(4):406.

203. Kennedy GA, Seymour JF, Wolf M, et al. Treatment of patients with advanced mycosis fungoides and Sezary syndrome with alemtuzumab. Eur J Haematol 2003;71(4):250–6.

204. Thachil J, Jadhav V, Gautam M, et al. The development of sarcoidosis with the use of alemtuzumab - clues to T-cell immune reconstitution. Br J Haematol 2007;138(4):559–60.

205. Faguer S, Launay F, Ysebaert L, et al. Acute cutaneous T-cell lymphoma transformation during treatment with alemtuzumab. Br J Dermatol 2007; 157(4):841–2.

206. Janssens A, Berth M, De Paepe P, et al. EBV negative Richter's syndrome from a coexistent clone after salvage treatment with alemtuzumab in a CLL patient. Am J Hematol 2006;81(9):706–12.

207. Andre MC, Pacheco D, Antunes J, et al. Generalized skin drug eruption to natalizumab in a patient with multiple sclerosis. Dermatol Online J 2010; 16(6):14.

208. Gutwinski S, Erbe S, Münch C, et al. Severe cutaneous Candida infection during natalizumab therapy in multiple sclerosis. Neurology 2010; 74(6):521–3.

209. Bergamaschi R, Montomoli C. Melanoma in multiple sclerosis treated with natalizumab: causal association or coincidence? Mult Scler 2009; 15(12):1532–3.

210. Castela E, Lebrun-Frenay C, Laffon M, et al. Evolution of nevi during treatment with natalizumab: a prospective follow-up of patients treated with natalizumab for multiple sclerosis. Arch Dermatol 2011;147(1):72–6.

211. Ismail A, Kemp J, Sharrack B. Melanoma complicating treatment with natalizumab (tysabri) for multiple sclerosis. J Neurol 2009;256(10):1771–2.

212. Mullen JT, Vartanian TK, Atkins MB. Melanoma complicating treatment with natalizumab for multiple sclerosis. N Engl J Med 2008;358(6): 647–8.

213. Vavricka BM, Baumberger P, Russmann S, et al. Diagnosis of melanoma under concomitant natalizumab therapy. Mult Scler 2011;17(2):255–6.

214. Larouche N, Larouche K, Béliveau A, et al. Transcriptional regulation of the alpha 4 integrin subunit gene in the metastatic spread of uveal melanoma. Anticancer Res 1998;18(5A):3539–47.

215. Holzmann B, Gosslar U, Bittner M. Alpha 4 integrins and tumor metastasis. Curr Top Microbiol Immunol 1998;231:125–41.

216. Kazatchkine MD, Kaveri SV. Immunomodulation of autoimmune and inflammatory diseases with intravenous immune globulin. N Engl J Med 2001; 345(10):747–55.

217. Katz U, Achiron A, Sherer Y, et al. Safety of intravenous immunoglobulin (IVIG) therapy. Autoimmun Rev 2007;6(4):257–9.

218. Misbah SA, Chapel HM. Adverse effects of intravenous immunoglobulin. Drug Saf 1993;9(4):254–62.

219. Brannagan TH 3rd, Nagle KJ, Lange DJ, et al. Complications of intravenous immune globulin treatment in neurologic disease. Neurology 1996; 47(3):674–7.

220. Orbach H, Katz U, Sherer Y, et al. Intravenous immunoglobulin: adverse effects and safe administration. Clin Rev Allergy Immunol 2005;29(3): 173–84.

221. Dalakas MC. Intravenous immune globulin therapy for neurologic diseases. Ann Intern Med 1997; 126(9):721–30.

222. Cohen Aubart F, Barete S, Amoura Z, et al. Intravenous immunoglobulins-induced eczematous eruption: a long-term follow-up study. Eur J Intern Med 2009;20(1):70–3.

223. Gerstenblith MR, Antony AK, Junkins-Hopkins JM, et al. Pompholyx and eczematous reactions associated with intravenous immunoglobulin therapy. J Am Acad Dermatol 2011;66(2):312–6.

224. Lin WL, Lin WC, Chang YC, et al. Intravenous immunoglobulin-induced, non-eczematous, vesiculobullous eruptions in Stevens-Johnson syndrome. Am J Clin Dermatol 2009;10(5):339–42.

225. Maetzke J, Sperfeld AD, Scharffetter-Kochanek K, et al. Vesicular and bullous eczema in response to intravenous immunoglobulins (IVIG). Allergy 2006;61(1):145–6.

226. Smith KJ, Dutka AL, Skelton HG. Lichenoid/interface cutaneous eruptions to IVIg with the primary infusion may be related to the re-regulation of anti-idiotype network. J Cutan Med Surg 1998; 3(2):96–101.

227. Sorensen PS, Wanscher B, Jensen CV, et al. Intravenous immunoglobulin G reduces MRI activity in relapsing multiple sclerosis. Neurology 1998; 50(5):1273–81.

228. Tada M, Tada M, Ishiguro H, et al. Eczematous reactions after intravenous immunoglobulin therapy in two patients with Guillain-Barré syndrome and a patient with Miller Fisher syndrome. No To Shinkei 2003;55(5):401–5 [in Japanese].

229. Uyttendaele H, Obadiah J, Grossman M. Dyshidrotic-like spongiotic dermatitis after intravenous immunoglobulin therapy. J Drugs Dermatol 2003; 2(3):337–41.

230. Vecchietti G, Kerl K, Prins C, et al. Severe eczematous skin reaction after high-dose intravenous immunoglobulin infusion: report of 4 cases and review of the literature. Arch Dermatol 2006; 142(2):213–7.

231. Barbaud A, Tréchot P, Granel F, et al. A baboon syndrome induced by intravenous human immunoglobulins: report of a case and immunological analysis. Dermatology 1999;199(3):258–60.

232. Guillet MH, Wierzbicka E, Guillet S, et al. A 3-year causative study of pompholyx in 120 patients. Arch Dermatol 2007;143(12):1504–8.

233. Iannaccone S, Wierzbicka E, Guillet S, et al. Pompholyx (vesicular eczema) after i.v. immunoglobulin

therapy for neurologic disease. Neurology 1999; 53(5):1154–5.

234. Ikeda K, Iwasaki Y, Ichikawa Y, et al. Pompholyx after IV immunoglobulin therapy for neurologic disease. Neurology 1879;54(9):2000.

235. Llombart M, Garcia-Abujeta JL, Sánchez-Pérez RM, et al. Pompholyx induced by intravenous immunoglobulin therapy. J Investig Allergol Clin Immunol 2007;17(4):277–8.

236. Rhee DY, Park GH, Chang SE, et al. Pompholyx after intravenous immunoglobulin therapy for treatment of Guillain-Barré syndrome. J Eur Acad Dermatol Venereol 2009;23(5):602–4.

237. Young PK, Ruggeri SY, Galbraith S, et al. Vesicular eczema after intravenous immunoglobulin therapy for treatment of Stevens-Johnson syndrome. Arch Dermatol 2006;142(2):247–8.

238. Sarmiento E, Micheloud D, Carbone J. Complement consumption associated with eczematous cutaneous reaction during infusions of high doses of intravenous immunoglobulin. Br J Dermatol 2004;151(3):721.

239. Whittam LR, Hay RJ, Hughes RA. Eczematous reactions to human immune globulin. Br J Dermatol 1997;137(3):481–2.

240. Hamdalla HH, Hawkes CH, Spokes EG, et al. Intravenous immunoglobulin in the Guillain-Barré syndrome. May cause severe adverse skin reactions. BMJ 1996;313(7069):1399–400.

241. Leclech C, Maillard H, Penisson-Besnier I, et al. Unusual skin reaction after intravenous infusion of polyvalent immunoglobulins: 3 case reports. Presse Med 1999;28(10):531 [in French].

242. Barucha C, McMillan JC. Eczema after intravenous infusion of immunoglobulin. Br Med J (Clin Res Ed) 1987;295(6606):1141.

243. Catteau B, Delaporte E, Piette F. Meningitis and skin reaction after intravenous immune globulin therapy. Ann Intern Med 1997;127(12):1130.

244. Lofgren SM, Warshaw EM. Dyshidrosis: epidemiology, clinical characteristics, and therapy. Dermatitis 2006;17(4):165–81.

245. Ferguson AC, Salinas FA. Elevated IgG immune complexes in children with atopic eczema. J Allergy Clin Immunol 1984;74(5):678–82.

246. Smed-Sorensen A, Moll M, Cheng TY, et al. IgG regulates the CD1 expression profile and lipid antigen-presenting function in human dendritic cells via FcgammaRIIa. Blood 2008;111(10):5037–46.

247. Hussein MR. Evaluation of Langerhans' cells in normal and eczematous dermatitis skin by CD1a protein immunohistochemistry: preliminary findings. J Cutan Pathol 2008;35(6):554–8.

248. Russano AM, Bassotti G, Agea E, et al. CD1-restricted recognition of exogenous and self-lipid antigens by duodenal gammadelta+ T lymphocytes. J Immunol 2007;178(6):3620–6.

249. Spada FM, Grant EP, Peters PJ, et al. Self-recognition of CD1 by gamma/delta T cells: implications for innate immunity. J Exp Med 2000;191(6):937–48.

250. Joyce S, Woods AS, Yewdell JW, et al. Natural ligand of mouse CD1d1: cellular glycosylphosphatidylinositol. Science 1998;279(5356):1541–4.

251. Dascher CC, Brenner MB. CD1 antigen presentation and infectious disease. Contrib Microbiol 2003;10:164–82.

252. Yockey SM, Ahmed I. Intravenous immunoglobulin-induced lichenoid dermatitis: a unique adverse reaction. Mayo Clin Proc 1997;72(12):1151–2.

253. Boyd AS, Neldner KH. Hydroxyurea therapy. J Am Acad Dermatol 1991;25(3):518–24.

254. Yarbro JW. Hydroxyurea in the treatment of refractory psoriasis. Lancet 1969;2(7625):846–7.

255. Leavell UW Jr, Yarbro JW. Hydroxyurea. A new treatment for psoriasis. Arch Dermatol 1970; 102(2):144–50.

256. Steinberg MH, Barton F, Castro O, et al. Effect of hydroxyurea on mortality and morbidity in adult sickle cell anemia: risks and benefits up to 9 years of treatment. JAMA 2003;289(13):1645–51.

257. Davies S, Olujohungbe A. Hydroxyurea for sickle cell disease. Cochrane Database Syst Rev 2001;(2):CD002202.

258. Kennedy BJ, Smith LR, Goltz RW. Skin changes secondary to hydroxyurea therapy. Arch Dermatol 1975;111(2):183–7.

259. Gropper CA, Don PC, Sadjadi MM. Nail and skin hyperpigmentation associated with hydroxyurea therapy for polycythemia vera. Int J Dermatol 1993;32(10):731–3.

260. O'Branski EE, Ware RE, Prose NS, et al. Skin and nail changes in children with sickle cell anemia receiving hydroxyurea therapy. J Am Acad Dermatol 2001;44(5):859–61.

261. Sigal M, Crickx B, Blanchet P, et al. Cutaneous lesions induced by long-term use of hydroxyurea. Ann Dermatol Venereol 1984;111(10):895–900 [in French].

262. Burns DA, Sarkany I, Gaylarde P. Effects of hydroxyurea therapy on normal skin: a case report. Clin Exp Dermatol 1980;5(4):447–9.

263. Richard M, Truchetet F, Friedel J, et al. Skin lesions simulating chronic dermatomyositis during long-term hydroxyurea therapy. J Am Acad Dermatol 1989;21(4 Pt 1):797–9.

264. Perrot JL, Cambazard F. A case for diagnosis: hydrea pseudo-dermatomyositis. Ann Dermatol Venereol 1994;121(6–7):499–500 [in French].

265. Kelly RI, Bull RH, Marsden A. Cutaneous manifestations of long-term hydroxyurea therapy. Australas J Dermatol 1994;35(2):61–4.

266. Senet P, Aractingi S, Porneuf M, et al. Hydroxyurea-induced dermatomyositis-like eruption. Br J Dermatol 1995;133(3):455–9.

267. Weber L, Schick E, Merkel M, et al. Dermatomyositis-like skin changes with long-term hydroxyurea (Litalir) therapy. Hautarzt 1995;46(10):717–21 [in German].

268. Bahadoran P, Castanet J, Lacour JP, et al. Pseudo-dermatomyositis induced by long-term hydroxyurea therapy: report of two cases. Br J Dermatol 1996;134(6):1161–3.

269. Marie I, Joly P, Levesque H, et al. Pseudo-dermatomyositis as a complication of hydroxyurea therapy. Clin Exp Rheumatol 2000;18(4):536–7.

270. Rocamora V, Puig L, Alomar A. Dermatomyositis-like eruption following hydroxyurea therapy. J Eur Acad Dermatol Venereol 2000;14(3):227–8.

271. Vassallo C, Passamonti F, Merante S, et al. Mucocutaneous changes during long-term therapy with hydroxyurea in chronic myeloid leukaemia. Clin Exp Dermatol 2001;26(2):141–8.

272. Oskay T, Kutluay L, Ozyilkan O. Dermatomyositis-like eruption after long-term hydroxyurea therapy for polycythemia vera. Eur J Dermatol 2002;12(6):586–8.

273. Dacey MJ, Callen JP. Hydroxyurea-induced dermatomyositis-like eruption. J Am Acad Dermatol 2003;48(3):439–41.

274. Oh ST, Lee DW, Lee JY, et al. Hydroxyurea-induced melanonychia concomitant with a dermatomyositis-like eruption. J Am Acad Dermatol 2003;49(2):339–41.

275. Elliott R, Davies M, Harmse D. Dermatomyositis-like eruption with long-term hydroxyurea. J Dermatolog Treat 2006;17(1):59–60.

276. Slobodin G, Lurie M, Munichor M, et al. Gottron's papules-like eruption developing under hydroxyurea therapy. Rheumatol Int 2006;26(8):768–70.

277. Janerowicz D, Czarnecka-Operacz M, Stawny M, et al. Dermatomyositis-like eruption induced by hydroxyurea: a case report. Acta Dermatovenerol Alp Panonica Adriat 2009;18(3):131–4.

278. Daoud MS, Gibson LE, Pittelkow MR. Hydroxyurea dermopathy: a unique lichenoid eruption complicating long-term therapy with hydroxyurea. J Am Acad Dermatol 1997;36(2 Pt 1):178–82.

279. Haniffa MA, Speight EL. Painful leg ulcers and a rash in a patient with polycythaemia rubra vera. Diagnosis: hydroxyurea-induced leg ulceration and dermatomyositis-like skin changes. Clin Exp Dermatol 2006;31(5):733–4.

280. Kirby B, Gibson LE, Rogers S, et al. Dermatomyositis-like eruption and leg ulceration caused by hydroxyurea in a patient with psoriasis. Clin Exp Dermatol 2000;25(3):256–7.

281. Martorell-Calatayud A, Requena C, Nagore-Enguidanos E, et al. Multiple, painful, treatment-resistant leg ulcers associated with dermatomyositis-like lesions over the interphalangeal joints induced by hydroxyurea. Actas Dermosifiliogr 2009;100(9):804–7 [in Spanish].

282. Suehiro M, Kishimoto S, Wakabayashi T, et al. Hydroxyurea dermopathy with a dermatomyositis-like eruption and a large leg ulcer. Br J Dermatol 1998;139(4):748–9.

283. Varma S, Lanigan SW. Dermatomyositis-like eruption and leg ulceration caused by hydroxyurea in a patient with psoriasis. Clin Exp Dermatol 1999;24(3):164–6.

284. Bohn J, Hansen JP, Menne T. Ulcerative lichen planus-like dermatitis due to long-term hydroxyurea therapy. J Eur Acad Dermatol Venereol 1998;10(2):187–9.

285. Renfro L, Kamino H, Raphael B, et al. Ulcerative lichen planus-like dermatitis associated with hydroxyurea. J Am Acad Dermatol 1991;24(1):143–5.

286. Velez A, Lopez-Rubio F, Moreno JC. Chronic hydroxyurea-induced dermatomyositis-like eruption with severe dermal elastosis. Clin Exp Dermatol 1998;23(2):94–5.

287. Inhoff O, Peitsch WK, Paredes BE, et al. Simvastatin-induced amyopathic dermatomyositis. Br J Dermatol 2009;161(1):206–8.

288. Rodriguez-Garcia JL, Serrano Commino M. Lovastatin-associated dermatomyositis. Postgrad Med J 1996;72(853):694.

289. Khattak FH, Morris IM, Branford WA. Simvastatin-associated dermatomyositis. Br J Rheumatol 1994;33(2):199.

290. Carroll GJ, Will RK, Peter JB, et al. Penicillamine induced polymyositis and dermatomyositis. J Rheumatol 1987;14(5):995–1001.

291. Kass E, Straume S, Munthe E. Dermatomyositis after B.C.G. vaccination. Lancet 1978;1(8067):772.

292. Akiyama C, Osada A, Sou K, et al. A case of dermatomyositis triggered by tegafur. Acta Derm Venereol 1997;77(6):490.

293. Ruiz-Genao DP, Sanz-Sánchez T, Bartolomé-Gonzalez B, et al. Dermatomyositis-like reaction induced by chemotherapeutical agents. Int J Dermatol 2002;41(12):885–7.

294. Kumar B, Saraswat A, Kaur I. Mucocutaneous adverse effects of hydroxyurea: a prospective study of 30 psoriasis patients. Clin Exp Dermatol 2002;27(1):8–13.

295. Iversen OH. Hydroxyurea enhances methylnitrosourea skin tumorigenesis when given shortly before, but not after, the carcinogen. Carcinogenesis 1982;3(8):891–4.

296. Disdier P, Harle JR, Grob JJ, et al. Rapid development of multiple squamous-cell carcinomas during chronic granulocytic leukemia. Dermatologica 1991;183(1):47–8.

297. Papi M, Didona B, DePità O, et al. Multiple skin tumors on light-exposed areas during long-term

treatment with hydroxyurea. J Am Acad Dermatol 1993;28(3):485–6.

298. Stasi R, Cantonetti M, Abruzzese E, et al. Multiple skin tumors in long-term treatment with hydroxyurea. Eur J Haematol 1992;48(2):121–2.

299. Angeli-Besson C, Koeppel MC, Jacquet P, et al. Multiple squamous-cell carcinomas of the scalp and chronic myeloid leukemia. Dermatology 1995; 191(4):321–2.

300. Grange F, Couilliet D, Audhuy B, et al. Multiple keratosis induced by hydroxyurea. Ann Dermatol Venereol 1995;122(1–2):16–8 [in French].

301. Callot-Mellot C, Bodemer C, Chosidow O, et al. Cutaneous carcinoma during long-term hydroxyurea therapy: a report of 5 cases. Arch Dermatol 1996;132(11):1395–7.

302. De Simone C, Guerriero C, Guidi B, et al. Multiple squamous cell carcinomas of the skin during long-term treatment with hydroxyurea. Eur J Dermatol 1998;8(2):114–5.

303. Salmon-Ehr V, Grosieux C, Potron G, et al. Multiple actinic keratosis and skin tumors secondary to hydroxyurea treatment. Dermatology 1998;196(2):274.

304. Best PJ, Petitt RM. Multiple skin cancers associated with hydroxyurea therapy. Mayo Clin Proc 1998;73(10):961–3.

305. Salmon-Ehr V, Leborgne G, Bilque JP, et al. Secondary cutaneous effects of hydroxyurea: prospective study of 26 patients from a dermatologic consultation. Rev Med Interne 2000;21(1): 30–4 [in French].

306. Esteve E, Georgescu V, Heitzmann P, et al. Multiple skin and mouth squamous cell carcinomas related to long-term treatment with hydroxyurea. Ann Dermatol Venereol 2001;128(8–9):919–21 [in French].

307. Aste N, Fumo G, Biggio P. Multiple squamous epitheliomas during long-term treatment with hydroxyurea. J Eur Acad Dermatol Venereol 2001; 15(1):89–90.

308. Saraceno R, Teoli M, Chimenti S. Hydroxyurea associated with concomitant occurrence of diffuse longitudinal melanonychia and multiple squamous cell carcinomas in an elderly subject. Clin Ther 2008;30(7):1324–9.

309. Sanchez-Palacios C, Guitart J. Hydroxyurea-associated squamous dysplasia. J Am Acad Dermatol 2004;51(2):293–300.

310. Bouldouyre MA, Avril MF, Gaulierk A, et al. Association of cutaneous side-effects of hydroxyurea and neuroendocrine carcinoma. Eur J Dermatol 2005; 15(4):268–70.

311. Francis AA, Blevins RD, Carrier WL, et al. Inhibition of DNA repair in ultraviolet-irradiated human cells by hydroxyurea. Biochim Biophys Acta 1979; 563(2):385–92.

312. Yarbro JW. Mechanism of action of hydroxyurea. Semin Oncol 1992;19(3 Suppl 9):1–10.

313. Jonason AS, Kunala S, Price GJ, et al. Frequent clones of p53-mutated keratinocytes in normal human skin. Proc Natl Acad Sci U S A 1996; 93(24):14025–9.

314. Zhang W, Remenyik E, Zelterman D, et al. Escaping the stem cell compartment: sustained UVB exposure allows p53-mutant keratinocytes to colonize adjacent epidermal proliferating units without incurring additional mutations. Proc Natl Acad Sci U S A 2001;98(24):13948–53.

315. Kalajian AH, Cely SJ, Malone JC, et al. Hydroxyurea-associated dermatomyositis-like eruption demonstrating abnormal epidermal p53 expression: a potential premalignant manifestation of chronic hydroxyurea and UV radiation exposure. Arch Dermatol 2010;146(3):305–10.

316. Weinlich G, Schuler G, Greil R, et al. Leg ulcers associated with long-term hydroxyurea therapy. J Am Acad Dermatol 1998;39(2 Pt 2):372–4.

317. Dissemond J, Hoeft D, Knab J, et al. Leg ulcer in a patient associated with hydroxyurea therapy. Int J Dermatol 2006;45(2):158–60.

318. Saravu K, Velappan P, Lakshmi N, et al. Hydroxyurea induced perimalleolar ulcers. J Korean Med Sci 2006;21(1):177–9.

319. Nguyen TV, Margolis DJ. Hydroxyurea and lower leg ulcers. Cutis 1993;52(4):217–9.

320. Best PJ, Daoud MS, Pittelkow MR, et al. Hydroxyurea-induced leg ulceration in 14 patients. Ann Intern Med 1998;128(1):29–32.

321. Disla E, D'Eamour L, Cioriou M. Hydroxyurea-associated leg ulceration. Ann Intern Med 1998;129(3): 252–3.

322. Kennedy BJ. Hydroxyurea-associated leg ulceration. Ann Intern Med 1998;129(3):252–3.

323. Young HS, Kirby B, Stewart EJ. Aggressive, extensive, vasculitic leg ulceration associated with hydroxyurea therapy and a fatal outcome. Clin Exp Dermatol 2001;26(8):664–7.

324. Demircay Z, Comert A, Adiguzel C. Leg ulcers and hydroxyurea: report of three cases with essential thrombocythemia. Int J Dermatol 2002;41(12):872–4.

325. Friedrich S, Raff K, Landthaler M, et al. Cutaneous ulcerations on hands and heels secondary to long-term hydroxyurea treatment. Eur J Dermatol 2004; 14(5):343–6.

326. Hwang SW, Hong SK, Kim SH, et al. A hydroxyurea-induced leg ulcer. Ann Dermatol 2009; 21(1):39–41.

327. Sirieix ME, Debure C, Baudot N, et al. Leg ulcers and hydroxyurea: forty-one cases. Arch Dermatol 1999;135(7):818–20.

328. Karincaoglu Y, Kaya E, Esrefoglu M, et al. Development of large genital ulcer due to hydroxyurea treatment in a patient with chronic myeloid leukemia and Behcet's disease. Leuk Lymphoma 2003;44(6):1063–5.

329. Yasuda N, Ohmori S, Usui T. Hydroxyurea-induced gangrene of the toes in a patient with chronic myelogenous leukemia. Am J Hematol 2000; 63(2):103–4.

330. Kido M, Tago O, Fujiwara H, et al. Leg ulcer associated with hydroxyurea treatment in a patient with chronic myelogenous leukaemia: successful treatment with prostaglandin E1 and pentoxifylline. Br J Dermatol 1998;139(6):1124–6.

331. Stagno F, Guglielmo P, Consoli U, et al. Successful healing of hydroxyurea-related leg ulcers with topical granulocyte-macrophage colony-stimulating factor. Blood 1999;94(4):1479–80.

332. Flores F, Eaglstein WA, Kirsner RS. Hydroxyurea-induced leg ulcers treated with Apligraf. Ann Intern Med 2000;132(5):417–8.

333. Aragane Y, Okamoto T, Yajima A, et al. Hydroxyurea-induced foot ulcer successfully treated with a topical basic fibroblast growth factor product. Br J Dermatol 2003;148(3):599–600.

334. Romanelli M, Dini V, Romanelli P. Hydroxyurea-induced leg ulcers treated with a protease-modulating matrix. Arch Dermatol 2007;143(10): 1310–3.

335. Zaccaria E, Cozzani E, Parodi A. Secondary cutaneous effects of hydroxyurea: possible pathogenetic mechanisms. J Dermatolog Treat 2006; 17(3):176–8.

336. Velez A, Garcia-Aranda JM, Moreno JC. Hydroxyurea-induced leg ulcers: is macroerythrocytosis a pathogenic factor? J Eur Acad Dermatol Venereol 1999;12(3):243–4.

337. Engstrom KG, Lofvenberg E. Treatment of myeloproliferative disorders with hydroxyurea: effects on red blood cell geometry and deformability. Blood 1998;91(10):3986–91.

338. Wirth K, Schoepf E, Mertelsmann R, et al. Leg ulceration with associated thrombocytosis: healing of ulceration associated with treatment of the raised platelet count. Br J Dermatol 1998;138(3): 533–5.

339. Weinlich G, Fritsch P. Leg ulcers in patients treated with hydroxyurea for myeloproliferative disorders: what is the trigger? Br J Dermatol 1999;141(1): 171–2.

340. Guillot B, Bessis D, Dereure O. Mucocutaneous side effects of antineoplastic chemotherapy. Expert Opin Drug Saf 2004;3(6):579–87.

341. Payne AS, James WD, Weiss RB. Dermatologic toxicity of chemotherapeutic agents. Semin Oncol 2006;33(1):86–97.

342. Wyatt AJ, Leonard GD, Sachs DL. Cutaneous reactions to chemotherapy and their management. Am J Clin Dermatol 2006;7(1):45–63.

343. James WD, Berger TG, Elston DM, editors. Andrews' diseases of the skin: clinical dermatology. 10th edition. Philadelphia: Saunders Elsevier; 2006.

344. Volcy J, Nzerue CM, Oderinde A, et al. Cocaine-induced acute renal failure, hemolysis, and thrombocytopenia mimicking thrombotic thrombocytopenic purpura. Am J Kidney Dis 2000; 35(1):E3.

345. Keung YK, Morgan D, Cobos E. Cocaine-induced microangiopathic hemolytic anemia and thrombocytopenia simulating thrombotic thrombocytopenia purpura. Ann Hematol 1996;72(3):155–6.

346. Chevalier X, Rostoker G, Larget-Piet B, et al. Schoenlein-Henoch purpura with necrotizing vasculitis after cocaine snorting. Clin Nephrol 1995;43(5):348–9.

347. Koury MJ. Thrombocytopenic purpura in HIV-seronegative users of intravenous cocaine. Am J Hematol 1990;35(2):134–5.

348. Savona S, Nardi MA, Lennette ET, et al. Thrombocytopenic purpura in narcotics addicts. Ann Intern Med 1985;102(6):737–41.

349. Drug Intelligence Brief. Cocaine containing levamisole adversely affecting drug users in the United States [DEA-10001-levamisole]. Drug Enforcement Administration, Intelligence Production Unit. United States Department of Justice, Washington, DC.

350. Buchanan JA, Heard K, Burbach C, et al. Prevalence of levamisole in urine toxicology screens positive for cocaine in an inner-city hospital. JAMA 2011;305(16):1657–8.

351. Krendel DA, Ditter SM, Frankel MR, et al. Biopsy-proven cerebral vasculitis associated with cocaine abuse. Neurology 1990;40(7):1092–4.

352. Fredericks RK, Lefkowitz DS, Challa VR, et al. Cerebral vasculitis associated with cocaine abuse. Stroke 1991;22(11):1437–9.

353. Morrow PL, McQuillen JB. Cerebral vasculitis associated with cocaine abuse. J Forensic Sci 1993; 38(3):732–8.

354. Merkel PA, Koroshetz WJ, Irizarry MC, et al. Cocaine-associated cerebral vasculitis. Semin Arthritis Rheum 1995;25(3):172–83.

355. Fiala M, Gan XH, Zhang L, et al. Cocaine enhances monocyte migration across the blood-brain barrier. Cocaine's connection to AIDS dementia and vasculitis? Adv Exp Med Biol 1998;437:199–205.

356. Enriquez R, Palacios FO, González CM, et al. Skin vasculitis, hypokalemia and acute renal failure in rhabdomyolysis associated with cocaine. Nephron 1991;59(2):336–7.

357. Kumar PD, Smith HR. Cocaine-related vasculitis causing upper-limb peripheral vascular disease. Ann Intern Med 2000;133(11):923–4.

358. Hofbauer GF, Burg G, Nestle FO. Cocaine-related Stevens-Johnson syndrome. Dermatology 2000; 201(3):258–60.

359. Chen SC, Jang MY, Wang CS, et al. Cocaine-related vasculitis causing scrotal gangrene. Ann Pharmacother 2009;43(2):375–8.

360. Orriols R, Muñoz X, Ferrer J, et al. Cocaine-induced Churg-Strauss vasculitis. Eur Respir J 1996;9(1):175–7.

361. Gertner E, Hamlar D. Necrotizing granulomatous vasculitis associated with cocaine use. J Rheumatol 2002;29(8):1795–7.

362. Marder VJ, Mellinghoff IK. Cocaine and Buerger disease: is there a pathogenetic association? Arch Intern Med 2000;160(13):2057–60.

363. Friedman DR, Wolfsthal SD. Cocaine-induced pseudovasculitis. Mayo Clin Proc 2005;80(5):671–3.

364. Armstrong M Jr, Shikani AH. Nasal septal necrosis mimicking Wegener's granulomatosis in a cocaine abuser. Ear Nose Throat J 1996;75(9):623–6.

365. Rachapalli SM, Kiely PD. Cocaine-induced midline destructive lesions mimicking ENT-limited Wegener's granulomatosis. Scand J Rheumatol 2008; 37(6):477–80.

366. Rowshani AT, Schot LJ, ten Berge IJ. c-ANCA as a serological pitfall. Lancet 2004;363(9411):782.

367. Wiesner O, Russell KA, Lee AS, et al. Antineutrophil cytoplasmic antibodies reacting with human neutrophil elastase as a diagnostic marker for cocaine-induced midline destructive lesions but not autoimmune vasculitis. Arthritis Rheum 2004; 50(9):2954–65.

368. Neynaber S, Mistry-Burchardi N, Rust C, et al. PR3-ANCA-positive necrotizing multi-organ vasculitis following cocaine abuse. Acta Derm Venereol 2008;88(6):594–6.

369. Rosenthal M, Beysse Y, Dixon AS, et al. Levamisole and agranulocytosis. Lancet 1977;1(8017):904–5.

370. Macfarlane DG, Bacon PA. Levamisole-induced vasculitis due to circulating immune complexes. Br Med J 1978;1(6110):407–8.

371. Scheinberg MA, Bezerra JB, Almeida FA, et al. Cutaneous necrotising vasculitis induced by levamisole. Br Med J 1978;1(6110):408.

372. Rongioletti F, Ghio L, Ginevri F, et al. Purpura of the ears: a distinctive vasculopathy with circulating autoantibodies complicating long-term treatment with levamisole in children. Br J Dermatol 1999; 140(5):948–51.

373. Amery WK, Bruynseels JP. Levamisole, the story and the lessons. Int J Immunopharmacol 1992; 14(3):481–6.

374. Farhat EK, Muirhead TT, Chaffins ML, et al. Levamisole-induced cutaneous necrosis mimicking coagulopathy. Arch Dermatol 2010;146(11):1320–1.

375. Walsh NM, Green PJ, Burlingame RW, et al. Cocaine-related retiform purpura: evidence to incriminate the adulterant, levamisole. J Cutan Pathol 2010;37(12):1212–9.

376. Waller JM, Feramisco JD, Alberta-Wszolek L, et al. Cocaine-associated retiform purpura and neutropenia: is levamisole the culprit? J Am Acad Dermatol 2010;63(3):530–5.

377. Fthenakis A, Klein PA. Retiform purpura in a patient with a history of cocaine use. Dermatol Online J 2011;17(4):12.

378. Bradford M, Rosenberg B, Moreno J, et al. Bilateral necrosis of earlobes and cheeks: another complication of cocaine contaminated with levamisole. Ann Intern Med 2010;152(11):758–9.

379. Muirhead TT, Eide MJ. Images in clinical medicine. Toxic effects of levamisole in a cocaine user. N Engl J Med 2011;364(24):e52.

380. Chung C, Tumeh PC, Birnbaum R, et al. Characteristic purpura of the ears, vasculitis, and neutropenia—a potential public health epidemic associated with levamisole-adulterated cocaine. J Am Acad Dermatol 2011;65(4):722–5.

381. Buchanan JA, Vogel JA, Eberhardt AM. Levamisole-induced occlusive necrotizing vasculitis of the ears after use of cocaine contaminated with levamisole. J Med Toxicol 2011;7(1):83–4.

382. Lung D, Lynch K, Agrawal S, et al. Images in emergency medicine. Adult female with rash on lower extremities. Vasculopathic purpura and neutropenia caused by levamisole-contaminated cocaine. Ann Emerg Med 2011;57(3):307, 311.

383. Ullrich K, Koval R, Koval E, et al. Five consecutive cases of a cutaneous vasculopathy in users of levamisole-adulterated cocaine. J Clin Rheumatol 2011;17(4):193–6.

384. Han C, Sreenivasan G, Dutz JP. Reversible retiform purpura: a sign of cocaine use. CMAJ 2011;183(9):E597–600.

385. Geller L, Whang TB, Mercer SE, et al. Retiform purpura: a new stigmata of illicit drug use? Dermatol Online J 2011;17(2):7.

386. Quesada JR, Hersh EM, Manning J, et al. Treatment of hairy cell leukemia with recombinant alpha-interferon. Blood 1986;68(2):493–7.

387. Quesada JR, Reuben J, Manning JT, et al. Alpha interferon for induction of remission in hairy-cell leukemia. N Engl J Med 1984;310(1):15–8.

388. Krown SE, Real FX, Vadhan-Raj S, et al. Kaposi's sarcoma and the acquired immune deficiency syndrome. Treatment with recombinant interferon alpha and analysis of prognostic factors. Cancer 1986;57(Suppl 8):1662–5.

389. Krown SE, Real FX, Cunningham-Rundles S, et al. Preliminary observations on the effect of recombinant leukocyte A interferon in homosexual men with Kaposi's sarcoma. N Engl J Med 1983; 308(18):1071–6.

390. Georgiou S, Monastirli A, Pasmatzi E, et al. Efficacy and safety of systemic recombinant interferon-alpha in Behcet's disease. J Intern Med 1998; 243(5):367–72.

391. Zouboulis CC, Orfanos CE. Treatment of Adamantiades-Behcet disease with systemic interferon alfa. Arch Dermatol 1998;134(8):1010–6.

392. O'Brien SG, Guilhot J, Larson RA, et al. Imatinib compared with interferon and low-dose cytarabine for newly diagnosed chronic-phase chronic myeloid leukemia. N Engl J Med 2003;348(11):994–1004.

393. Preudhomme C, Guilhot J, Nicolini FE, et al. Imatinib plus peginterferon alfa-2a in chronic myeloid leukemia. N Engl J Med 2010;363(26):2511–21.

394. Marcellin P, Lau GK, Bonino F, et al. Peginterferon alfa-2a alone, lamivudine alone, and the two in combination in patients with HBeAg-negative chronic hepatitis B. N Engl J Med 2004;351(12):1206–17.

395. McHutchison JG, Lawitz EJ, Mitchell L, et al. Peginterferon alfa-2b or alfa-2a with ribavirin for treatment of hepatitis C infection. N Engl J Med 2009; 361(6):580–93.

396. Hill NO, Pardue A, Khan A, et al. Interferon and cimetidine for malignant melanoma. N Engl J Med 1983;308(5):286.

397. Borgstrom S, von Eyben FE, Flodgren P, et al. Human leukocyte interferon and cimetidine for metastatic melanoma. N Engl J Med 1982;307(17):1080–1.

398. Eron LJ, Judson F, Tucker S, et al. Interferon therapy for condylomata acuminata. N Engl J Med 1986;315(17):1059–64.

399. Maurtua MA, Moscinski LC, Messina J, et al. Type III hypersensitivity reaction with the use of interferon-alpha. Am J Hematol 1997;55(1):53–4.

400. Detmar U, Agathos M, Nerl C. Allergy of delayed type to recombinant interferon alpha 2c. Contact Dermatitis 1989;20(2):149–50.

401. Milkiewicz P, Yim C, Pache I, et al. Diffuse skin reaction in patient with hepatitis B, treated with two different formulations of pegylated interferon. Can J Gastroenterol 2005;19(11):677–8.

402. Krainick U, Kantarjian H, Broussard S, et al. Local cutaneous necrotizing lesions associated with interferon injections. J Interferon Cytokine Res 1998; 18(10):823–7.

403. Rosina P, Girolomoni G. Cutaneous necrosis complicating the injection of pegylated interferon alpha-2b in a patient with chronic hepatitis C. Acta Dermatovenerol Croat 2008;16(1):35–7.

404. Funk J, Langeland T, Schrumpf E, et al. Psoriasis induced by interferon-alpha. Br J Dermatol 1991; 125(5):463–5.

405. Wolfe JT, Singh A, Lessin SR, et al. De novo development of psoriatic plaques in patients receiving interferon alfa for treatment of erythrodermic cutaneous T-cell lymphoma. J Am Acad Dermatol 1995;32(5 Pt 2):887–93.

406. Wolfer LU, Goerdt S, Schröder K, et al. Interferon-alpha-induced psoriasis vulgaris. Hautarzt 1996; 47(2):124–8 [in German].

407. Nguyen C, Misery L, Tigaud JD, et al. Psoriasis induced by interferon-alpha. Apropos of a case. Ann Med Interne (Paris) 1996;147(7):519–21 [in French].

408. Taylor C, Burns DA, Wiselka MJ. Extensive psoriasis induced by interferon alfa treatment for chronic hepatitis C. Postgrad Med J 2000; 76(896):365–7.

409. Ketikoglou I, Karatapanis S, Elefsiniotis I, et al. Extensive psoriasis induced by pegylated interferon alpha-2b treatment for chronic hepatitis B. Eur J Dermatol 2005;15(2):107–9.

410. Horev A, Halevy S. New-onset psoriasis following treatment with pegylated interferon-alpha 2b and ribavirin for chronic hepatitis C. Isr Med Assoc J 2009;11(12):760–1.

411. Kusec R, Ostojić S, Planinc-Peraica A, et al. Exacerbation of psoriasis after treatment with alpha-interferon. Dermatologica 1990;181(2):170.

412. Quesada JR, Gutterman JU. Psoriasis and alpha-interferon. Lancet 1986;1(8496):1466–8.

413. Georgetson MJ, Yarze JC, Lalos AT, et al. Exacerbation of psoriasis due to interferon-alpha treatment of chronic active hepatitis. Am J Gastroenterol 1993; 88(10):1756–8.

414. Pauluzzi P, Kokelj F, Perkan V, et al. Psoriasis exacerbation induced by interferon-alpha. Report of two cases. Acta Derm Venereol 1993;73(5):395.

415. Downs AM, Dunnill MG. Exacerbation of psoriasis by interferon-alpha therapy for hepatitis C. Clin Exp Dermatol 2000;25(4):351–2.

416. Cervoni JP, Serfaty L, Picard O, et al. The treatment of hepatitis B and C with interferon-alpha can induce or aggravate psoriasis. Gastroenterol Clin Biol 1995;19(3):324–5 [in French].

417. Ladoyanni E, Nambi R. Psoriasis exacerbated by interferon-alpha in a patient with chronic myeloid leukemia. J Drugs Dermatol 2005;4(2):221–2.

418. Erkek E, Karaduman A, Akcan Y, et al. Psoriasis associated with HCV and exacerbated by interferon alpha: complete clearance with acitretin during interferon alpha treatment for chronic active hepatitis. Dermatology 2000;201(2):179–81.

419. Besisik SK, Kocabey G, Caliskan Y. Major depression and psoriasis activation due to interferon-alpha in a patient with chronic myeloid leukemia; "overlooked and/or misdiagnosed adverse reaction in malignant disease". Am J Hematol 2003; 74(3):224.

420. Yurci A, Guven K, Torun E, et al. Pyoderma gangrenosum and exacerbation of psoriasis resulting from pegylated interferon alpha and ribavirin treatment of chronic hepatitis C. Eur J Gastroenterol Hepatol 2007;19(9):811–5.

421. Nestle FO, Conrad C, Tun-Kyi A, et al. Plasmacytoid predendritic cells initiate psoriasis through interferon-alpha production. J Exp Med 2005; 202(1):135–43.

422. Eriksen KW, Lovato P, Skov L, et al. Increased sensitivity to interferon-alpha in psoriatic T cells. J Invest Dermatol 2005;125(5):936–44.

423. Boyman O, Hefti HP, Conrad C, et al. Spontaneous development of psoriasis in a new animal model shows an essential role for resident T cells and tumor necrosis factor-alpha. J Exp Med 2004; 199(5):731–6.

424. Nestle FO, Gilliet M. Defining upstream elements of psoriasis pathogenesis: an emerging role for interferon alpha. J Invest Dermatol 2005;125(5):xiv–xxv.

425. Tekin NS, Ustundag Y, Tekin IO, et al. Early administration of ultraviolet treatment is effective in pegylated interferon alpha-induced severe acute exacerbation of psoriasis: a case report and short review of the literature. Int J Clin Pract 2010; 64(1):101–3.

426. Ohhata I, Ochi T, Kurebayashi S, et al. A case of subcutaneous sarcoid nodules induced by interferon-alpha. Nihon Kyobu Shikkan Gakkai Zasshi 1994;32(10):996–1000 [in Japanese].

427. Yavorkovsky LL, Carrum G, Bruce S, et al. Cutaneous sarcoidosis in a patient with Philadelphia-positive chronic myelogenous leukemia treated with interferon-alpha. Am J Hematol 1998;58(1): 80–1.

428. Savoye G, Goria O, Herve S, et al. Probable cutaneous sarcoidosis associated with combined ribavirin and interferon-alpha therapy for chronic hepatitis C. Gastroenterol Clin Biol 2000;24(6–7): 679 [in French].

429. Neglia V, Sookoian S, Herrera M, et al. Development of cutaneous sarcoidosis in a patient with chronic hepatitis C treated with interferon alpha 2b. J Cutan Med Surg 2001;5(5):406–8.

430. Cogrel O, Doutre MS, Marliére V, et al. Cutaneous sarcoidosis during interferon alfa and ribavirin treatment of hepatitis C virus infection: two cases. Br J Dermatol 2002;146(2):320–4.

431. Nawras A, Alsolaiman MM, Mehboob S, et al. Systemic sarcoidosis presenting as a granulomatous tattoo reaction secondary to interferon-alpha treatment for chronic hepatitis C and review of the literature. Dig Dis Sci 2002;47(7):1627–31.

432. Leclerc S, Myers RP, Moussalli J, et al. Sarcoidosis and interferon therapy: report of five cases and review of the literature. Eur J Intern Med 2003; 14(4):237–43.

433. Rogers CJ, Romagosa R, Vincek V. Cutaneous sarcoidosis associated with pegylated interferon alfa and ribavirin therapy in a patient with chronic hepatitis C. J Am Acad Dermatol 2004;50(4):649–50.

434. Toulemonde A, Quereux G, Dreno B. Sarcoidosis granuloma on a tattoo induced by interferon alpha. Ann Dermatol Venereol 2004;131(1 Pt 1):49–51 [in French].

435. Werchniak AE, Cheng SX, Dhar AD, et al. Sarcoidosis presenting as tattoo changes in a patient undergoing treatment with interferon-alpha and ribavirin. Clin Exp Dermatol 2004;29(5):547–8.

436. Guilabert A, Bosch X, Juliá M, et al. Pegylated interferon alfa-induced sarcoidosis: two sides of the same coin. Br J Dermatol 2005;152(2):377–9.

437. Alonso-Perez A, Ballestero-Diez M, Fraga J, et al. Cutaneous sarcoidosis by interferon therapy in a patient with melanoma. J Eur Acad Dermatol Venereol 2006;20(10):1328–9.

438. Benali S, Boustiére C, Castellani P, et al. Sarcoidosis following pegylated interferon therapy: two cases. Gastroenterol Clin Biol 2006;30(4):615–9 [in French].

439. Sanchez-Ruano JJ, Artaza-Varasa T, Gómez-Rodriguez R, et al. Cutaneopulmonary sarcoidosis during pegylated interferon plus ribavirin therapy. Gastroenterol Hepatol 2006;29(3):150 [in Spanish].

440. Fischer J, Metzler G, Schaller M. Cosmetic permanent fillers for soft tissue augmentation: a new contraindication for interferon therapies. Arch Dermatol 2007;143(4):507–10.

441. Honsova E, Sticova E, Sperl J. Cutaneous sarcoidosis during pegylated interferon alpha and ribavirin treatment of chronic hepatitis C—a case report. Cesk Patol 2007;43(1):27–30 [in Czech].

442. Pelletier F, Manzoni P, Jacoulet P, et al. Pulmonary and cutaneous sarcoidosis associated with interferon therapy for melanoma. Cutis 2007;80(5):441–5.

443. Perez-Gala S, Delgado-Jimenez Y, Goiriz R, et al. Cutaneous sarcoidosis limited to scars following pegylated interferon alfa and ribavirin therapy in a patient with chronic hepatitis C. J Eur Acad Dermatol Venereol 2007;21(3):393–4.

444. Descamps V, Landry J, Francés C, et al. Facial cosmetic filler injections as possible target for systemic sarcoidosis in patients treated with interferon for chronic hepatitis C: two cases. Dermatology 2008;217(1):81–4.

445. Fantini F, Padalino C, Gualdi G, et al. Cutaneous lesions as initial signs of interferon alpha-induced sarcoidosis: report of three new cases and review of the literature. Dermatol Ther 2009;22(Suppl 1): S1–7.

446. Martins EV, Gaburri AK, Gaburri D, et al. Cutaneous sarcoidosis: an uncommon side effect of pegylated interferon and ribavirin use for chronic hepatitis C. Case Rep Gastroenterol 2009;3(3):366–71.

447. Monsuez JJ, Carcelain G, Charniot JC, et al. T cells subtypes in a patient with interferon-alpha induced sarcoidosis. Am J Med Sci 2009;337(1):60–2.

448. Shinohara MM, Davis C, Olerud J. Concurrent antiphospholipid syndrome and cutaneous [corrected] sarcoidosis due to interferon alfa and ribavirin treatment for hepatitis C. J Drugs Dermatol 2009; 8(9):870–2.

449. Shuja F, Kavoussi SC, Mir MR, et al. Interferon induced sarcoidosis with cutaneous involvement along lines of venous drainage in a former intravenous drug user. Dermatol Online J 2009;15(12):4.

450. Dhaille F, Viseux V, Caudron A, et al. Cutaneous sarcoidosis occurring during anti-TNF-alpha treatment: report of two cases. Dermatology 2010; 220(3):234–7.

451. Faurie P, Broussolle C, Zoulim F, et al. Sarcoidosis and hepatitis C: clinical description of 11 cases. Eur J Gastroenterol Hepatol 2010;22(8):967–72.

452. Gayet AR, Plaisance P, Bergmann JF, et al. Development of sarcoidosis following completion of treatment for hepatitis C with pegylated interferon-{alpha}2a and ribavirin: a case report and literature review. Clin Med Res 2010;8(3–4):163–7.

453. Heinzerling LM, Anliker MD, Müller J, et al. Sarcoidosis induced by interferon-alpha in melanoma patients: incidence, clinical manifestations, and management strategies. J Immunother 2010; 33(8):834–9.

454. Lee YB, Lee JI, Park HJ, et al. Interferon-alpha induced sarcoidosis with cutaneous involvement along the lines of venous drainage. Ann Dermatol 2011;23(2):239–41.

455. Lopez V, Molina I, Monteagudo C, et al. Cutaneous sarcoidosis developing after treatment with pegylated interferon and ribavirin: a new case and review of the literature. Int J Dermatol 2011;50(3): 287–91.

456. North J, Mully T. Alpha-interferon induced sarcoidosis mimicking metastatic melanoma. J Cutan Pathol 2011;38(7):585–9.

457. Atluri D, Iduru S, Veluru C, et al. A levitating tattoo in a hepatitis C patient on treatment. Liver Int 2010; 30(4):583–4.

458. Ramos-Casals M, Mañá J, Nardi N, et al. Sarcoidosis in patients with chronic hepatitis C virus infection: analysis of 68 cases. Medicine (Baltimore) 2005;84(2):69–80.

459. Akahoshi M, Ishihara M, Remus N, et al. Association between IFNA genotype and the risk of sarcoidosis. Hum Genet 2004;114(5):503–9.

460. Chen H, Wang LW, Huang YQ, et al. Interferon-alpha induces high expression of APOBEC3G and STAT-1 in vitro and in vivo. Int J Mol Sci 2010;11(9):3501–12.

461. Rosenbaum JT, Pasadhika S, Crouser ED, et al. Hypothesis: sarcoidosis is a STAT1-mediated disease. Clin Immunol 2009;132(2):174–83.

462. Iannuzzi MC, Rybicki BA, Teirstein AS. Sarcoidosis. N Engl J Med 2007;357(21):2153–65.

463. Roberts SD, Kohli LL, Wood KL, et al. CD4+CD28- T cells are expanded in sarcoidosis. Sarcoidosis Vasc Diffuse Lung Dis 2005;22(1):13–9.

464. Menon Y, Cucurull E, Reisin E, et al. Interferon-alpha-associated sarcoidosis responsive to infliximab therapy. Am J Med Sci 2004;328(3):173–5.

465. Zissel G, Prasse A, Muller-Quernheim J. Sarcoidosis—immunopathogenetic concepts. Semin Respir Crit Care Med 2007;28(1):3–14.

466. Segawa F, Shimizu Y, Saito E, et al. Behcet's disease induced by interferon therapy for chronic myelogenous leukemia. J Rheumatol 1995;22(6): 1183–4.

467. Budak-Alpdogan T, Demircay Z, Alpdogan O, et al. Behcet's disease in patients with chronic myelogenous leukemia: possible role of interferon-alpha treatment in the occurrence of Behcet's symptoms. Ann Hematol 1997;74(1):45–8.

468. Budak-Alpdogan T, Demircay Z, Alpdogan O, et al. Skin hyperreactivity of Behcet's patients (pathergy reaction) is also positive in interferon alpha-treated chronic myeloid leukaemia patients, indicating similarly altered neutrophil functions in both disorders. Br J Rheumatol 1998;37(11):1148–51.

469. Dalekos GN, Christodoulou D, Kistis KG, et al. A prospective evaluation of dermatological side-effects during alpha-interferon therapy for chronic viral hepatitis. Eur J Gastroenterol Hepatol 1998; 10(11):933–9.

470. Rebora A. Skin diseases associated with hepatitis C virus: facts and controversies. Clin Dermatol 2010;28(5):489–96.

471. Grossmann S de M, Teixeira R, de Aguiar MC, et al. Exacerbation of oral lichen planus lesions during treatment of chronic hepatitis C with pegylated interferon and ribavirin. Eur J Gastroenterol Hepatol 2008;20(7):702–6.

472. Arrue I, Saiz A, Ortiz-Romero PL, et al. Lupus-like reaction to interferon at the injection site: report of five cases. J Cutan Pathol 2007;34(Suppl 1):18–21.

473. Berger L, Descamps V, Marck Y, et al. Alpha interferon-induced eczema in atopic patients infected by hepatitis C virus: 4 case reports. Ann Dermatol Venereol 2000;127(1):51–5 [in French].

474. Veldt BJ, Schalm SW, Janssen HL. Severe allergic eczema due to pegylated alpha-interferon may abate after switching to daily conventional alpha-interferon. J Clin Gastroenterol 2007;41(4):432.

475. Dereure O, Raison-Peyron N, Larrey D, et al. Diffuse inflammatory lesions in patients treated with interferon alfa and ribavirin for hepatitis C: a series of 20 patients. Br J Dermatol 2002; 147(6):1142–6.

476. Kerl K, Negro F, Lubbe J. Cutaneous side-effects of treatment of chronic hepatitis C by interferon alfa and ribavirin. Br J Dermatol 2003;149(3):656.

477. Vazquez-López F, Manjón-Haces JA, Pérez-Alvarez R, et al. Eczema-like lesions and disruption of therapy in patients treated with interferon-alfa and ribavirin for chronic hepatitis C: the value of an interdisciplinary assessment. Br J Dermatol 2004;150(5):1046–7, author reply 1047.

478. Girard C, Bessis D, Blatire V, et al. Meyerson's phenomenon induced by interferon-alfa plus ribavirin in hepatitis C infection. Br J Dermatol 2005; 152(1):182–3.

479. Conde-Taboada A, de la Torre C, Feal C, et al. Meyerson's naevi induced by interferon alfa plus ribavirin combination therapy in hepatitis C infection. Br J Dermatol 2005;153(5):1070–2.

480. Krischer J, Pechére M, Salomon D, et al. Interferon alfa-2b-induced Meyerson's nevi in a patient with dysplastic nevus syndrome. J Am Acad Dermatol 1999;40(1):105–6.

481. Radha Krishna Y, Itha S. What caused this lingual hyperpigmentation in a patient with chronic hepatitis C? Liver Int 2010;30(3):416.

482. Gurguta C, Kauer C, Bergholz U, et al. Tongue and skin hyperpigmentation during PEG-interferon-alpha/ribavirin therapy in dark-skinned non-Caucasian patients with chronic hepatitis C. Am J Gastroenterol 2006;101(1):197–8.

483. Torres HA, Bull L, Arduino RC, et al. Tongue hyperpigmentation in a caucasian patient coinfected with HIV and hepatitis C during peginterferon alfa-2b and ribavirin therapy. Am J Gastroenterol 2007;102(6):1334–5.

484. Sood A, Midha V, Bansal M, et al. Lingual hyperpigmentation with pegylated interferon and ribavirin therapy in patients with chronic hepatitis C. Indian J Gastroenterol 2006;25(6):324.

485. Willems M, Munte K, Vrolijk JM, et al. Hyperpigmentation during interferon-alpha therapy for chronic hepatitis C virus infection. Br J Dermatol 2003;149(2):390–4.

486. Lin J, Lott JP, Amorosa VK, et al. Iatrogenic hyperpigmentation in chronically infected hepatitis C patients treated with pegylated interferon and ribavirin. J Am Acad Dermatol 2009;60(5):882–3.

487. Kartal ED, Alpat SN, Ozgunes I, et al. Reversible alopecia universalis secondary to PEG-interferon alpha-2b and ribavirin combination therapy in a patient with chronic hepatitis C virus infection. Eur J Gastroenterol Hepatol 2007;19(9):817–20.

488. Taliani G, Biliotti E, Capanni M, et al. Reversible alopecia universalis during treatment with PEG-interferon and ribavirin for chronic hepatitis C. J Chemother 2005;17(2):212–4.

489. Demirturk N, Aykin N, Demirdal T, et al. Alopecia universalis: a rare side effect seen on chronic hepatitis C treatment with peg-IFN and ribavirin. Eur J Dermatol 2006;16(5):579–80.

490. Shafa S, Borum ML, Igiehon E. A case of irreversible alopecia associated with ribavirin and peg-interferon therapy. Eur J Gastroenterol Hepatol 2010;22(1):122–3.

491. Montoto S, Bosch F, Estrach T, et al. Pyoderma gangrenosum triggered by alpha2b-interferon in a patient with chronic granulocytic leukemia. Leuk Lymphoma 1998;30(1–2):199–202.

492. Sanders S, Busam K, Tahan SR, et al. Granulomatous and suppurative dermatitis at interferon alfa injection sites: report of 2 cases. J Am Acad Dermatol 2002;6(4):611–6.

493. Delecluse J, de Bast C, Achten G. Pyoderma gangrenosum with altered cellular immunity and dermonecrotic factor. Br J Dermatol 1972;87:529–32.

Histopathologic Patterns Associated with External Agents

Luis Requena, MD[a],*, Lorenzo Cerroni, MD[b],
Heinz Kutzner, MD[c]

KEYWORDS

- Foreign substance • Foreign-body granuloma • Multinucleate giant cells • External particles

KEY POINTS

- A large list of foreign substances may penetrate the skin due to both voluntary and involuntary reasons.
- Histopathologically, most of these substances induce a foreign-body granuloma with multinucleate giant cells.
- The microscopic morphology of the external particles is helpful in recognizing specifically the involved foreign substance.

A large number of foreign substances may penetrate the skin for both voluntary and involuntary reasons. The voluntary group includes the particulate materials used in tattoos and cosmetic fillers, whereas the involuntary group is almost always caused by accidental inclusion of external substances secondary to cutaneous trauma. **Table 1** summarizes the most common foreign bodies found in cutaneous biopsies. Histopathologically, most of these substances induce a foreign-body granuloma with multinucleate giant cells, involving the dermis, and often extend to the subcutaneous tissue. Sometimes secondary infection occurs in the preexisting foreign-body granuloma. The foreign substance may or may not be refringent when sections are examined under polarized light. Cutaneous foreign-body granulomas may also develop secondary to endogenous material that has become altered in such a way that it is recognized as a foreign substance, as in the case of calcium deposits, urate, oxalate, keratin, and hair shafts. These endogenous materials are not discussed in this article. Herein, the authors focus on the histopathologic findings seen in cutaneous reactions to exogenous agents, with special emphasis on the microscopic morphology of the external particles in recognizing specifically the involved substance (something that is becoming increasingly important in the event of litigation).

TATTOO PIGMENTS

Most tattoos have cosmetic purposes and are created by mechanical introduction of insoluble pigments in the dermis. In recent years, cosmetic tattooing has also been used as permanent makeup in adult women for lips, eyelids, and eyebrows. Occasionally pigment is traumatically introduced in the skin by accident during work or sports activities. **Box 1** summarizes the main components of

The authors do not have any conflict of interest to declare.
The authors do not have any financial support for this article.
[a] Department of Dermatology, Fundación Jiménez Díaz, Universidad Autónoma, Avenida Reyes Católicos 2, Madrid 28040, Spain; [b] Department of Dermatology, Medical University of Graz, Auenbruggerplatz 8, A-8036, Graz, Austria; [c] Dermatopathologie Friedrichshafen, Siemensstrasse 6/1, D-88048, Friedrichshafen, Germany
* Corresponding author.
E-mail address: lrequena@fjd.es

Dermatol Clin 30 (2012) 731–748
http://dx.doi.org/10.1016/j.det.2012.06.006

derm.theclinics.com

Table 1
Foreign substances that may be found in the skin

Substance	Histopathology
Tattoo pigments	Sarcoidal or foreign-body granulomas. Pseudolymphoma. Pigmented granules of several colors according to the composition of the tattoo
Cosmetic fillers	Foreign-body granulomas containing particles of variable morphology (see **Table 2**)
Drugs and medications	Tuberculoid or foreign-body granulomas. Ferruginated collagen fibers with Monsel solution Banana-like collagen fibers in exogenous ochronosis. Foreign-body granuloma with numerous lymphoid aggregates at the site of injection of aluminum-adsorbed vaccines. Mostly lobular panniculitis at the site of injection of several drugs
Silica	Sarcoidal granulomas containing birefringent particles
Beryllium	Sarcoidal granulomas with central fibrinoid necrosis
Zirconium	Sarcoidal granulomas
Glass	Foreign-body granulomas containing birefringent particles
Starch	Suppurative granulomas
Talc	Suppurative granulomas containing Maltese-cross birefringent granules
Graphite	Foreign-body granuloma around black polygonal particles with birefringent borders
Paraffin	Mostly lobular panniculitis with Swiss-cheese appearance
Shrapnel	Foreign-body or suppurative granulomas
Suture material	Foreign-body granuloma. Each type of suture shows a characteristic appearance and birefringence pattern
Arthropods	Dermal eosinophilic granulomas
Sea urchin spines	Sarcoidal granulomas
Cactus spine	Suppurative granulomas
Vegetable oil	Suppurative granulomas
Wood splinter	Suppurative granulomas
Mineral oil	Sclerosing lipogranulomas
Food particles	So-called pulsed granulomas containing small hyaline rings. Sometimes hyaline perivascular rings (hyaline angiopathy)

the most commonly used substances for tattooing according to the wanted color. In recent years, the incidence of complications secondary to tattoos is becoming rarer, owing to better hygiene during the tattooing process and because of the declining use of strong irritant substances, such as mercury salts. However, infections, allergic reactions, photosensitivity, cutaneous diseases localized to tattoos as a Koebner phenomenon, tumors within preexisting tattoos, and miscellaneous reactions are still sporadically reported as complications resulting from tattoos (**Box 2**).[1] Temporary henna tattoos are nowadays very common, especially among teenagers, and they induce frequent local irritant and allergic reactions at the applied site.

Histopathologically, tattoo pigments usually are easily visualized in hematoxylin-eosin–stained sections. The pigment is mostly localized around the blood vessels of the upper and mid dermis, and most pigment is seen as extracellular deposits between collagen bundles, although small amounts of pigmented particles may be also visualized within the cytoplasm of macrophages. In many instances, the pigment is seen lying free in the

Box 1
Composition of the tattoo pigments according to color

- Black: Coal and graphite
- Red: Mercury salts, ferric hydrate, cadmium selenide
- Yellow: Cadmium sulfide
- Green: Chromium compounds
- Blue: Cobalt compounds
- Purple: Manganese compounds

Box 2
Complications from tattoos

- Infectious
  - Staphylococcal and streptococcal infections
  - Syphilis
  - Leprosy
  - Tuberculosis
  - Tetanus
  - Chancroid
  - Verrucae
  - Vaccinia
  - Herpes simplex and herpes zoster
  - Molluscum contagiosum
  - Viral hepatitis B and C
  - Dermatophytoses
- Dermatoses as Koebner phenomenon
  - Psoriasis
  - Lichen planus
  - Darier disease
  - Discoid lupus erythematosus
  - Sarcoidosis
  - Granuloma annulare
  - Necrobiosis lipoidica
- Allergic reactions
- Photosensitivity reactions
- Leukocytoclastic vasculitis
- Hypertophic scars and keloids
- Neoplasms in preexisting tattoos
  - Solitary reticulohistiocytoma
  - Basal cell carcinoma
  - Keratoacanthoma
  - Squamous cell carcinoma
  - Kaposi sarcoma
  - Cutaneous lymphomas
  - Melanoma

dermis without apparent inflammatory response (Fig. 1). Often the pigment is slightly refractile, but not doubly refractile. In general, traumatic implanted pigments during work or sport accidents are larger and more variable in size and shape when compared with the relatively small and homogeneous size and shape of the pigment particles used in decorative tattoos. Histopathologic patterns vary according to the composition of the used pigment. Hypersensitivity reactions include the development of a diffuse lymphohistiocytic infiltrate involving the full thickness of the dermis,[2] lichenoid reactions (which seem to be more frequent with red pigments) (Fig. 2),[3] sarcoidal granulomas (Fig. 3),[4] granuloma annulare–like reaction,[5] necrobiosis lipoidica,[6] perforating granulomatous dermatitis,[7] vasculitis,[8] a pseudolymphomatous pattern (Fig. 4),[9] and a morphea-like reaction.[10] The overlying epidermis is usually normal, although spongiosis and pseudoepitheliomatous hyperplasia have been described.

COSMETIC FILLERS

Numerous agents are currently injected or surgically implanted into the dermis and subcutaneous tissue for correction of cosmetic defects or soft-tissue augmentation. Adverse reactions to these substances are uncommon, but they have been recently reviewed.[11] **Table 2** summarizes the most common fillers currently used, classified into 2 main categories: (1) transitory biodegradable or resorbable within months and years, respectively, and (2) permanent or nonresorbable. **Fig. 5** illustrates the light microscopic morphology of the particles of the most commonly injected cosmetic fillers.

Bovine collagen has been used as transitory injectable filler to correct depressed scars, deep nasolabial folds, age-related rhytides, and soft-tissue augmentation. The duration of the effect from an injection of bovine collagen is usually less than 6 months. Skin tests are required before injection of these products, because 3% of the population develop a delayed hypersensitivity response. Although some investigators report antibovine collagen antibodies after injections, most reactions to bovine collagen are due to delayed hypersensitivity, and serum antibodies are usually not present. Histopathology of these hypersensitivity reactions include the formation of foreign-body granulomas,[12] palisading granulomas resembling granuloma annulare at the test-site injection,[13] and cyst or abscess formation.[14] Rare examples of disseminated and recurrent sarcoid-like granulomatous panniculitis caused by bovine collagen injection have also been described.[15] More uncommon side effects include bruising, reactivation of herpetic infection, verified bacterial infection, and local necrosis. The latter is mostly seen with bovine collagen injected at the glabellar area caused by vascular interruption, and injections should thus be avoided in this region. Histopathologically bovine collagen appears different from human collagen, because bundles of bovine collagen are thicker and show a homogeneous appearance nearly devoid of

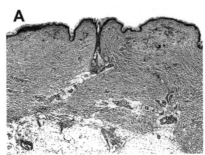
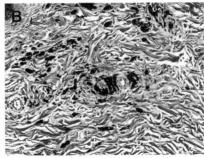

Fig. 1. Histopathology of a coal tattoo. (*A*) Low-power view showing black pigment in superficial dermis. (*B*) The pigment is disposed in perivascular and interstitial fashion (Hematoxylin-eosin, original magnifications: *A* ×20; *B* ×200).

spaces between them (see **Fig. 5**A). Furthermore, human collagen is birefringent under polarized light and stains green with Masson trichrome stain, whereas bovine collagen is not birefringent with polarized light and stains with a pale gray-violet color with Masson trichrome. The inflammatory infiltrate around the implant is denser when the bovine collagen is injected into the deep reticular dermis or partially infiltrates the subcutaneous fat, but panniculitis is not usually seen when the implant is confined to the dermis.

To avoid the hypersensitivity adverse reaction to bovine collagen, human-based collagen implants have been produced in recent years. No skin tests for hypersensitivity reactions are required with human-derived collagen products. Local adverse reactions include bruising, erythema, and swelling at the site of injection. However, there also have been a few reported cases of granulomatous reaction at the site of the injection[16] or at a skin-test site after injection of acellular human collagen.[17]

Injections of hyaluronic acid gel are now used as a resorbable filler for filling out wrinkles of the face, soft-tissue augmentation, and correction of all types of defects, such as scars and facial lipoatrophy. The longevity of the injected gel is about 6 months. Hyaluronic acid has no organ or species specificity, and thus in theory there is no risk of

an allergic reaction. Very few adverse hypersensitivity reactions secondary to injection of hyaluronic acid used as a filler have been reported. Histopathologically they consisted of a granulomatous foreign-body reaction, with abundant multinucleated giant cells surrounding an extracellular basophilic amorphous material (see **Fig. 5**B), which was the injected hyaluronic acid gel.[18,19] Scant amounts of hyaluronic acid may be also seen within multinucleated giant cells. Hyaluronic acid stains positively for Alcian blue at a pH of 2.7 and is negative when examined under polarized light. Rare described histopathologic findings at the sites of injection of hyaluronic acid included a prominent eosinophilic granulomatous reaction[20] and suppurative granuloma without evidence of infection.[21] A mixture of nonanimal-stabilized hyaluronic acid and dextranomer microspheres has been also used as a resorbable filler, with a single case report of foreign-body granuloma caused by this filler described. Histopathology of this case demonstrated a suppurative granuloma surrounding the hyaluronic acid and spherical dark-bluish particles (see **Fig. 5**C) that represented the dextranomer microparticles.[22]

Poly-L-lactic acid is a resorbable filler that has been used to correct the signs of lipoatrophy in patients infected with human immunodeficiency

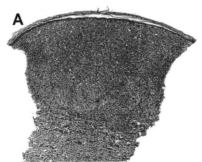
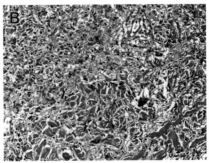

Fig. 2. Histopathology of a red tattoo reaction. (*A*) Scanning power showing dense inflammatory infiltrates in superficial and mid dermis. (*B*) Particles of red pigment are seen among the inflammatory cells (Hematoxylin-eosin, original magnifications: *A* ×20; *B* ×200).

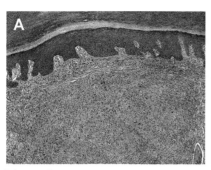
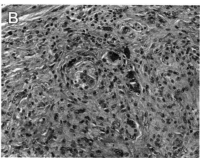

Fig. 3. Sarcoidal granuloma against tattoo pigment. (*A*) The infiltrate is composed of aggregates of histiocytes. (*B*) Higher magnification of the black particles of the tattoo within the cytoplasm of multinucleated giant cells (Hematoxylin-eosin, original magnifications: *A* ×40; *B* ×200).

virus (HIV) receiving antiprotease treatment, as well as for facial cosmetic augmentation. Poly-ʟ-lactic acid induces tissue augmentation that lasts up to at least 24 months. This filler frequently results in nodules at the site of injection, which are palpable but generally not visible. Histopathologically the nodules show foreign-body granuloma, with numerous multinucleated giant cells around translucent particles of different sizes, most of them showing a fusiform, oval, or spiky shape (see **Fig.** 5D), which are birefringent on examination with polarized light.[23]

Calcium hydroxylapatite is another resorbable filler composed of calcium hydroxylapatite microspheres that stimulate the endogenous production of collagen. These microspheres induce almost no foreign-body reaction, and appear with bluish color and round or oval shape. When this agent is injected into the lips, it tends to be associated with a high incidence of nodules. In some patients, however, calcium hydroxylapatite microspheres may induce a foreign-body granulomatous reaction, seen as blue-gray microspheres in the extracellular matrix or within multinucleated giant cells (see **Fig.** 5E).[19]

A single case of granulomatous reaction to a new resorbable filler consisting of the purified polysaccharide alginate (Novabel) has been described at the site of injection for an intradermal test with this filler. Histopathologically the granulomatous reaction was confined to the deep dermis and subcutaneous fat, which were involved by numerous multinucleated giant cells and histiocytes. Within this granulomatous reaction, a nonpolarizing exogenous material was identified consisting of slightly bluish deposits of variable size and shape, some of which were well delineated, others with a blurred or spiky perimeter, and frequently showing retraction in a clear vacuole. These particles of purified polysaccharide alginate reacted weakly with periodic acid-Schiff (PAS) and Alcian blue, but were intensely stained with toluidine blue.[24]

Paraffin is no longer used as a filler because of its frequent adverse reactions, but as it is a nonresorbable material, it is still possible to see granulomatous reactions secondary to injections performed many years ago. These granulomatous reactions, also named paraffinomas, consist histopathologically of a mostly lobular panniculitis, in which the subcutaneous fat exhibits a Swiss-cheese appearance (see **Fig.** 5F), with cystic spaces of variable size and shape surrounded by foamy histiocytes and multinucleated giant cells.[25] Sclerosing lipogranuloma is a specific form of paraffinoma that results from injection of paraffin in

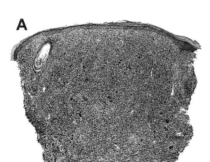
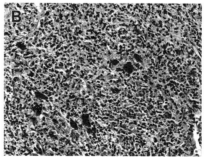

Fig. 4. Pseudolymphoma-like reaction against tattoo pigment. (*A*) Scanning power showing a diffuse inflammatory infiltrate involving the full thickness of the dermis. (*B*) Particles of black pigment are seen among the lymphoid infiltrate (Hematoxylin-eosin, original magnifications: *A* ×20; *B* ×200).

Table 2
The most common fillers used for augmentation of soft tissue

Category	Chemical Composition	Trademark	Microscopic Appearance of Particles
Resorbable within months	Bovine collagen	Zyderm, Zyplast	Eosinophilic thick, nonbirefringent collagen
	Human-derived collagen	Autologen, Cosmoderm, Cosmoplast, Cymetra	Normal birefringent human collagen
	Hyaluronic acid	Hylaform, Restylane, Juvederm, Perlane, Macrolane	Extracellular nonbirefringent basophilic amorphous material
	Purified polysaccharide alginate	Novabel	Bluish nonbirefringent particles with spiky perimeter
Resorbable within years	Hyaluronic acid + dextranomer microparticles	Matridex, Reviderm intra	Spherical dark-bluish nonbirefringent particles
	Poly-L-lactic acid microspheres + sodium carboxymethylcellulose, nonpyrogenic mannitol, sterile water	Sculptra, New Fill	Oval birefringent particles
	Calcium hydroxylapatite + carboxymethylcellulose and glycerine	Radiance, Radiesse	Spherical nonbirefringent bluish particles
Permanent	Paraffin		Lobular panniculitis with Swiss-cheese appearance
	Silicone oil	Silikon 1000, Silskin	Round empty nonbirefringent vacuoles of different sizes
	Silicone gel	MDX 4-4011, Dow Corning	
	Silicone elastomer particles + polyvinylpyrrolidone	Bioplastique	Popcorn-like nonbirefringent particles
	Polymethylmethacrylate microspheres and bovine collagen	Artecoll, Arteplast, Artefill	Round nonbirefringent particles with uniform size
	Hydroxyethylmethacrylate/ ethylmethacrylate fragments and hyaluronic acid	Dermalive, Dermadeep	Polygonal, pink translucent nonbirefringent particles
	Polyacrylamide hydrogel	Aquamid, Interfall, OutLine, Royamid, Formacryl, Argiform, Amazing gel, Bio-Formacryl, Kosmogel	Basophilic multivacuolated nonbirefringent material
	Polyalkylimide gel	Bio-Alcamid	Basophilic nonbirefringent granular material
	Polyvinylhydroxide microspheres + polyacrylamide gel	Evolution	Translucent nonbirefringent microspheres

the penis, causing fibrosis and deformity of the penis body.[26]

Silicone has been in the last decades the most widely used filler material for soft-tissue augmentation. Recently it has also been injected as a filler to circumvent facial lipoatrophy in HIV-infected patients receiving antiprotease treatment. Silicone gel is capable of migrating to distant sites, where it may give rise to an inflammatory reaction and hamper clinical diagnosis. In the past decade there has been considerable controversy in the literature about the relationship between systemic scleroderma and other connective-tissue diseases and the use of breast implants containing silicone gel. There appears to be little scientific basis for any association between silicone breast implants and

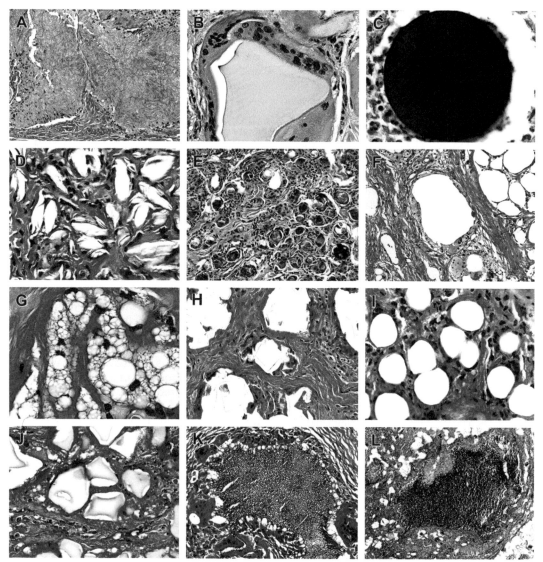

Fig. 5. Light microscopic appearance of the particles of the most common fillers. (*A*) Bovine collagen. (*B*) Hyaluronic acid. (*C*) Dextranomer microspheres. (*D*) Polylactic acid. (*E*) Calcium hydroxylapatite. (*F*) Paraffin. (*G*) Silicone. (*H*) Bioplastique. (*I*) Artecoll. (*J*) Dermalive. (*K*) Aquamid. (*L*) Bio-Alcamid (Hematoxylin-eosin, original magnifications: *A* ×200; *B* ×400; *C* ×400; *D* ×400; *E* ×200; *F* ×200; *G* ×400; *H* ×200; *I* ×400; *J* ×400; *K* ×200; *L* ×200).

any well-defined connective tissue disease. Histopathologic findings in local reactions to implants of silicone are variable, depending mainly on the form of the injected silicone. Solid elastomer silicone induces an exuberant foreign-body granulomatous reaction, whereas silicone oil and gel induce a sparser inflammatory response.[27] Silicone particles appear as groups of round empty vacuoles of different sizes between collagen bundles or within macrophages (see **Fig. 5**G), and the particles are not birefringent under polarized light.

A permanent filler, composed of particles of polymerized silicone elastomer dispersed in a carrier of polyvinylpyrrolidone (Bioplastique), has been recently introduced for correction of facial rhytides and lip augmentation. Granulomas secondary to this filler are uncommon, but when they develop consist of irregularly shaped cystic spaces containing translucent, jagged popcorn-like, nonbirefringent particles of varying size (see **Fig. 5**H) dispersed in a sclerotic stroma, surrounded by abundant multinucleated foreign-body giant cells.[28]

Another permanent biphasic filler, composed of polymethylmethacrylate microspheres suspended in a degradable bovine collagen solution as a carrier (Artecoll), is used mostly in Europe as a cosmetic microimplant for correction of facial wrinkles and furrows, perioral lines, small scars, and other subdermal defects. Because it contains bovine collagen, it is mandatory to perform an intradermal test before the first use of this filler. Histopathologically, adverse reactions to this filler show a nodular or diffuse granulomatous infiltrate surrounding rounded vacuoles of similar shape and size (see **Fig. 5I**), which mimic normal adipocytes and correspond to the implanted polymethylmethacrylate microspheres.[29] The microspheres may be distinguished from normal adipocytes because they are markedly homogeneous in size and shape.

Another permanent biphasic filler is composed of ethylmethacrylate and hydroxyethylmethacrylate particles suspended in hyaluronic acid gel (Dermalive). Histopathologically, granulomatous reactions to this filler consist of nodular infiltrates of macrophages and multinucleated giant cells with numerous pseudocystic structures of different sizes and shapes containing polygonal, pink, translucent (see **Fig. 5J**), nonbirefringent foreign bodies.[30] Transepidermal elimination of the product may occur.[28]

An injected hydrophilic gel of polyacrylamide (Aquamid) has been used in large quantities mostly in China, Ukraine, and the former Soviet Union for breast, buttock, and calf augmentation. More recently, it has been used in European countries for treatment of antiretroviral-related facial lipoatrophy in HIV-infected patients as well as for correction of acquired or congenital malformations with depressed skin. This permanent filler may cause nodules after the injections that frequently develop secondary localized bacterial infection.[31] Granulomas secondary to this filler are composed of macrophages, foreign-body giant cells, lymphocytes, and red cells surrounding a basophilic multivacuolated nonbirefringent material (see **Fig. 5K**), which corresponds to the polyacrylamide hydrogel. This material shows some histopathologic similarity to hyaluronic acid, although granulomas secondary to hyaluronic acid usually show a less dense inflammatory infiltrate than those secondary to polyacrylamide hydrogel. Polyacrylamide hydrogel is positive with Alcian blue stain and is not birefringent under polarizing microscopy.

Bio-Alcamid is a permanent translucent gel filler made of a hydrophilic biopolymer composed of sterile water and polyalkylimide polymer. It has been used to increase volume in the cheeks in HIV-infected patients with facial lipoatrophy related to antiretroviral therapy, as well as for buttock augmentation, correction of scar depressions, and posttraumatic subcutaneous atrophy.

The few histopathologic studies describing adverse reactions to this filler have reported basophilic amorphous material corresponding to the implanted material (see **Fig. 5L**) surrounded by epithelioid histiocytes, foreign-body multinucleated giant cells, neutrophils, and red blood cells.[32]

DRUGS AND MEDICATIONS

Some medications, such as polyvinylpyrrolidone, which was used in the past as a plasma expander, may show dermal deposits as cutaneous expression of the polyvinylpyrrolidone storage disease.[33] Cutaneous histopathology shows perivascular histiocytes, involving superficial and deep dermal plexus, containing cytoplasmic bluish-gray vacuoles (**Fig. 6**). These vacuoles are positive for mucicarmine, colloidal iron, and Congo red stain, but they do not stain with PAS or Alcian blue.

Tuberculoid or foreign-body granulomatous reactions after topical application of several substances as well as local panniculitis secondary to injection of different drugs and medications have been described (**Table 3**). The exact mechanism of these reactions is not known, but they probably occur as a consequence of a multifactorial etiopathogenesis, whereby vasoconstriction with tissue ischemia, inflammatory response to precipitated drug in the tissue, trauma and hypersensitivity reactions after repeated injections are implicated. Some of them show specific histopathologic findings that allow identification of the applied or injected medication. For example, application of Monsel solution (20% ferric subsulfate) for hemostasis to wounds caused by superficial excisions of the skin causes ferrugination of dermal collagen, which appears coated with a slightly refractile, gray-brown substance strongly positive with Perl reaction for iron (**Fig. 7**). Some of the ferruginated collagen fibers may become calcified and eliminated through the epidermis. These fibers act as foreign bodies to elicit a granulomatous reaction.[34] Topical application of hydroquinone creams for bleaching skin can induce discoloration, mostly in dark-skinned individuals, predominantly on malar areas. This condition is known as exogenous ochronosis, histopathologically characterized by striking discoloration of the collagen bundles of the upper dermis, which appear stout, with yellow color and crescentic, vermiform, or banana shapes (**Fig. 8**).[35] Sometimes a foreign-body granuloma develops around these banana-shaped bodies and, in rare instances, transepidermal elimination of these altered collagen bundles has been described. The local cutaneous reaction after immunization with aluminum-adsorbed vaccines consists of deep dermal or subcutaneous nodules,

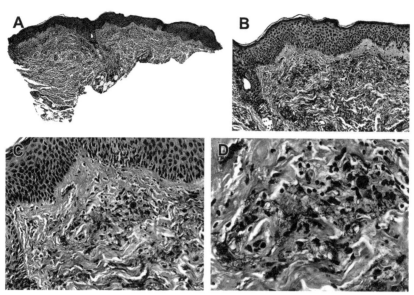

Fig. 6. Polyvinylpyrrolidone dermal deposits. The product was used as a plasma expander. (*A*) Scanning power. (*B*) Perivascular histiocytes, involving superficial and deep dermal plexus, containing cytoplasm bluish-gray vacuoles. (*C*) Bluish material is seen within the perivascular histiocytes. (*D*) Higher magnification of the polyvinylpyrrolidone deposit (Hematoxylin-eosin, original magnifications: *A* ×10; *B* ×40; *C* ×200; *D* ×400). (*Courtesy of* Dr T.T. Kuo, Department of Pathology, Chang Gung Memorial Hospital, Kwei San, Tao Yuan, Taiwan.)

histopathologically characterized by a central zone of degenerated collagen surrounded by a rim of histiocytes with granular cytoplasm and lymphoid aggregates, some of them with germinal center formation, and abundant eosinophils (**Fig. 9**).[36] The aluminum composition of the bluish granules within the cytoplasm of the histiocytes may be confirmed by the solochrome-azurine stain, which stains the crystals of aluminum salts a deep gray-blue color, or by x-ray microanalyisis.[37] Hemostatic agents containing aluminum chloride are sometimes used for minor surgical procedures, and after their application there are descriptions of macrophages with abundant cytoplasm containing aluminum particles.[38] Localized panniculitis to subcutaneous glatiramer acetate injections for treatment of multiple sclerosis is histopathologically characterized by a mostly lobular panniculitis of lipophagic granuloma, with scattered neutrophils and eosinophils both in the septa and the fat lobules (**Fig. 10**). Connective tissue septa show widening, fibrosis, and frequent lymphoid follicles with germinal center formation. Immunohistochemistry demonstrates that the inflammatory infiltrate involving the fat lobule is mostly composed of CD68-positive histiocytes and suppressor/cytotoxic T lymphocytes. By contrast, lymphoid follicles at the septa are mainly composed of B lymphocytes.[39] Injections of substances containing phosphatidylcholine to treat fat accumulation and lipomas induce lobular neutrophilic panniculitis with necrotic adipocytes,

whereas the connective tissue septa show thickening and a pseudocapsule surrounding the inflamed area (**Fig. 11**).[40] Palisading granulomas with necrobiosis have been also described, with the foreign material introduced through the use of a lubricating agent containing a copolymer (Carbopol 934) for liposuction.[41] Pentazocine injections cause sclerodermoid plaques at the sites of injection secondary to thrombosis of small vessels and endarteritis, with subsequent granulomatous inflammation, necrosis of adipocytes, lipophagic granuloma, and pronounced fibrosis of the dermis and septa of the subcutaneous tissue.[42] Vitamin K1 injections also cause sclerosis of the connective tissue septa of subcutaneous fat and an inflammatory infiltrate composed of lymphocytes and plasma cells, closely resembling the histopathologic findings of deep morphea.[43]

Other drug-induced granulomas include sarcoidal granulomas at the sites of injection of interferon-β1b for multiple sclerosis[44] and interferon-α2a for hepatitis C,[45] tuberculoid granulomas at the site of injection of zinc-containing insulin,[46] necrobiotic palisading granulomas at the injection sites of hepatitis B vaccine[47] and disodium clodronate,[48] mixed granulomatous reaction combining sarcoidal and foreign-body granulomas after depot injections of leuprorelin acetate for the treatment of prostatic cancer,[49] and granulomas at the base of the penis after injection of acyclovir tablets dissolved in hydrogen peroxidase as self-treatment for recurrent genital herpes.[50] Ophthalmologic

Table 3
Local cutaneous reactions to drugs and medications

Drug or Medication	Histopathology
Foreign-Body and Tuberculoid Granulomas	
Application of Monsel solution (20% ferric subsulfate) for hemostasis to superficial wounds	Ferrugination of dermal collagen
Exogenous ochronosis secondary to applications of hydroquinone creams	Banana-like collagen fibers
Zinc-containing insulin	Tuberculoid granulomas
Granulomas in tribal scars containing long-standing burnt carbon and after injections of highly active antiretroviral therapy (HAART) for human immunodeficiency virus infection as expression of immune reconstitution inflammatory syndrome (IRIS)	Foreign-body granulomas
Immunization with aluminum-adsorbed vaccines	Foreign-body granulomas and lymphoid aggregates
Mantoux test and BCG vaccination	Foreign-body granulomas
Injections of depot formulations of leuprorelin acetate for prostate carcinoma	Granulomatous reaction of mixed foreign-body and sarcoidal types
Injections of phosphatidylcholine-containing substances for lipolysis of lipomas or fat accumulation	Neutrophilic panniculitis with lipophagic granulomas
Local Panniculitis at the Sites of Injections	
Opiaceous alkaloids: pethidine, pentazocine, methadone	Sclerosing panniculitis with fat necrosis
Povidone	Lobular panniculitis, focal hemorrhage, fat necrosis
Gold salts: aurothioglucose	Erythema nodosum–like panniculitis
Phytonadione (vitamin K1)	Sclerotic septa with plasma cells mimicking deep morphea
Glatiramer acetate for multiple sclerosis	Lobular panniculitis with lymphoid aggregates at the septa
Tetanus antioxidant vaccination	Granulomatous panniculitis with lymphoid aggregates
Antihepatitis vaccination	Erythema nodosum–like panniculitis
Anticancer vaccine reactions: gangliosides for melanoma, carcinoembryonic antigen, and MUC1 for pancreatic cancer	Septal panniculitis with numerous eosinophils
Interferon-β	Mostly lobular panniculitis with secondary lipoatrophy
Granulocyte colony-stimulating factor	Neutrophilic lobular panniculitis
Interleukin-2	Neutrophilic lobular panniculitis

drops containing sodium bisulfite may induce facial papules, histopathologically characterized by sarcoidal granulomas containing black-brown pigment within the cytoplasm of multinucleated giant cells.[51]

MINERAL, METALLIC, AND OTHER PARTICLES

Silica is a frequent contaminant of skin wounds after sports or motor traffic accidents. Silica particles appear as dirt, sand, rock, or glass, and induce papules and nodules at the sites of trauma.

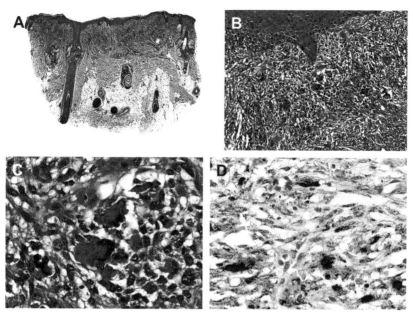

Fig. 7. Granulomatous reaction to Monsel solution. (*A*) Scanning power showing a band-like inflammatory infiltrate in the superficial dermis. (*B*) Brown pigment of Monsel solution surrounded by histiocytes and some multinucleated giant cell. (*C*) Higher magnification of the pigment of Monsel solution. (*D*) Strong positivity with Perl reaction for iron (*A, B* and *C* Hematoxylin-eosin; *D*, Perl reaction. Original magnifications: *A* ×10; *B* ×40; *C* ×400; *D* ×200).

Histopathologically, silica particles included in the skin induce sarcoidal granulomas, with abundant numbers of Langhans or foreign-body multinucleated giant cells, where the determinant particles are difficult to see with routine microscopy. However, silica particles are easily identified with polarized light microscopy, because they are strongly birefringent (**Fig. 12**).[52] Histopathologic differential diagnosis with authentic cutaneous sarcoidosis may be difficult and, moreover, it has been suggested that particles of foreign material may serve as a trigger for granuloma formation in true sarcoidosis.[53] Silica granulomas are interpreted as a response to colloidal silica particles rather than as a result of a hypersensitivity reaction.[54]

Sarcoidal granulomas have been also described as an uncommon complication of piercing in the ear lobule and other sites. These lesions are not due to trauma or scarring, but develop as a consequence of contact allergy to nickel and other metals contained in the rings. Histopathologically they consist of sarcoidal granulomas involving the entire thickness of the dermis but, in contrast to true sarcoidosis, a dense lymphoid infiltrate surrounds the aggregates of epithelioid histiocytes (**Fig. 13**).[55] Usually no foreign material is identified with routine microscopy and polarized light. In one reported case, the granulomatous reaction developed against the titanium alloy used in the ear piercing.[56]

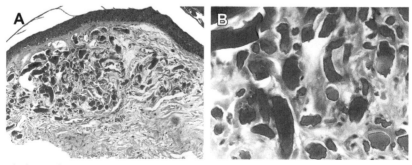

Fig. 8. Histopathology of exogenous ochronosis secondary to topical application of hydroquinone creams. (*A*) Striking discoloration of the collagen bundles of the upper dermis, which appear stout, with yellow color and crescentic, vermiform, or banana shapes. (*B*) These banana bodies induce sparse inflammatory response (Hematoxylin-eosin, original magnifications: *A* ×20; *B* ×400).

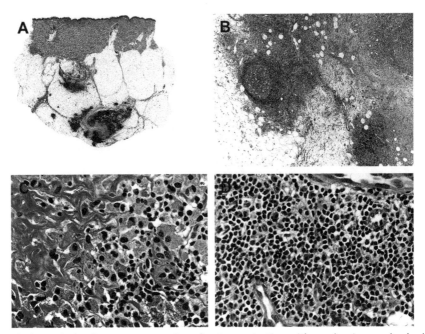

Fig. 9. Histopathology of a local cutaneous reaction after immunization with an aluminum-adsorbed vaccine. (*A*) Scanning power showing subcutaneous nodular infiltrate. (*B*) Numerous lymphoid aggregates with germinal center formation. (*C*) Histiocytes with granular cytoplasm containing particles of aluminum. (*D*) Numerous lymphocytes and eosinophils are also present in the infiltrate (Hematoxylin-eosin, original magnifications: *A* ×10; *B* ×40; *C* ×200; *D* ×200).

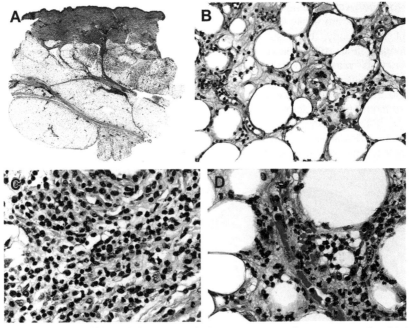

Fig. 10. Localized panniculitis at the site of injection of glatiramer acetate for treatment of multiple sclerosis. (*A*) Scanning power showing a mostly lobular panniculitis. (*B*) Lipophagic granuloma involving the fat lobule. (*C*) Numerous lymphocytes, plasma cells, and eosinophils are present in the infiltrate. (*D*) Higher power magnification of the infiltrate showing numerous eosinophils (Hematoxylin-eosin, original magnifications: *A* ×10; *B* ×40; *C* ×200; *D* ×400).

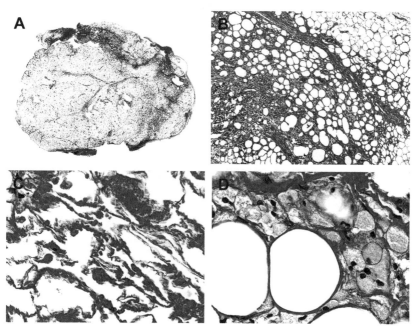

Fig. 11. Inflammatory reaction of a lipoma injected with substances containing phosphatidylcholine. (*A*) Scanning power showing inflammatory infiltrate mostly at the periphery of the lesion. (*B*) Necrotic adipocytes lacking nuclei. (*C*) Histopathologic features of lipomembranous or membranocystic panniculitis. (*D*) Higher magnification showing lipophagic granuloma around the adipocytes (Hematoxylin-eosin, original magnifications: *A* ×10; *B* ×40; *C* ×200; *D* ×400).

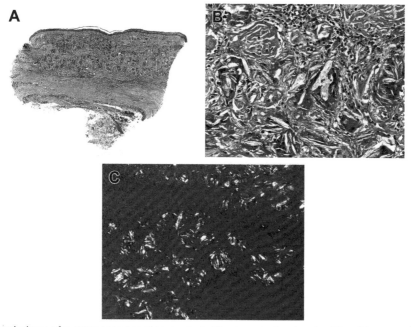

Fig. 12. Histopathology of a cutaneous reaction against silica as a contaminant of the skin wound in a patient after a motorcycle traffic accident. (*A*) Scanning power showing infiltrate in the superficial and mid dermis. (*B*) Higher magnification showing granulomatous reaction with foreign-body multinucleated giant cells around the silica particles. (*C*) Particles of silica are strongly birefringent (Hematoxylin-eosin, original magnifications: *A* ×10; *B* ×200; *C* ×40).

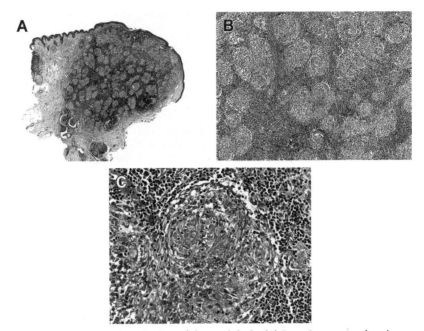

Fig. 13. Granulomatous reaction against piercing of the ear lobule. (*A*) Scanning power showing numerous granulomas involving the full thickness of the dermis. (*B*) The granulomas are surrounded by a dense lymphocytic infiltrate. (*C*) The granulomas are composed of aggregates of epithelioid histiocytes (Hematoxylin-eosin, original magnifications: *A* ×10; *B* ×40; *C* ×200).

Many HIV-infected patients initiating antiretroviral therapy develop immune reconstitution inflammatory syndrome (IRIS). IRIS is defined as a paradoxic clinical worsening caused by a subclinical opportunistic pathogen (unmasking IRIS) or a previously known treated, completed, or ongoing opportunistic infection (paradoxic IRIS). Several noninfective cutaneous diseases have also been described as an expression of IRIS. One of these consisted of multiple, linear nodular lesions that develop at cutaneous intravenous drug-injection sites and that may mimic polyarteritis nodosa, false aneurysms, and lymphatic spread of infection.[57] Histopathologically these lesions show a sarcoidal granulomatous reaction to extravasated suspended drug particles, in which inert material has been identified.[57] An IRIS-associated foreign-body granulomatous reaction has also been described in tattoos and tribal scars containing long-standing burnt carbon.[58] It has been hypothesized that a highly active antiretroviral therapy–augmented T-helper response with macrophage activation via interleukin-2 and interferon-δ is responsible for these granulomatous reactions as an expression of IRIS.[58]

Chronic beryllium disease is a granulomatous disorder characterized by a cell-mediated immune response to beryllium. Most reports of chronic beryllium disease describe pulmonary involvement. However, occupational chronic beryllium

cutaneous diseases have also been reported, including irritant contact dermatitis, allergic contact dermatitis, cutaneous ulcers, and allergic granulomas. These granulomas were histopathologically characterized by sarcoid-like granulomas with areas of central fibrinoid necrosis.[59]

Zirconium compounds used as topical deodorants may induce granulomas identical to those of sarcoidosis at the sites of application, and therefore axillary folds are the most common location.[60,61] These granulomas seem to develop by allergic mechanism and therefore only appear in previously sensitized individuals.[60]

Pulse granulomas, also named hyalin angiopathy, are rare granulomatous reactions to particles of food that have been described in the oral mucosa and in the skin around fistulae involving the gastrointestinal tract. Histopathologically these granulomas consist of amorphous eosinophilic material within and around blood vessels, intermingled with chronic inflammation and numerous epithelioid histiocytes and multinucleated giant cells.[62–65]

Suppurative granulomas secondary to mercury have been described at the sites of soft-tissue trauma from a broken thermometer. Usually large black spheres of mercury are easily identified within the neutrophilic aggregates at the center of the granulomas.[66] A large variety of disparate foreign substances may induce different types of

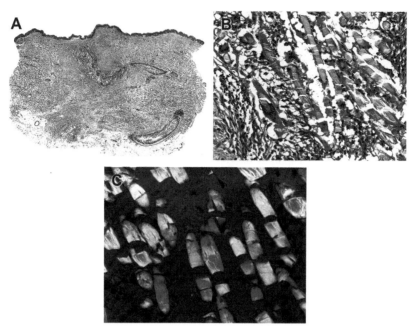

Fig. 14. Granulomatous reaction to suture. (*A*) Scanning power view showing a vertical scar involving the dermis with cystic areas. (*B*) Higher magnification showing the suture filaments surrounded by histiocytes and multinucleated giant cells. (*C*) The suture material is strongly birefringent under polarized light (Hematoxylin-eosin, original magnifications: *A* ×10; *B* ×200; *C* ×200).

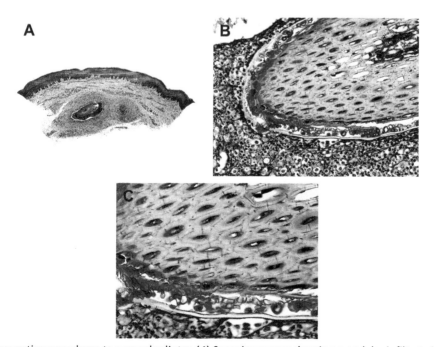

Fig. 15. Suppurative granuloma to a wood splinter. (*A*) Scanning power showing a nodular infiltrate in the deep dermis. (*B*) Numerous neutrophils surrounding the wood splinter. (*C*) Higher magnification of the wood splinter. Numerous hyphae are also seen at the periphery of the wood splinter (Giemsa stain, original magnifications: *A* ×10; *B* ×200; *C* ×400).

granulomas in the skin, including starch,[67] talc,[68] suture (Fig. 14),[69,70] acrylic or nylon fibers,[71] cactus bristles,[72,73] plant, wood (Fig. 15) and steel splinters,[74] fragments of a chainsaw blade,[75] sea urchin spines,[76] wheat stubble,[77] pencil graphite,[78,79] artificial hair,[80] golf club graphite,[81] and insect fragments after arthropod bites[82]; and at the points of entry of needles coated with silicone for acupuncture, catheters, and venipunctures,[83–85] and retained epicardial pacing wires.[86,87]

In conclusion, a large list of disparate exogenous materials may penetrate the skin. These exogenous materials usually induce a foreign-body granuloma composed of epithelioid histiocytes and multinucleate giant cells. The foreign body may or may not be birefringent when examined under polarized light, but in most cases the morphology of the foreign particles is specific enough to identify microscopically the nature of the material that has penetrated the skin.

REFERENCES

1. Goldstein N. IV. Complications from tattoos. J Dermatol Surg Oncol 1979;5:869–78.
2. Goldstein AP. VII. Histologic reactions in tattoos. J Dermatol Surg Oncol 1979;5:896–900.
3. Mortimer NJ, Chave TA, Johnson GA. Red tattoo reactions. Clin Exp Dermatol 2003;28:508–10.
4. Morales-Callaghan AM Jr, Aguilar-Bernier M, Martínez-Garcia G, et al. Sarcoid granuloma on black tattoo. J Am Acad Dermatol 2006;55:S71–3.
5. Bagwan IN, Walker M, Theaker JM. Granuloma annulare-like tattoo reaction. J Cutan Pathol 2007; 34:804–5.
6. Bethune GC, Miller RA, Murray SJ, et al. A novel inflammatory reaction in a tattoo: challenge. Am J Dermatopathol 2011;33:740–1, 749.
7. Sweeney SA, Hicks LD, Ranallo N, et al. Perforating granulomatous dermatitis reaction to exogenous tattoo pigment: a case report and review of the literature. Am J Dermatopathol 2011. [Epub ahead of print].
8. Kluger N, Jolly M, Guillot B. Tattoo-induced vasculitis. J Eur Acad Dermatol Venereol 2008;22:643–4.
9. Blumental G, Okun MR, Ponitch JA. Pseudolymphomatous reaction to tattoos. J Am Acad Dermatol 1982;6:485–8.
10. Mahalingman M, Kim E, Bhawan J. Morphea-like tattoo reaction. Am J Dermatopathol 2002;24:392–5.
11. Requena L, Requena C, Christensen L, et al. Adverse reactions to injectable soft tissue fillers. J Am Acad Dermatol 2011;64:1–34.
12. Barr RJ, Stegman SJ. Delayed skin test reaction to injectable collagen implant (Zyderm). J Am Acad Dermatol 1984;10:652–8.
13. Barr RJ, King DF, McDonald RM, et al. Necrobiotic granulomas associated with bovine collagen test site injections. J Am Acad Dermatol 1982;6:867–9.
14. McCoy JP Jr, Schade WJ, Siegle RJ, et al. Characterization of the humoral immune response to bovine collagen implants. Arch Dermatol 1985;121:990–4.
15. Garcia-Domingo MI, Alijotas Rey J, Cistero-Bahima A, et al. Disseminated and recurrent sarcoid-like granulomatous panniculitis due to bovine collagen injection. J Investig Allergol Clin Immunol 2000;10:107–9.
16. Sclafani A, Romo T, Jacono AA, et al. Evaluation of acellular dermal graft in sheet (Alloderm) and injectable (micronized Alloderm) forms for soft tissue augmentation: clinical observations and histologic findings. Arch Facial Plast Surg 2000;2:130–6.
17. Moody BR, Sengelmann RD. Self-limited adverse reaction to human-derived collagen injectable product. Dermatol Surg 2000;26:936–8.
18. Ghislanzoni M, Bianchi F, Barbareschi M, et al. Cutaneous granulomatous reaction to injectable hyaluronic acid gel. Br J Dermatol 2006;154:755–8.
19. Dadzie OE, Mahalingam M, Parada M, et al. Adverse reactions to soft tissue fillers—a review of the histological features. J Cutan Pathol 2008;35:536–48.
20. Okada S, Okuyama R, Tagami H, et al. Eosinophilic granulomatous reaction after intradermal injection of hyaluronic acid. Acta Derm Venereol 2008;88: 69–70.
21. Fernandez Aceñero MJ, Zamora E, Borbujo J. Granulomatous foreign body reaction against hyaluronic acid: report of a case after lip augmentation. Dermatol Surg 2003;29:1225–6.
22. Massone C, Horn M, Kerl H, et al. Foreign body granuloma due to Matridex injection for cosmetic purposes. Am J Dermatopathol 2009;31:197–9.
23. Dijkema SJ, van der Lei B, Kibbelaar RE. New-fill injections may induce late-onset foreign body granulomatous reaction. Plast Reconstr Surg 2005;115: 76e–8e.
24. Moulonguet I, de Goursac V, Plantier F. Granulomatous reaction after injection of a new resorbable filler Novabel. Am J Dermatopathol 2011;33: 710–1.
25. Darsow U, Bruckbauer H, Worret WI, et al. Subcutaneous oleomas induced by self-injection of sesame seed oil for muscle augmentation. J Am Acad Dermatol 2000;42:292–4.
26. Claudy A, Garcier F, Schmitt D. Sclerosing lipogranuloma of the male genitalia: ultrastructural study. Br J Dermatol 1981;105:451–5.
27. Morgan AM. Localized reactions to injected therapeutic materials. Part 2. Surgical agents. J Cutan Pathol 1995;22:289–303.
28. Zimmermann US, Clerici TJ. The histological aspects of fillers complications. Semin Cutan Med Surg 2004;23:241–50.

29. Rudolph CM, Soyer HP, Schuller-Petrovic S, et al. Foreign body granulomas due to injectable aesthetic microimplants. Am J Surg Pathol 1999; 23:113–7.

30. Requena C, Izquierdo MJ, Navarro M, et al. Adverse reactions to injectable aesthetic microimplants. Am J Dermatopathol 2001;23:197–202.

31. Christensen L, Breiting V, Vuust J, et al. Adverse reactions following injection with a permanent facial filler polyacrylamide hydrogel (Aquamid): causes and treatment. Eur J Plast Surg 2006;28:464–71.

32. Gómez-de la Fuente E, Alvarez-Fernández JG, Pinedo F, et al. Reacción cutánea tras implante con Bio-Alcamid. Actas Dermosifiliogr 2007;98:271–5.

33. Kuo TT, Hu S, Huang CL, et al. Cutaneous involvement in polyvinylpyrrolidone storage disease: a clinicopathologic study of five patients, including two patients with severe anemia. Am J Surg Pathol 1997;21:1361–7.

34. Amazon K, Robinson MJ, Rywlin AM. Ferrugination caused by Monsel's solution. Clinical observation and experimentations. Am J Dermatopathol 1980; 2:197–205.

35. Snider RL, Thiers BH. Exogenous ochronosis. J Am Acad Dermatol 1993;28:662–4.

36. Fawcett HA, Smith NP. Injection-site granuloma due to aluminium. Arch Dermatol 1984;120:1318–22.

37. Slater DN, Underwood JC, Durrant TE, et al. Aluminium hydroxide granulomas: light and electron microscopic studies and X-ray microanalysis. Br J Dermatol 1982;107:103–8.

38. Del Rosario RN, Barr RJ, Graham BS, et al. Exogenous and endogenous cutaneous anomalies and curiosities. Am J Dermatopathol 2005; 27:259–67.

39. Soares Almeida LM, Requena L, Kutzner H, et al. Localized panniculitis secondary to subcutaneous glatiramer acetate injections for the treatment of multiple sclerosis: a clinicopathologic and immunohistochemical study. J Am Acad Dermatol 2006;55: 968–74.

40. Bechara F, Sand M, Hoffman K, et al. Fat tissue after lipolysis of lipomas: a histopathological and immunohistochemical study. J Cutan Pathol 2007;34: 552–7.

41. Shanesmith RP, Vogiatzis PI, Binder SW, et al. Unusual palisading and necrotizing granulomas associated with a lubricating agent used in lipoplasty. Am J Dermatopathol 2010;32:448–52.

42. Palestine RF, Millns JL, Spigel GT, et al. Skin manifestations of pentazocine abuse. J Am Acad Dermatol 1980;2:47–55.

43. Pujol RM, Puig L, Moreno A, et al. Pseudoscleroderma secondary to phytonadione (vitamin K1) injections. Cutis 1989;43:365–8.

44. Mehta CL, Tyler RJ, Cripps DJ. Granulomatous dermatitis with focal sarcoidal features associated with recombinant interferon β-1b injections. J Am Acad Dermatol 1988;39:1024–8.

45. Eberlein-Köning B, Hein R, Abeck D, et al. Cutaneous sarcoid foreign body granulomas developing at sites of previous skin injury after systemic interferon-alpha treatment for chronic hepatitis C. Br J Dermatol 1999;140:370–2.

46. Jordaan HF, Sandler M. Zinc-induced granuloma—a unique complication of insulin therapy. Clin Exp Dermatol 1989;14:227–9.

47. Ajithkumar K, Anand U, Pulimood S, et al. Vaccine-induced necrobiotic granulomas. Clin Exp Dermatol 1998;23:222–4.

48. Lalinga AV, Pellegrino M, Laurini L, et al. Necrobiotic palisading granuloma at injection site of disodium clodronate: a case report. Dermatology 1999;198: 394–5.

49. Yasukawa K, Sawamura D, Sugawara H, et al. Leuprorelin acetate granulomas: case reports and review of the literature. Br J Dermatol 2005;152:1045–7.

50. Porter WM, Grabczynska S, Francis N, et al. The perils and pitfalls of penile injections. Br J Dermatol 1999;141:736–8.

51. Carlson JA, Schutzer P, Pattison T, et al. Sarcoidal foreign-body granulomatous dermatitis associated with ophthalmic drops. Am J Dermatopathol 1998; 20:175–8.

52. Mowry RG, Sams WM Jr, Caufield JB. Cutaneous silica granuloma. Arch Dermatol 1991;127:692–4.

53. Walsh NM, Hanly JG, Tremaine R, et al. Cutaneous sarcoidosis and foreign bodies. Am J Dermatopathol 1993;15:203–7.

54. Shelley WB, Hurley HJ. The pathogenesis of silica granulomas in man: a non-allergic colloidal phenomenon. J Invest Dermatol 1960;34:107–23.

55. Casper C, Groth W, Hunzelmann N. Sarcoidal-type allergic contact granuloma. A rare complication of ear piercing. Am J Dermatopathol 2004;26: 59–62.

56. High WA, Ayers RA, Adams JR, et al. Granulomatous reaction to titanium alloy: an unusual reaction to ear piercing. J Am Acad Dermatol 2006;55:716–20.

57. Fernández-Casado A, Martin-Ezquerra G, Yébenes M, et al. Progressive supravenous granulomatous nodular eruption in a human immunodeficiency virus-positive intravenous drug user treated with highly active antiretroviral therapy. Br J Dermatol 2008;158: 145–9.

58. Farrant P, Higgins E. A granulomatous response to tribal medicine as a feature of the immune reconstitution syndrome. Clin Exp Dermatol 2004; 29:366–8.

59. Berlin JM, Taylor JS, Sigel JE, et al. Beryllium dermatitis. J Am Acad Dermatol 2003;49:939–41.

60. Shelley WB, Hurley HJ. Allergic origin of zirconim deodorant granuloma. Br J Dermatol 1958;70: 75–101.

61. Skelton HG III, Smith KJ, Johnson FB, et al. Zirconium granuloma resulting from an aluminum zirconium complex: a previously unrecognized agent in development of hypersensitivity granulomas. J Am Acad Dermatol 1993;28:874–6.

62. Martin RW III, Lumadue JA, Corio RL, et al. Cutaneous giant cell hyalin angiopathy. J Cutan Pathol 1993;20:356–8.

63. Rhee DD, Wu ML. Pulse granulomas detected in gallbladder, fallopian tube, and skin. Arch Pathol Lab Med 2006;130:1839–42.

64. Beer TW, Cole JM. Cutaneous pulse granulomas. Arch Pathol Lab Med 2007;131:1513–4.

65. Tschen JA, Tschen JA. Pulse granuloma in a rectocutaneous fistula. J Cutan Pathol 2008;35: 343–5.

66. Rachman R. Soft-tissue injury by mercury from a broken thermometer. A case report and review of the literature. Am J Clin Pathol 1974;61: 296–300.

67. Leonard DD. Starch granulomas. Arch Dermatol 1973;107:101–3.

68. Tye MJ, Hashimoto K, Fox F. Talc granulomas of the skin. JAMA 1966;198:1370–2.

69. Postlethwait RW, Willigan DA, Ulin AW. Human tissue reaction to sutures. Ann Surg 1975;181:144–50.

70. Holzheimer RG. Adverse events of sutures: possible interactions of biomaterials? Eur J Med Res 2005;10: 521–6.

71. Pimentel JC. Sarcoidal granulomas of the skin produced by acrylic and nylon fibers. Br J Dermatol 1977;96:673–7.

72. Gutiérrez MC, Martín L, Arias D, et al. Granulomas faciales por espinas de cactus. Med Cut ILA 1990; 18:197–200 [in Spanish].

73. Madkan VK, Abraham T, Lesher JL Jr. Cactus spine granuloma. Cutis 2007;79:208–10.

74. Zinder RA, Schwartz RA. Cactus bristle implantation. Report of an unusual case initially seen with rows of yellow hairs. Arch Dermatol 1983;119: 152–4.

75. Osawa R, Abe R, Inokuma D, et al. Chain saw blade granuloma: reaction to deeply embedded metal fragment. Arch Dermatol 2006;142:1079–80.

76. De La Torre C, Toribio J. Sea-urchin granuloma: histologic profile. A pathologic study of 50 biopsies. J Cutan Pathol 2001;28:223–8.

77. Pimentel JC. The "wheat-stubble sarcoid granuloma": a new epithelioid granuloma of the skin. Br J Dermatol 1972;87:444–9.

78. Hatano Y, Asada Y, Komada S, et al. A case of pencil core granuloma with unusual temporal profile. Dermatology 2000;201:151–3.

79. Gormley RH, Kovach SJ 3rd, Zhang PJ. Role for trauma in inducing pencil "lead" granuloma in the skin. J Am Acad Dermatol 2010;62:1074–5.

80. Peluso AM, Fanti PA, Monti M, et al. Cutaneous complications of artificial hair implantation: a pathological study. Dermatology 1992;184:129–32.

81. Young PC, Smack DP, Sau P, et al. Golf club granuloma. J Am Acad Dermatol 1995;32:1047–8.

82. Allen AC. Persistent "insect bites" (dermal eosinophilic granulomas) simulating lymphoblastomas, histiocytes, and squamous cell carcinomas. Am J Pathol 1948;24:367–75.

83. Yanagihara M, Fujii T, Wakamatu N, et al. Silicone granuloma on the entry points of acupuncture, venepuncture and surgical needles. J Cutan Pathol 2000;27:301–5.

84. Kenmochi A, Satoh T, Igawa K, et al. Silica granuloma induced by indwelling catheter. J Am Acad Dermatol 2007;57:S54–5.

85. Alani RM, Busam K. Acupuncture granulomas. J Am Acad Dermatol 2001;45:S225–6.

86. Matwiyoff GN, McKinlay JR, Miller CH, et al. Transepidermal migration of external cardiac pacing wire presenting as a cutaneous nodule. J Am Acad Dermatol 2000;42:865–6.

87. Gilaberte M, Delclós J, Yebenés M, et al. Delayed foreign body granuloma secondary to an abandoned cardiac pacemaker wire. J Eur Acad Dermatol Venereol 2007;21:107–9.

Current Understanding of Cutaneous Lymphoma
Selected Topics

Janyana M.D. Deonizio, MD[a], Joan Guitart, MD[a,b],*

KEYWORDS

- Cutaneous T-cell lymphomas • γδ cutaneous T-cell lymphomas • T follicular helper cells
- Cutaneous CD30 + T-cell lymphoproliferative disorders

KEY POINTS

- The World Health Organization-European Organization for Research and Treatment of Cancer classification of cutaneous lymphomas is the result of a consensus among dermatologists, dermatopathologists, and hematopathologists and reflects the unique characteristics of skin lymphomas.
- Subcutaneous panniculitis-like T-cell lymphoma is often preceded by a nondiagnostic lymphoid infiltrate of the subcutaneous fat, which may share features with lupus profundus.
- Marginal zone lymphoma is an indolent condition, which can present with a marked plasmacytic differentiation. These cases need to be differentiated from plasmacytomas, which are often associated with multiple myeloma.
- Cutaneous γδ lymphomas can present with a variety of pathologic patterns, ranging from a lichenoid superficial pattern to a deep necrotizing panniculitic process.
- Follicular T-helper cells may be the cell of origin to certain skin lymphomas, including d'emblée presentation of MF and small/medium pleomorphic T-cell lymphomas.
- There is some clinical and pathologic overlap between pediatric lymphomatoid papulosis and pityriasis lichenoides acuta, especially when the infiltrate is primarily CD8 positive.

Recent epidemiology studies have identified a steady increase in the incidence of cutaneous lymphomas over the past few decades. A study by Bradford and colleagues[1] using 16 tumor registries from the SEER (Surveillance Epidemiology and End Results) program noted an increase over the past 25 years from 5.0 to 12.7 new patients per million inhabitants per year. This increase in cancer incidence is at a time when the incidence of many other malignancies is in decline. Although possible explanations for this increased incidence include heightened awareness of these conditions as well as a more refined diagnostic acuity by dermatologists and pathologists, an increase secondary to environmental factors cannot be discounted.

Our understanding of cutaneous lymphomas keeps evolving, as shown by the marked increase of scientific literature in all areas related to cutaneous lymphomas. Consequently, our present knowledge and understanding of cutaneous lymphomas requires reconsideration of past

The authors have nothing to disclose.
[a] Department of Dermatology, Northwestern University, 676 North Saint Clair Suite 1765, Chicago, IL 60611, USA; [b] Dermatology Department, Unit and Cutaneous Lymphoma Clinic at Northwestern University, 676 North Saint Clair Suite 1765, Chicago, IL 60611, USA
* Corresponding author. Department of Dermatology, Northwestern University, 676 North Saint Clair Suite 1765, Chicago, IL 60611.
E-mail address: j-guitart@northwestern.edu

Dermatol Clin 30 (2012) 749–761
http://dx.doi.org/10.1016/j.det.2012.06.002

dogma and critical revision of the new proposals. In this article, some hot topics and important new findings in the field are reviewed.

EUROPEAN ORGANIZATION FOR RESEARCH AND TREATMENT OF CANCER/WORLD HEALTH ORGANIZATION CLASSIFICATION OF CUTANEOUS LYMPHOMAS: A WORK IN PROGRESS

The classification of cutaneous lymphomas has evolved and become more complex over the years, reflecting the contemporary understanding of these conditions. This trend will most certainly continue in the future as we continue to gain knowledge of the field. The current classification, established in 2005, is based on a consensus of the European Organization for Research and Treatment of Cancer (EORTC) and World Health Organization (WHO) as the result of a remarkable effort to find common ground between European dermatologists and American hematopathologists.[2] The essence of this classification was incorporated in the most recent lymphoma classification update from WHO in 2008 (**Tables 1** and **2**).[3] For the first time, distinct cutaneous entities that in the past would had been diagnosed and classified differently depending on specialty and location of the physician are now broadly recognized by the scientific community as specific entities. This consensus was the result of an unprecedented meeting of minds at which extensive discussions took place between hematopathologists, dermatologists, and dermatopathologists. On reviewing their extensive experiences and taking into consideration morphologic, immunophenotypical, and molecular evidence, the experts assigned distinct skin lymphoma entities based on the unique characteristics of skin lymphomas even as compared with the same morphologic conditions in primary lymphoid organs. For instance, primary cutaneous follicle center cell lymphoma, unlike the nodal counterpart, lacks the typical t(11;14) translocation and diffuse large B-cell lymphoma, leg-type (DLBL-LT) became the first skin lymphoma to incorporate an anatomic site in the name. However, this new lymphoma subtype, as is discussed later, is still a debatable entity for some experts. Finally, we

Table 1
WHO classification 2008 for mature T-cell and NK cell neoplasms

Mature T-Cell and NK Cell Neoplasms	Cutaneous Involvement
T-cell prolymphocytic leukemia	Rare
T-cell large granular lymphocytic leukemia	Rare
Chronic lymphoproliferative disorder of NK-cells[a]	Rare
Aggressive NK cell leukemia	Rare
Systemic EBV T-cell lymphoproliferative disease of childhood	Rare
Hydroa vacciniforme-like lymphoma	Yes
Adult T-cell leukemia/lymphoma	Yes
Extranodal NK/T-cell lymphoma, nasal type	Common
Enteropathy-associated T-cell lymphoma	Rare
Hepatosplenic T-cell lymphoma	No
Subcutaneous panniculitis-like T-cell lymphoma	Yes
Mycosis fungoides	Yes
Sézary syndrome	Yes
Primary cutaneous CD30+ T-cell lymphoproliferative disorder (LyP and PCALCL)	Yes
PC aggressive epidermotropic CD8+ cytotoxic T-cell lymphoma[a]	Yes
PC γδ T-cell lymphoma	Yes
PC small to medium-size CD4+ T-cell lymphoma[a]	Yes
Angioimmunoblastic T-cell lymphoma	Rare
ALK+	Rare
ALK−[a]	Common

Abbreviations: ALK, anaplastic lymphoma kinase; EBV, Epstein-Barr virus; LyP, lymphomatoid papulosis; NK, natural killer; PC, primary cutaneous; PCALCL, primary cutaneous anaplastic large-cell lymphoma.
[a] These neoplasms represent provisional entities or provisional subtypes of other neoplasms.

Table 2
WHO classifications 2008 for mature B-cell neoplasms

Mature B-Cell Neoplasms	Cutaneous Involvement
Chronic lymphocytic leukemia/small lymphocytic lymphoma	Common
B-cell prolymphocytic leukemia	Rare
Splenic marginal zone lymphoma	No
Hairy cell leukemia	Rare
Splenic lymphoma/leukemia, unclassifiable[a]	No
Lymphoplasmacytic lymphoma (Waldenström macroglobulinemia)	Rare
Heavy chain diseases (α, γ, μ)	No
Plasma cell myeloma	Rare
Solitary plasmacytoma of bone	No
Extraosseous plasmacytoma	Rare
Extranodal marginal zone B-cell lymphoma of mucosa-associated lymphoid tissue	Common
Nodal marginal zone B-cell lymphoma	No
Follicular lymphoma	Rare
Primary cutaneous follicle center lymphoma	Yes
Mantle cell lymphoma	Rare
Diffuse large B-cell lymphoma (DLBL)	Common
Lymphomatoid granulomatosis	Common
Primary mediastinal (thymic) large B-cell lymphoma	Rare
Intravascular large B-cell lymphoma	Common
Primary cutaneous DLBL, leg-type	Yes
Anaplastic large-cell lymphoma kinase+ large B-cell lymphoma	Rare
Plasmablastic lymphoma	Rare
Primary effusion lymphoma	Rare
Large B-cell lymphoma arising in human herpesvirus 8–associated multicentric Castleman disease	Rare
Burkitt lymphoma	Rare
B-cell lymphoma, unclassifiable	Rare
Hodgkin lymphomas (classified separately)	Rare

Abbreviation: DLBL, diffuse large B-cell lymphoma.
[a] These neoplasms represent provisional entities or provisional subtypes of other neoplasms.

can use a cutaneous lymphoma classification that makes sense to the clinical dermatologists from a prognostic point of view and is accepted by the pathology community. Although the WHO-EORTC classification of cutaneous lymphomas represents a major advancement over previous classifications, several issues remain unsolved. There are provisional entities like primary cutaneous aggressive epidermotropic CD8+ T-cell lymphoma (often referred to as Berti lymphoma), which as we learn more about these rare conditions, should eventually become a definitive entity. There are other entities like CD4+ small to medium-sized pleomorphic T-cell lymphoma (CD4+SMPTCL) and probably lymphomatoid papulosis that in our opinion may be overdiagnosed because reactive conditions

can mimic these conditions and also because the defining criteria as described in the consensus publications are imprecise and prone to misinterpretation. SMPTCL is diagnosed at our center to comply with classification standards. However, we believe that they should be diagnosed as a cutaneous lymphoid hyperplasia or pseudolymphoma. Most if not all patients presenting with unilesional CD4+SMPTCL have an entirely indolent course, regardless of the presence or absence of T-cell clonality. This indolent course has been confirmed by a large cohort from the Graz group that suggested an undeterminate significance, although none of their patients showed tumor progression.[4] Cetinozman and colleagues[5] have also reported that the lesions currently diagnosed as CD4+SMPTCL express a follicular T-helper phenotype that is identical to lesions reported as pseudolymphoma in the past. Lymphomatoid papulosis as a subtype of CD30 lymphoproliferative disorder also remains poorly defined, and as a consequence, patients with brief papular episodes of unclear nature but focal CD30 expression may be misdiagnosed as suffering from a lymphoproliferative disorder. To further complicate this entity, patients may be diagnosed with the so-called lymphomatoid papulosis type B with complete absence of CD30 expression. The classification of cutaneous lymphomas also includes conditions that are often systemic from their onset, like adult T-cell leukemia/lymphoma or extranodal natural killer (NK)/T-cell lymphoma.

Perhaps the most controversial entity in the WHO-EORTC classification is the designation of a specific entity to a distinct anatomic site. DLBL-LT has been mostly described on the leg of elderly patients, especially women. Two reasons for the specific entity designation include the site of presentation and the poor prognosis reported, which contrasts with the indolent course of most other primary skin B-cell lymphomas. However, there are several arguments that should be considered against this entity. First, 10% to 20% of the cases present at sites other than the legs. Second, even T-cell lymphomas presenting on the leg are recalcitrant to therapies and carry a worse prognosis compared with similar T-cell lymphomas presenting at other anatomic regions.[6] The advanced age of the patients may also contribute to the poor prognosis, although the 50% 5-year survival was reported as being disease-specific, older patients have a low reserve or worse performance status and are more vulnerable to succumb to a relatively lower tumor burden than a younger patient population. The best argument to eliminate this subcategory is the recent recognition in hematopathology of a similar molecular counterpart in the lymph node, which is referred to as DLBLs with activated phenotype.[7,8] Like DLBL-LT, this subtype of nodal lymphoma is characterized by the expression of multiple myeloma (MM) oncogene 1 and forkhead box protein 1 (FOXP1), as well as bcl-2 and bcl-6.

The expression of FOXP1 is characteristic of most nodal activated phenotype as well as DLBL-LT and connotes a less favorable prognosis. The mechanism involved in FOXP1 expression deregulation is not completely understood. Even though FOXP1 gene rearrangements have been reported in extranodal DLBL, recent studies failed to find it in DLBL-LT.[7] High frequency of aberrant gene expression of the cyclin-dependent kinase inhibitor gene CDKN2A localized on chromosome 9p21 has been found in DLBL-LT. This gene encodes p16 (INK4A), and inactivation of p16 is associated with a worse prognosis in primary DLBL-LT.[9] Although it is important to recognize the worse prognosis associated with most large-cell lymphomas involving the leg and to check these prognostically significant immunomarkers, we believe the inaccuracy of the terminology and the lack of scientific rationale for a distinct entity are strong arguments to reconsider its position in future cutaneous lymphoma classifications. Other newly described conditions like Epstein-Barr virus (EBV)+ B-cell lymphoma seen in elderly patients, posttransplant, methotrexate, and other immune suppression conditions have not yet been incorporated and need to be considered in future classifications.

ATYPICAL LYMPHOCYTIC LOBULAR PANNICULITIS, LUPUS PANNICULITIS, AND SUBCUTANEOUS PANNICULITIS-LIKE T-CELL LYMPHOMA

The concept of cutaneous lymphoid dyscrasia assumes that some lymphomas are preceded by a chronic phase characterized by a clonal or oligoclonal lymphoid-rich infiltrate, but otherwise not fulfilling histopathologic criteria for the diagnosis of a lymphoma.[10] Although this theory is controversial, the diagnostic dilemma of an inflammatory process versus a lymphoma is a constant preoccupation for dermatopathologists. Cutaneous lymphoid dyscrasia presenting with a pattern of panniculitis was first reported by Magro and colleagues.[11] Since then, other reports of inflammatory panniculitis preceding a subcutaneous panniculitis-like T-cell lymphoma (SPTCL) have been published.[12] Pincus and colleagues[12] reported overlapping features between lupus panniculitis with clinical criteria for systemic lupus erythematosus evolving to SPTCL.

Clinically, atypical lymphocytic lobular panniculitis (ALLP) is similar to SPTCL, presenting with deep plaques in young women often with positive lupus serology.[11] The plaques tend to involve the lower extremities and can be tender, but do not ulcerate. Fever, fatigue, and other systemic symptoms are rarely noted.

Morphologically, ALLP shows a lobular infiltrate with small to intermediate-sized lymphocytes without significant nuclear atypia. Interstitial prominent histiocytes tend to accompany the lymphoid infiltrate. Dermal mucin deposits and an interface process at the dermal-epidermal junction may indicate in some cases a frank overlap with lupus panniculitis. Moreover, in some of the cases reported as overlap between lupus and SPTCL, aggregates of B cells and clusters of plasmacytoid dendritic cells, as seen in lupus panniculitis, were reported.[12] Overall, the infiltrate is less dense, and rimming around adipocytes or lipid vacuoles is not as prominent as in SPTCL. Cytotoxic features like hemorrhage, karyorrhexis, or vasculitis are more typical of SPTCL and for the most part are absent in these cases. Like in SPTCL, the lymphoid infiltrate may be characterized by a low CD4/CD8 ratio, but the overwhelming CD8 profile of the SPTCL infiltrate is not seen. This process is chronic and may resolve spontaneously or with antiinflammatory therapy, only rarely evolving to frank SPTCL.

When should we consider the term ALLP? If all the criteria of lupus profundus mentioned earlier are present, one is compelled to diagnose lupus panniculitis. Even if this diagnosis may rarely precede SPTCL, we embrace the concept of ALLP as a variant of cutaneous lymphoid dyscrasia seen only in exceptional cases when the infiltrate is atypical for lupus yet there are insufficient morphologic criteria to diagnose a lymphoma. The concept of ALLP helps us categorize these unresolved cases in need of close follow-up, and provides a well-defined reference that can be presented and discussed with the patient and their relatives. This concept is not broadly accepted and other pathologists may prefer a descriptive noncommittal diagnosis like nonspecific panniculitis.

SPTCL was considered as a distinct entity for the first time in the WHO-EORTC classification for cutaneous lymphomas in 2005.[2] This lymphoma entity is limited to T-cell lymphomas expressing the $\alpha\beta$ T-cell receptor (TCR) heterodimer. Patients typically present with multiple indurated nonulcerated and asymptomatic nodules, mostly involving the lower extremities. Unlike the so-called unilesional mycosis fungoides (MF), which has an excellent prognosis, we and others have observed SPTCL presenting with a single lesion, yet with eventual progression to advanced stages or with abnormal blood and imaging results at the initial staging workup. The age of presentation is wide, but approximately 20% of the patients are younger than 20 years, with numerous case reports involving children.[13] Approximately half of the patients have constitutional symptoms and laboratory anomalies, including frequent mild cytopenias and positive autoimmune serology are often noted. There is a strong association of SPTCL with autoimmune conditions, primarily lupus erythematosus but also Sjögren syndrome and rheumatoid arthritis.[14] The possible iatrogenic effect of immunosuppression associated with the treatment of rheumatic conditions in the lymphomagenesis of SPTCL is unknown, but case reports of SPTCL developing during pregnancy and human immunodeficiency virus (HIV) infection suggest an etiologic role of immunosuppression in some SPTCL cases.[15] Besides numerous case reports and epidemiologic evidence linking SPTCL with lupus erythematous, a link between SPTCL and so-called cytophagic histiocytic panniculitis has also been suggested.[16] However, the existence of this entity is in question, because it lacks a distinct pathomechanism and emperipolesis can be observed in benign and malignant conditions characterized by an activated cytotoxic lymphoid infiltrate like SPTCL, $\gamma\delta$ lymphomas, or viral-induced panniculitis.

Autoimmunity and chronic inflammation may play a role in the lymphomagenesis of SPTCL. It remains to be determined if the relationship with autoimmunity arises from a common constitutional defect in the immune system or perhaps iatrogenic immunosuppressive therapy may predispose to these lymphomas. We have observed a young woman with Crohn disease developing SPTCL after a long course on azathioprine. In some cases, the disease presents or progresses while on steroids or other immunosuppressive therapy for rheumatic diseases,[17] whereas other SPTCL or ambiguous cases may resolve with steroids, methotrexate, or cyclosporine.[18] Taking into consideration that cyclosporine and other potent immunosuppressors tend to accelerate tumor progression in cutaneous T-cell lymphoma (CTCL), this observation is counterintuitive and intriguing.

SPTCL has been reported in a young patient with mutations of the perforin gene.[19] Mutations of the perforin gene, which are commonly associated with hemophagocytic syndrome (HPS), may dysregulate homoeostasis, favoring the uncontrolled proliferation of atypical lymphocytes. A report of 2 siblings developing SPTCL in childhood, both of them complicated with HPS, is also supportive of congenital gene defects predisposing to this condition.[20]

Nodal or other systemic involvement is rarely detected in SPTCL. Paratrabecular lymphoid aggregates as typically seen in bone marrow involved by systemic lymphomas are not seen in SPTCL. However, we have observed in several patients subtle atypical lymphocytes rimming around the marrow adipocytes in a manner similar to that seen in the subcutaneous tissue.

The infiltrate in SPTCL is dense and centered around the subcutaneous fat lobules. The tumor cells display adipotropism, with rimming of atypical intermediate-size lymphocytes around adipocytes and empty lipid vacuoles. However, rimming is not unique to SPTCL and has been noted in other lymphomas involving the subcutaneous tissue.[21]

Small reactive lymphocytes and many histiocytes are also typically present, with some cases showing a plasma cell component. Fat necrosis and karyorrhexis are focally present, but without the extensive hemorrhage and liquefactive necrosis seen in other cytotoxic lymphomas.[22] T-cell clonality is detected in most cases and the immunophenotype is positive for CD3, CD8, TIA-1, granzyme B, and βF1. Ki-67 (MIB-1) shows a high proliferative index, but EBER shows no evidence of EBV infection and CD56 is typically negative.

The prognosis of SPTCL is fairly good, with a 5-year survival of 85%, and a notable poor prognosis for patients who developed HPS.[13] The clinical and histologic comparison between ALLP and SPTCL is summarized in **Table 3**.

IMMUNOCYTOMA OR PLASMACYTOMA

The dilemma is a skin biopsy with a rich infiltrate composed of monotypical plasma cells without significant nuclear atypia, blastic changes, or mitotic activity. The prognosis varies widely depending on the diagnosis, which could be a primary cutaneous marginal zone B-cell lymphoma (MZL) with extensive plasmacytic differentiation, a systemic B-cell lymphoma (lymphoplasmacytic lymphoma or small lymphocytic lymphoma) with plasmacytic differentiation, or a plasmacytoma secondary to MM. Although the cellular element of all these tumors can be similar, the former has an excellent prognosis, whereas the latter has a poor one. Cutaneous or other extramedullary spread of MM indicates an aggressive process and portends a poor prognosis.[23]

As a neoplasia of postgerminal center B cells, MZL can display an array of cellular elements, ranging from monocytoid or centrocyte-like small cells to plasma cells. Although small aggregates of plasma cells are commonly seen in primary cutaneous MZL, only rarely the tumor is composed predominantly of mature plasma cells. The plasmacytic variant of MZL with extensive plasmacytic differentiation has been previously reported in the literature as immunocytomas as well as primary cutaneous plasmacytoma, which accentuates the confusion of this topic. The reason why certain MZL cases display plasmacytic morphology is unknown, but unlike the conventional MZL seen in young patients, the plasmacytic variant is more common in elderly patients. Besides advanced age, the plasmacytic variant has also been observed after rituximab therapy for extracutaneous MZL, which may indicate that morphology is influenced by the immune status.[24] However, unlike other immunosuppression-related B-cell lymphoproliferative disorders, viral agents like EBV or human herpesvirus 8 have not been identified.

Morphologically, the infiltrate in MM is purely plasmacytic, with fewer scattered lymphocytes, and the cells tend to show other features like nuclear atypia, multinucleation, Dutcher bodies, and often mitotic activity. Amyloid deposits can also be observed in MM-related plasmacytoma or other systemic lymphoplasmacytic lymphomas, but are rarely seen in primary cutaneous MZL. Nevertheless, a definitive diagnosis exclusively based on morphology is rarely made, often relying on ancillary tests like immunohistochemistry or flow cytometry. A few immune markers can help solve the quandary. MZL express B-cell markers like CD20 and CD19 as well as the common lymphocyte antigen CD45R. In contrast, MM-related plasmacytoma should be mostly negative for all 3 markers CD19/CD20/CD45. In addition, tumor cells often express the NK cell marker

Table 3 Comparison between ALLP and SPTCL		
	Atypical Lymphocytic Lobular Panniculitis	**Subcutaneous Panniculitis-Like T-Cell Lymphoma**
Constitutional symptoms	Rare	Common (50%)
Nuclear atypia	–	+
Infiltrate	Less dense	Dense, rimming around adipocytes or lipids vacuoles
Lymphocytes	Small to intermediate-sized	Intermediate-sized
Cytotoxic features	No	Occasionally
CD4/CD8 ratio	Normal to low	Low. Overwhelming CD8 profile
Prognosis	Good	85% (5-y survival)

CD56 and CD117.[23] Weaker bcl-2 expression and absence of cyclinD1 expression have also been reported to help distinguish extramedullary plasmacytomas, which is the same as MZL with extensive plasma cell differentiation, from MM- related plasmacytomas.[23]

The distinction between the plasma cell variant of MZL and other neoplastic mature B-cell neoplasms may also be challenging. Although CD23 may be expressed in some cases, one often needs to rely on clinical staging data to exclude a systemic lymphoma.

Flow cytometry studies of MZL of various anatomic sites have shown weak surface light chain expression and CD20 as well as negative CD56, CD138, and CD38. In contrast, plasmacytomas in patients with MM were positive for CD38 and CD56. The investigators concluded that these plasmacytic MZL cases are neoplasms of plasma cell precursors, which are distinct from the more mature plasma cell stage in cases of MM.[25,26]

THE MANY FACES OF γδ CUTANEOUS T-CELL LYMPHOMAS

Cutaneous γδ T-cell lymphoma (CGDTL) is a rare condition, which is no longer considered a provisional entity in the latest WHO classification of cutaneous lymphomas.[3,27] CGDTL has been poorly characterized because of the lack of reliable immunomarkers. Historically, the diagnosis of CGDTL from paraffin-embedded material was a presumptive diagnosis, relying on the absence of αβ TCR heterodimer expression on the tumor cells. The diagnosis of a CGDTL could be established with certainty only by flow cytometry of tissue samples or on frozen sections by immunohistochemistry. Recently, a new method to identify the γ chain of the γδ TCR heterodimer in paraffin-embedded tissue was reported.[28] We recently analyzed the clinical, pathologic, and immunophenotypic features of a cohort of CGDTL using this method. The diagnosis of CGDTL was based on expression of the γδ heterodimer on the tumor cells by immunohistochemistry or flow cytometry. In most cases, the monoclonal antibody γ M1 (clone γ3.20, Thermo/Fisher Scientific, Waltham, MA) was used according to the retrieval method described by Roullet and colleagues.[28]

Most of the 45 patients with CGDTL were white, with a median age of 60 years (range 7–91 years) and male/female ratio of 2:1. Although most patients had generalized involvement (T3), a subset of patients had localized disease (T1) presenting with a single or a cluster of lesions resembling cellulitis, hematoma, pyoderma, or an arthropod bite reaction. Some of these lesions were deep, involving the subcutaneous soft tissue or underlying structures like salivary glands. The legs were more often involved than the torso, arms, or head and neck region. Mucosal lesions were observed in only 2 patients. Most patients presented with large and deep indurated plaques with a panniculitic appearance. The plaques were eroded at presentation or eventually became ulcerated, with a hemorrhagic and necrotic appearance in 60% of the patients. Ten patients presented with chronic scaly erythematous patches resembling psoriasis or MF, often with superimposed superficial erosive features. Constitutional symptoms were reported in 54% of the patients at the time of presentation, including some patients with limited skin involvement.

Comorbidities at the time of presentation were common, including 5 patients with other lymphoproliferative disorders, 4 patients with systemic carcinomas, and 2 patients with hepatitis C. Concurrent illness associated with immune dysregulation was also noted in several patients, including Hashimoto thyroiditis, Crohn disease, temporal arteritis, alopecia areata, celiac disease/uveitis/arthritis, and sarcoidosis. Four patients carried the diagnosis of lupus panniculitis, which for the most part was directly related to the lesions eventually diagnosed as CGDTL with a panniculitic pattern. None of the patients had a history of immunosuppression from either HIV infection, post–organ transplant, or other causes. Lymphadenopathy was rare and was noted in only 3 patients at presentation. Serum lactose dehydrogenase (LDH) levels were increased at the time of presentation in 55% of the patients. Bone marrow biopsies were mostly negative, with 21% reported as positive, including 4 patients with signs of hemophagocytosis. One patient progressed with tumor involvement in the testes and 3 patients developed mental status changes with confirmation of tumor by brain imaging and cerebrospinal fluid involvement by flow cytometry. Three patients had lymphomatous involvement of the gastrointestinal tract concurrently or after the skin lymphoma was diagnosed. Follow-up information was available on 47 patients, with a median follow-up time of 18 months (range 1–107 months). Twenty-six patients (57%) died of disease or complications of treatment, including 4 patients with HPS and complications of central nervous system involvement in 3 patients. The 5-year overall survival rate was 21.3%.

The pattern of the lymphoid infiltrate was variable, ranging from a pagetoid pattern to cases with exclusive subcutaneous tissue involvement. In some patients diverse patterns were noted in biopsies obtained simultaneously or at different times. Most cases had a dense infiltrate, with partial involvement of epidermal, dermal, and subcutaneous compartments. The epidermal component was predominantly a junctional lymphoid infiltrate, often accompanied by superficial hemorrhage and subtle exocytosis of erythrocytes. The initial biopsy in some of the cases resembled MF or an interface dermatitis with exocytosis of atypical lymphocytes, vacuolar degeneration of the basal cell layer, and scattered necrotic keratinocytes. Variable acanthosis and hyperkeratosis was noted, but Pautrier microabscesses were not observed in any cases. Three cases had significant pagetoid features, with atypical lymphocytes involving the entire epidermal thickness. Cytotoxic features, including hemorrhage, fat necrosis with karyorrhexis, and vasculitic pattern with fibrinoid necrosis, were occasionally noted. Rare cases had a histiocyte-rich infiltrate, with some granulomatous features. The cytologic detail of these lymphomas was monomorphous and consisted predominantly of medium-sized lymphocytes, with a few cases characterized by a predominantly large-cell infiltrate.

All cases analyzed by immunohistochemistry were CD3 positive and βF1 negative. The null phenotype CD4−/CD8− seen in 29 cases was more common than CD8+ or CD4+. CD30 was mostly negative. γδ T-cell phenotype was inferred in all cases by the absence of βF1 expression or by the expression of γ M1. CD56 was positive in 35% of the cases and CD5 was positive in only 12% of the cases.

Based on our experience, CGDTL tends to present with extensive and deep indurated plaques on the extremities, which may resemble inflammatory panniculitis. However, unlike inflammatory panniculitis, the process is usually more extensive, with a tendency to ulcerate during the course of the disease. Another subset of cases characterized by solitary or multiple lesions confined to 1 anatomic region was often associated with constitutional symptoms and high LDH levels and carried an equally poor prognosis. Therefore, unlike other cutaneous lymphomas, the skin tumor burden does not seem to correlate with prognosis. We identified a third subset of patients presenting with chronic erythematous and scaly patches resembling MF or psoriasis. Although some of these patients evolved into a more aggressive phase, with extensive ulceration of the patches and tumor formation, the overall survival of this group was significantly better and some patients have remained with indolent patch lesions for several years of follow-up. With the exception of a few cases presenting with a pagetoid pattern,

these patches differ from MF by the absence of Pautrier microabscesses and the frequent association with scattered necrotic keratinocytes.

Several of our patients had comorbidities associated with immune suppression, including other lymphoproliferative conditions, immune dysregulation, other malignancies, and pregnancy. Chronic antigenic stimulation has been hypothesized to play a role in the pathogenesis of CGDTCL.[29] This premise is supported by the clonal expansion of γδ T cells, which has been observed in patients with celiac disease, Crohn disease, renal allografts, lupus erythematosus, rheumatoid arthritis, multiple sclerosis, and Hodgkin lymphoma.[30–32] There are also reports of γδ T-cell lymphomas associated with opportunistic infections occurring in patients in congenital and acquired immune suppression and autoimmunity.[30,33–35] We also noted comorbidity with lupus erythematosus, an association that has also been reported in patients with αβ-SCPLTCL.[12] Some of these initial skin biopsies in our cases showed dermal mucin deposits and an interface vacuolar reaction. An interface pattern in CGDTCL resembling lupus erythematosus was also noted by Massone and colleagues.[36] The pathomechanistic connection between these precursor biopsies resembling lupus and CGDTCL has not been elucidated. Likewise, a panniculitic precursor resembling lupus profundus was observed in 1 of our patients. Another case report of a patient with an ALLP for 15 years with eventual progression into an aggressive CGDTCL emphasizes the disparity of presentations and the fact that although many patients have a rapid aggressive course, others may have a prolonged cutaneous lymphoid process that is difficult to categorize.[37] As previously noted,[38,39] an atypical lymphoid infiltrate involving the dermis and subcutaneous tissue is an important clue for the diagnosis of CGDTCL. A pure panniculitic pattern, as seen in αβ-SCPLTCL, was rarely observed in our cohort. We observed variable patterns of the lymphoma infiltrate (ie, superficial vs deep subcutaneous), even when simultaneous biopsies were obtained from different anatomic sites of the same patient. This inconsistency of histopathologic patterns noted in CGDTCL suggests that multiple skin biopsies may be required for proper evaluation.

Chronic EBV infection and viral integration may play an etiologic role in a subset of CGDTCL cases. The first case of EBV-induced GDTCL was recently reported by Caudron and colleagues.[40] Five of our cases showed strong EBV expression in the tumor cells, including a child with hydroa vacciniforme-like lymphoproliferative disorder and 2 adults, 1 of whom had an angiotropic lymphoma and another who developed nasopharynx involvement on follow-up. Similar cases overlapping with NK/T-cell lymphoma have been reported. Occasionally GDTCL can express 1 or more NK cell markers (CD16, CD56, CD57) and there is evidence that normal NK/T cells comprise subsets of $\gamma\delta$ T cells. Therefore, clinical and pathologic overlap with NK/T-cell lymphomas may be observed in exceptional cases.[29,32,34]

In our experience, the lack of CD5 expression is associated with the $\gamma\delta$ phenotype, but CD56 expression was often negative and hence not reliable to define $\gamma\delta$ T cells. Although CD4/CD8 double negative was the most common immunophenotype, we observed numerous CD8-positive and rare CD4-positive cases, as previously reported.[40,41] This immunophenotypic model may replicate the distribution of normal human $\gamma\delta$ T cells, which are mostly double negative, with fewer cells expressing CD8 and only rare cells expressing CD4.[42] We also noted a switch of phenotype from CD4 to CD8 at the time of tumor progression in 1 of our patients.

For the most part, all therapies have shown modest effectiveness. Neither radiation, nor immune therapy, nor multiagent chemotherapy has resulted in sustained remissions. Only 1 of 4 patients treated with myeloablative allogeneic hematopoietic stem cell transplantation (AHSCT) was alive with a partial remission at the end of the study. However, a case with complete remission for 23 months after AHSCT was recently reported.[43] Cytarabine combined with platinum-containing dose-intensive chemotherapy consolidated with AHSCT has been suggested as the best therapeutic option for eligible patients.[29]

T FOLLICULAR HELPER CELLS

The T follicular helper (Tfh) has been recently reported as a subset of CD4+ T cells that plays a role in B-cell recruitment and maturation. They participate in all stages of antigen-specific B-cell development. On first contact with antigen-primed B cells, pregerminal center effector Tfh cells promote B-cell clonal expansion, antibody isotype switch, plasma cell differentiation, and the induction of germinal centers.[44]

The expression signature of these cells consists of CXCR5, CXCL13, PD-1 (programmed cell death 1), BCL6, SAP (signaling lymphocytic activation molecule-associated protein), ICOS (inducible T-cell costimulator)[2,45] and CD200 (OX-2 membrane glycoprotein).[46] In addition, Tfh cells express markers such as CD25, CD57, CD69, and CD95.[45] Tfh cells are considered the cell origin

of angioimmunoblastic T-cell lymphoma (AITL) and probably other rare systemic peripheral T-cell lymphomas presenting with a follicular growth pattern. AITL comprises about 18% of all T-cell lymphomas and is characterized by constitutional symptoms, lymphadenopathy, arthritis, anemia, high sedimentation rate, polyclonal hypergammaglobulinemia, and autoimmune manifestations.[3] In addition, nearly 50% of the patients have ill-defined skin rashes.[47] These eruptions are characterized by the presence of scattered EBV-positive immunoblast large cells intermingled with medium-sized cells with abundant clear cytoplasm. The infiltrate is often perivascular and there is a subtle increase in vascularity with prominent endothelial cells and rarely focal evidence of vasculitis.[47] The infiltrate is predominantly T cells with many mixed reactive B cells. Tumor cells are CD3, CD2, CD5, and CD7 positive. The CD4/CD8 ratio is not high because of the presence of numerous reactive T cells. Coexpression of CD3 (cytoplasmic pattern) and bcl-6 (nuclear pattern) may help identify the Tfh population. CD10 is also positive but the presence of marked background staining makes it less reliable. Most cases reveal a T-cell clone and a few cases may also show a dual B-cell clone.

A subset of CTCLs may derive from cells with Tfh phenotype. These Tfh have been described in B-cell–rich T-cell lymphomas, for example primary cutaneous CD4+ small/medium-sized pleomorphic cutaneous T-cell lymphoma (PCSMTCL)[48] and AITL.[49] PCSMTCL is still considered a provisional entity in the latest WHO classification of lymphoid tumors and as previously mentioned,[3,5,24] is a controversial entity because most unilesional cases were reported until recently as pseudolymphomas. The atypical cells in this entity express follicular helper T-cell markers such as PD-1, CXCL13 (chemokine involved in germinal center organization), and BCL-6 (protein involved in B-cell proliferation). In addition, these CD4+ T cells are seen in association with B cells in a rosette or cluster arrangement. This phenomenon is also found in lymphocyte-predominant Hodgkin lymphoma.[48,50] PD-1 is a receptor expressed by follicular helper T cells known to be a negative regulator of immune responses and participating in peripheral tolerance. The expression of PD-1 by Tfh cells is well documented in reactive lymphoid tissue and AITL.[50] It is possible that B-cell stimulation could play an important role in CTCLs. For instance, the expression of CXCL13 in large CD4+ cells in PCSMTCL suggests that this chemokine might contribute to chemotaxis and recruitment of B cells to the skin and be an explanation for the rich B-cell infiltrate in these cases.[48,50] We have observed a few patients with d'emblée presentation of CTCL without patches or plaques and mostly presenting with tumoral lesions in intertriginous areas and also expressing a similar Tfh immunophenotype. These patients were characterized by an aggressive course and in our opinion may represent the rare cases reported as PCSMTCL with a poor outcome. Therefore, we believe that most unilesional tumors often presenting in the head and neck region and presently diagnosed as PCSMTCL represent an indolent clonal but benign expansion of Tfh cells, which do not deserve to be categorized as lymphomas. Other terminology like cutaneous lymphoid hyperplasia or lymphomatoid folliculitis could be more appropriate for such cases. However, patients presenting with multiple often intertriginous tumors with similar pathologic findings are a distinct condition that clearly deserves the lymphoma designation.

RARE VARIANTS OF CD30-POSITIVE LYMPHOPROLIFERATIVE DISORDERS

Primary cutaneous CD30+ lymphoproliferative disorders (CD30+ LPD) represent the second most common types of CTCL.[2,51] The spectrum ranges from lymphomatoid papulosis with chronic, self-healing, benign papulonodular and papulonecrotic lesions to more stable nodules or tumors with large-cell anaplastic or pleomorphic morphology (cutaneous anaplastic large-cell lymphoma [CALCL]). Both entities may have overlapping histopathologic characteristics and may be accompanied by varying numbers of inflammatory cells such as reactive T cells, histiocytes, neutrophils, or eosinophils.[2,52]

Neutrophil-rich or eosinophil-rich variants of CALCL have been described in the literature.[53–55] Clinically, this variant could be manifest as multiple erythematous nodules, brownish indurated plaques, exophytic masses, or keratoacanthoma-like lesions with or without ulceration.[56–58] This type of CALCL should be differentiated from various infectious and reactive conditions, especially from nonneoplastic cutaneous CD30+ infiltrates rich in neutrophils and eosinophils such as persistent arthropod bite reactions, nodular scabies, herpetic folliculitis, hidradenitis, and resolving furuncles and dermal abscesses. In neutrophil/eosinophil-rich CD30+ LPD, the inflammatory cells tend to be intermingled with the atypical large cells, whereas in nonneoplastic infiltrates, neutrophils and eosinophils tend to be more compartmentalized in different fields from the CD30+ cells. In addition, a more complex polymorphous background of reactive cells including plasma cells and reactive

small lymphocytes is present in these nonneoplasic processes.[57]

Simultaneous eosinophil-rich and neutrophil-rich variants of CD30+ LPD can occasionally be associated with prominent pseudoepitheliomatous hyperplasia (PEH), also known as pseudocarcinomatous hyperplasia, a reactive epithelial proliferation with tongue-like projections into the dermis, found in an extensive variety of neoplastic, infectious, and inflammatory conditions.[55,56,59] Some CD30+ LPD with PEH may have a folliculocentric pattern with direct connection of the proliferating epithelium with the pilosebaceous units. In our experience, CD30+ LPD with PEH tend to present with exophytic eroded nodules that may resemble a pyogenic granuloma or a squamous cell carcinoma and histologically they can also mimic a keratoacanthoma or an infiltrating squamous cell carcinoma.

The definition of CALCL is based on histologic, clinical, immunophenotypic, and molecular features. The aberrant expression of anaplastic large-cell lymphoma kinase (ALK) such as ALK-1 is often used with the purpose of excluding a cutaneous metastasis of a systemic ALCL because more than 80% of the systemic cases are positive.[60] The t(2;5) translocation results in a fusion protein of ALK, a tyrosine kinase and an activating promoter that leads to an abrupt proliferative response.[52] There is recent evidence for a rare association between ALK-positive primary cutaneous ALCL and insect bites in 5 cases. The patients developed persistent skin lesions after reported single or multiple arthropod bites accompanied by regional adenopathy. The investigators noted a delay in diagnosis because of misinterpretation of the findings as a cutaneous reaction to the arthropod bite. All cases had a small population of cells expressing nuclear and cytoplasmic ALK, and the morphology of these tumors was also unconventional, with 3 histiocyte-rich cases and 2 cases with a significant small-cell tumoral population. The typical benign course of cutaneous ALCL was not observed in these patients, and 2 of them died of tumor progression or infection. It is possible that the patients had an occult nodal lymphoma and the insect-bite–associated antigens could result in an influx of T lymphocytes, including some bearing the translocation t(2;5). The subsequent release of cytokines at the site of the bite could elicit activation of these cells with expression of the oncogenic NPM-ALK fusion protein and uncontrolled proliferation in the skin.[61]

Although most lymphomatoid papulosis cases are composed of CD4+ T cells, a new variant commonly seen in children is reported to be composed of CD8+ T cells and to present with a pagetoid pattern resembling primary cutaneous aggressive CD8+ epidermotropic T-cell lymphoma. In our opinion, these cases, which are usually seen in children and morphologically composed of medium-size cells with a low percentage of CD30-positive cells, may overlap with pityriasis lichenoides acuta. The term LyP type D has been proposed for this unusual variant.[62] We and others have also observed patients with the clinicopathologic pattern of LyP but predominantly composed of γδ T cells; perhaps such cases could be called type E.[52]

SUMMARY

Our understanding of cutaneous lymphomas continues to evolve. This progress is driven by advances in basic sciences, lymphomagenesis, pathology, hematology/oncology, and dermatology. As a result of the developing skin lymphoma database and astute clinical and pathologic observations, new layers of complexity are continually added to our collective past experiences. These advances continue to crystallize in new and more precise classifications of cutaneous lymphomas, detailed descriptions of new entities and lymphoma subsets and novel observations that will affect our goal of improving patient care with more accurate diagnosis and consequently more effective therapeutic approaches for our patients.

REFERENCES

1. Bradford PT, Devesa SS, Anderson WF, et al. Cutaneous lymphoma incidence patterns in the United States: a population-based study of 3884 cases. Blood 2009;113(21):5064–73.
2. Willemze R, Jaffe ES, Burg G, et al. WHO-EORTC classification for cutaneous lymphomas. Blood 2005;105(10):3768–85.
3. Campo E, Swerdlow SH, Harris NL, et al. The 2008 WHO classification of lymphoid neoplasms and beyond: evolving concepts and practical applications. Blood 2011;117(19):5019–32.
4. Leinweber B, Beltraminelli H, Kerl H, et al. Solitary small- to medium-sized pleomorphic T-cell nodules of undetermined significance: clinical, histopathological, immunohistochemical and molecular analysis of 26 cases. Dermatology 2009;219(1):42–7.
5. Cetinozman F, Jansen PM, Willemze R. Expression of programmed death-1 in primary cutaneous CD4-positive small/medium-sized pleomorphic T-cell lymphoma, cutaneous pseudo-T-cell lymphoma, and other types of cutaneous T-cell lymphoma. Am J Surg Pathol 2012;36(1):109–16.
6. Grange F, Beylot-Barry M, Courville P, et al. Primary cutaneous diffuse large B-cell lymphoma, leg type: clinicopathologic features and prognostic analysis in 60 cases. Arch Dermatol 2007;143(9):1144–50.
7. Espinet B, Garcia-Herrera A, Gallardo F, et al. FOXP1 molecular cytogenetics and protein expression analyses in primary cutaneous large B cell lymphoma, leg-type. Histol Histopathol 2011;26(2):213–21.
8. Lossos IS, Czerwinski DK, Alizadeh AA, et al. Prediction of survival in diffuse large-B-cell lymphoma based on the expression of six genes. N Engl J Med 2004;350(18):1828–37.
9. Kaune KM, Neumann C, Hallermann C, et al. Simultaneous aberrations of single CDKN2A network components and a high Rb phosphorylation status can differentiate subgroups of primary cutaneous B-cell lymphomas. Exp Dermatol 2011;20(4):331–5.
10. Guitart J, Magro C. Cutaneous T-cell lymphoid dyscrasia: a unifying term for idiopathic chronic dermatoses with persistent T-cell clones. Arch Dermatol 2007;143(7):921–32.
11. Magro CM, Schaefer JT, Morrison C, et al. Atypical lymphocytic lobular panniculitis: a clonal subcutaneous T-cell dyscrasia. J Cutan Pathol 2008;35(10):947–54.
12. Pincus LB, LeBoit PE, McCalmont TH, et al. Subcutaneous panniculitis-like T-cell lymphoma with overlapping clinicopathologic features of lupus erythematosus: coexistence of 2 entities? Am J Dermatopathol 2009;31(6):520–6.
13. Willemze R, Jansen PM, Cerroni L, et al. Subcutaneous panniculitis-like T-cell lymphoma: definition, classification, and prognostic factors: an EORTC Cutaneous Lymphoma Group Study of 83 cases. Blood 2008;111(2):838–45.
14. Yokota K, Akiyama Y, Adachi D, et al. Subcutaneous panniculitis-like T-cell lymphoma accompanied by Sjogren's syndrome. Scand J Rheumatol 2009;38(6):494–5.
15. Reimer P, Rudiger T, Muller J, et al. Subcutaneous panniculitis-like T-cell lymphoma during pregnancy with successful autologous stem cell transplantation. Ann Hematol 2003;82(5):305–9.
16. Marzano AV, Berti E, Paulli M, et al. Cytophagic histiocytic panniculitis and subcutaneous panniculitis-like T-cell lymphoma: report of 7 cases. Arch Dermatol 2000;136(7):889–96.
17. Shi Q, Zheng WJ, Li J, et al. Clinical analysis of subcutaneous panniculitis-like T cell lymphoma misdiagnosed as rheumatic diseases: 8 cases report. Zhonghua nei ke za zhi 2009;48(12):1019–22 [in Chinese].
18. Al Zolibani AA, Al Robaee AA, Qureshi MG, et al. Subcutaneous panniculitis-like T-cell lymphoma with hemophagocytic syndrome successfully treated with cyclosporin A. Skinmed 2006;5(4):195–7.

19. Clementi R, Locatelli F, Dupre L, et al. A proportion of patients with lymphoma may harbor mutations of the perforin gene. Blood 2005;105(11):4424–8.

20. Gau JP, Yang CF, Liu JH, et al. Subcutaneous panniculitis-like T cell lymphoma: familial aggregation while different response to chemotherapy. Int J Hematol 2009;89(1):63–5.

21. Lozzi GP, Massone C, Citarella L, et al. Rimming of adipocytes by neoplastic lymphocytes: a histopathologic feature not restricted to subcutaneous T-cell lymphoma. Am J Dermatopathol 2006;28(1):9–12.

22. Hoque SR, Child FJ, Whittaker SJ, et al. Subcutaneous panniculitis-like T-cell lymphoma: a clinicopathological, immunophenotypic and molecular analysis of six patients. Br J Dermatol 2003;148(3):516–25.

23. Kremer M, Ott G, Nathrath M, et al. Primary extramedullary plasmacytoma and multiple myeloma: phenotypic differences revealed by immunohistochemical analysis. J Pathol 2005;205(1):92–101.

24. Cerroni L, Gatter KC, Kerl H. Skin lymphoma the illustrated guide. 3rd edition. Oxford (United Kingdom): Wiley Blackwell; 2009.

25. Seegmiller AC, Xu Y, McKenna RW, et al. Immunophenotypic differentiation between neoplastic plasma cells in mature B-cell lymphoma vs plasma cell myeloma. Am J Clin Pathol 2007;127(2):176–81.

26. Meyerson HJ, Bailey J, Miedler J, et al. Marginal zone B cell lymphomas with extensive plasmacytic differentiation are neoplasms of precursor plasma cells. Cytometry Part B Clin Cytom 2011;80(2):71–82.

27. Burg G, Kempf W, Cozzio A, et al. WHO/EORTC classification of cutaneous lymphomas 2005: histological and molecular aspects. J Cutan Pathol 2005;32(10):647–74.

28. Roullet M, Gheith SM, Mauger J, et al. Percentage of {gamma}{delta} T cells in panniculitis by paraffin immunohistochemical analysis. Am J Clin Pathol 2009;131(6):820–6.

29. Tripodo C, Iannitto E, Florena AM, et al. Gamma-delta T-cell lymphomas. Nat Rev Clin Oncol 2009;6(12):707–17.

30. Kelsen J, Dige A, Schwindt H, et al. Infliximab induces clonal expansion of gammadelta-T cells in Crohn's disease: a predictor of lymphoma risk? PLoS One 2011;6(3):e17890.

31. Volk HD, Reinke P, Neuhaus K, et al. Expansion of a CD 3+4-8- TCR alpha/beta- T lymphocyte population in renal allograft recipients. Transplantation 1989;47(3):556–8.

32. Belhadj K, Reyes F, Farcet JP, et al. Hepatosplenic gammadelta T-cell lymphoma is a rare clinicopathologic entity with poor outcome: report on a series of 21 patients. Blood 2003;102(13):4261–9.

33. Koens L, Senff NJ, Vermeer MH, et al. Cutaneous gamma/delta T-cell lymphoma during treatment with etanercept for rheumatoid arthritis. Acta Derm Venereol 2009;89(6):653–4.

34. Arnulf B, Copie-Bergman C, Delfau-Larue MH, et al. Nonhepatosplenic gammadelta T-cell lymphoma: a subset of cytotoxic lymphomas with mucosal or skin localization. Blood 1998;91(5):1723–31.

35. Toro JR, Beaty M, Sorbara L, et al. gamma delta T-cell lymphoma of the skin: a clinical, microscopic, and molecular study. Arch Dermatol 2000;136(8):1024–32.

36. Massone C, Chott A, Metze D, et al. Subcutaneous, blastic natural killer (NK), NK/T-cell, and other cytotoxic lymphomas of the skin: a morphologic, immunophenotypic, and molecular study of 50 patients. Am J Surg Pathol 2004;28(6):719–35.

37. Hosler GA, Liegeois N, Anhalt GJ, et al. Transformation of cutaneous gamma/delta T-cell lymphoma following 15 years of indolent behavior. J Cutan Pathol 2008;35(11):1063–7.

38. Toro JR, Liewehr DJ, Pabby N, et al. Gamma-delta T-cell phenotype is associated with significantly decreased survival in cutaneous T-cell lymphoma. Blood 2003;101(9):3407–12.

39. Salhany KE, Macon WR, Choi JK, et al. Subcutaneous panniculitis-like T-cell lymphoma: clinicopathologic, immunophenotypic, and genotypic analysis of alpha/beta and gamma/delta subtypes. Am J Surg Pathol 1998;22(7):881–93.

40. Caudron A, Bouaziz JD, Battistella M, et al. Two atypical cases of cutaneous gamma/delta T-cell lymphomas. Dermatology 2011;222(4):297–303.

41. Saito T, Matsuno Y, Tanosaki R, et al. Gamma delta T-cell neoplasms: a clinicopathological study of 11 cases. Ann Oncol 2002;13(11):1792–8.

42. Groh V, Porcelli S, Fabbi M, et al. Human lymphocytes bearing T cell receptor gamma/delta are phenotypically diverse and evenly distributed throughout the lymphoid system. J Exp Med 1989;169(4):1277–94.

43. Koch R, Jaffe ES, Mensing C, et al. Cutaneous gamma/delta T-cell lymphoma. J Dtsch Dermatol Ges 2009;7(12):1065–7.

44. McHeyzer-Williams LJ, Pelletier N, Mark L, et al. Follicular helper T cells as cognate regulators of B cell immunity. Curr Opin Immunol 2009;21(3):266–73.

45. Laurent C, Fazilleau N, Brousset P. A novel subset of T-helper cells: follicular T-helper cells and their markers. Haematologica 2010;95(3):356–8.

46. Dorfman DM, Shahsafaei A. CD200 (OX-2 membrane glycoprotein) is expressed by follicular T helper cells and in angioimmunoblastic T-cell lymphoma. Am J Surg Pathol 2011;35(1):76–83.

47. Balaraman B, Conley JA, Sheinbein DM. Evaluation of cutaneous angioimmunoblastic T-cell lymphoma. J Am Acad Dermatol 2011;65(4):855–62.

48. Rodríguez Pinilla SM, Roncador G, Rodríguez-Peralto JL, et al. Primary cutaneous CD4+ small/medium-sized pleomorphic T-cell lymphoma expresses follicular T-cell markers. Am J Surg Pathol 2009;33(1):81–90.

49. Piccaluga PP, Agostinelli C, Califano A, et al. Gene expression analysis of angioimmunoblastic lymphoma indicates derivation from T follicular helper cells and vascular endothelial growth factor deregulation. Cancer Res 2007;67(22):10703–10.

50. Ferenczi K. Could follicular helper T-cells play a role in primary cutaneous CD4+ small/medium-sized pleomorphic T-cell lymphomas? J Cutan Pathol 2009;36(6):717–8.

51. Guitart J, Querfeld C. Cutaneous CD30 lymphoproliferative disorders and similar conditions: a clinical and pathologic prospective on a complex issue. Semin Diagn Pathol 2009;26(3):131–40.

52. Duvic M. CD30+ neoplasms of the skin. Curr Hematol Malig Rep 2011;6(4):245–50.

53. Kato N, Mizuno O, Ito K, et al. Neutrophil-rich anaplastic large cell lymphoma presenting in the skin. Am J Dermatopathol 2003;25(2):142–7.

54. Burg G, Kempf W, Kazakov DV, et al. Pyogenic lymphoma of the skin: a peculiar variant of primary cutaneous neutrophil-rich CD30+ anaplastic large-cell lymphoma. Clinicopathological study of four cases and review of the literature. Br J Dermatol 2003;148(3):580–6.

55. Bittencourt AL, Rothers S, Boente P, et al. Primary cutaneous eosinophil-rich anaplastic large cell lymphoma: report of an unusual case and literature review. J Cutan Med Surg 2008;12(2):88–92.

56. Lin JH, Lee JY. Primary cutaneous CD30 anaplastic large cell lymphoma with keratoacanthoma-like pseudocarcinomatous hyperplasia and marked eosinophilia and neutrophilia. J Cutan Pathol 2004;31(6):458–61.

57. Kong YY, Dai B, Kong JC, et al. Neutrophil/eosinophil-rich type of primary cutaneous anaplastic large cell lymphoma: a clinicopathological, immunophenotypic and molecular study of nine cases. Histopathology 2009;55(2):189–96.

58. Martín JM, Ricart JM, Monteagudo C, et al. Primary cutaneous CD30+ anaplastic large-cell lymphomas mimicking keratoacanthomas. Clin Exp Dermatol 2007;32(6):668–71.

59. El-Khoury J, Kibbi AG, Abbas O. Mucocutaneous pseudoepitheliomatous hyperplasia: a review. Am J Dermatopathol 2012;34(2):165–75.

60. Jaffe ES. Anaplastic large cell lymphoma: the shifting sands of diagnostic hematopathology. Mod Pathol 2001;14(3):219–28.

61. Lamant L, Pileri S, Sabattini E, et al. Cutaneous presentation of ALK-positive anaplastic large cell lymphoma following insect bites: evidence for an association in five cases. Haematologica 2010;95(3):449–55.

62. Saggini A, Gulia A, Argenyi Z, et al. A variant of lymphomatoid papulosis simulating primary cutaneous aggressive epidermotropic CD8+ cytotoxic T-cell lymphoma. Description of 9 cases. Am J Surg Pathol 2010;34(8):1168–75.

Direct Immunofluorescence Testing in the Diagnosis of Immunobullous Disease, Collagen Vascular Disease, and Vascular Injury Syndromes

Cynthia M. Magro[a], Jennifer Roberts-Barnes[b], A. Neil Crowson[b,c,d,e,*]

KEYWORDS

- Direct immunofluorescence • Immunobullous disease • Collagen vascular disease
- Vascular injury syndromes

KEY POINTS

- Direct immunofluorescence is a key adjunct in the investigation and diagnosis of a variety of dermatoses.
- In particular, the evaluation of immunobullous and connective tissue disease and vasculitis is often incomplete without direct immunofluorescence testing.
- Immunofluorescence using knockout models can be used to map antibody specificities in some immunobullous disorders.
- The incubation of patient serum with human umbilical cord endothelia in indirect immunofluorescence assays using a linking antibody has a role in predicting the severity of disease and the distribution of organ system involvement in certain systemic connective tissue disease states.

INTRODUCTION

The 2 principal techniques used in immunofluorescence (IF) testing are direct IF (DIF) and indirect IF (IIF). DIF testing uses fluorescein-conjugated antibodies monospecific for immunoglobulin (Ig) G, IgM, and IgA and complement fractions including C3, C3d, C4d, and C1q directly overlaid on frozen sections of patient tissue. IIF by definition uses a linking antibody, and that term should be used irrespective of the test substrate, be it patient lesional tissue or nonhuman esophagus, skin, or bladder. However, in common terminology, IIF refers to the application of patient serum in concert with fluorescein-conjugated anti-IgG and a mucosal substrate such as guinea pig or monkey esophagus or rat bladder. The 3 main disease categories in which DIF may be a critical diagnostic adjunct are vesiculobullous disorders, vasculitis, and autoimmune connective tissue disease (CTD) (**Box 1**). The light microscopy

[a] Department of Pathology and Laboratory Medicine, Weill Medical College of Cornell University, New York, NY 10065, USA; [b] Department of Dermatology, University of Oklahoma, St John Medical Center, Tulsa, OK 74114, USA; [c] Department of Pathology, University of Oklahoma, St John Medical Center, Tulsa, OK 74114, USA; [d] Department of Surgery, University of Oklahoma, St John Medical Center, Tulsa, OK 74114, USA; [e] Regional Medical Laboratory, University of Oklahoma, St John Medical Center, Tulsa, OK 74114, USA
* Corresponding author. Regional Medical Laboratory, St John Medical Center, 4142 S Mingo Road, Tulsa, OK 74146.
E-mail address: ncrowson@sjmc.org

Dermatol Clin 30 (2012) 763–798
http://dx.doi.org/10.1016/j.det.2012.06.008

Box 1
Disorders with a positive immunofluorescent profile

Autoimmune vesiculobullous disorders:

Antibodies directed to components of the epidermal basement membrane zone

Bullous and cicatricial pemphigoid

Herpes gestationis

P200 pemphigoid

Linear IgA disease

Bullous systemic lupus erythematosus

Epidermolysis bullosa acquisita

Antibodies to intercellular components of the epidermis

Pemphigus foliaceus

Pemphigus vulgaris

IgA pemphigus

Drug-induced pemphigus

Paraneoplastic pemphigus

Diseases associated with an immune complex–based pattern of IF

Dermatitis herpetiformis

IgA vasculitis

Mixed cryoglobulinemic vasculitis

Urticarial vasculitis

Lupus erythematosus (specifically in the context of the positive lupus band test)

Diseases associated with antibodies to endothelium with C5b-9 as the critical effector mechanism of vascular injury

Lupus erythematosus associated with anti-Ro antibodies

Dermatomyositis

Antiphospholipid antibody syndrome

Bullous disorders unrelated to an autoimmune-based cause

Porphyria

Pseudoporphyria

Bullosa diabeticorum

Collagen vascular disease

Lupus erythematosus

Mixed connective tissue disease

Dermatomyositis

Sclerodermatomyositis

Vasculopathic disorders with distinctive immunofluorescent profiles

IgA vasculitis/Henoch-Schönlein purpura

Mixed cryoglobulinemic vasculitis

Antineutrophil cytoplasmic antibody–positive vasculitic syndromes

Hypocomplementemic urticarial vasculitis

Antiphospholipid antibody syndrome

of several other non–immune-based disorders can mimic certain of the conditions mentioned earlier, but most of these non–immune-based blistering diseases have nonspecific or negative DIF and IIF profiles (**Table 1**). This article focuses on the various conditions associated with diagnostic IF profiles and their pathophysiologic basis. The dominant focus is on the immunobullous diseases, bullous pemphigoid (BP), epidermolysis bullosa acquisita (EBA), cicatricial pemphigoid, P200 pemphigoid, linear IgA disease, dermatitis herpetiformis (DH), and bullous systemic lupus erythematosus (SLE). In addition, IF application in the evaluation of CTDs including lupus erythematosus, mixed connective tissue disease (MCTD), dermatomyositis (DM), and sclerodermatomyositis is discussed. Its value in the approach to cutaneous vasculitis is considered. The use of the antiendothelial cell antibody assay is also discussed, which may be used in concert with routine microscopy and DIF in evaluating for certain CTDs associated with microvascular injury, as exemplified by DM and MCTD. Immunofluorescent studies have also been used to elucidate the presence or absence of certain basement membrane zone (BMZ) components in geno dermatoses such as congenital epidermolysis bullosa and Alport syndrome. Consideration is also given to nondiagnostic DIF profiles that may be encountered in skin biopsy material.

AUTOIMMUNE CONDITIONS ASSOCIATED WITH ANTIBODIES TO COMPONENTS OF THE BMZ
Normal Constituents of the BMZ

The BMZ contains antigens that are the targets of antibodies in autoimmune bullous disorders (**Table 2**).[1] The uppermost zone is the dermal pole of the basal cell plasma membrane, which contains hemidesmosomes that in turn have an intracellular and extracellular portion.[1] The BMZ proper comprises the lamina lucida or lamina rara, which is traversed by anchoring filaments. The lamina densa surmounts the fibrous network of the sub-BMZ proper; this sub-basal lamina fibrillar network contains anchoring fibrils that are contiguous with the lamina densa and insert in the dermis.[1]

BP antigens

There are 2 BP antigens. One has an intracellular location and is associated with hemidesmosomes; it is designated BP Ag1 (230 kDa). Analysis of its amino acid sequence has revealed that it belongs to the same protein family as the desmosomal plaque protein desmoplakin; this homology accounts for the only known molecular relationship between hemidesmosomes and desmosomes. The genes that encode BPAg1 and desmoplakin are located on chromosome 6. The C-terminal domains are responsible for binding the cytokeratin filaments and are likely the major antigenic epitope. This protein is of major importance for tonofilament binding.

The other BP antigen has both intracellular and extracellular components and is designated BPAg2 (180 kDa). The gene that encodes this antigen is found on chromosome 10q. It is a transmembrane protein with an extracellular C terminus. Although the intracellular portion is basic and is part of the hemidesmosomal plaque, the longer extracellular portion contains collagenlike domains.

Table 1
Disorders in which the immunofluorescent profile is negative or nonspecific

Disorder with Negative/Nonspecific IF	Differential Excluded by Virtue of Negative IF
Subcorneal pustulosis	IgA pemphigus
Hailey-Hailey disease	Pemphigus
Bullous impetigo	Pemphigus
Darier disease	Pemphigus
Grover disease	Pemphigus
Acantholytic pityriasis rubra pilaris	Pemphigus
Bullous insect bite reaction	Bullous pemphigoid
Bullous drug reaction	Bullous pemphigoid
Lichen planopilaris	Discoid lupus erythematosus
Drug-induced lichenoid photodermatitis	Subacute cutaneous lupus erythematosus
Non–IgA-associated vasculitis	IgA vasculitis/Henoch-Schönlein purpura

Table 2
Basement membrane constituents identified in the dermoepidermal junction and their ultrastructural locations

Component	Location in DEJ
Type IV collagen	Lamina densa
Laminin	Lamina lucida
Heparan sulfate proteoglycan	In clusters on either side of the lamina densa
BP antigen	Basal cell plasma membrane
EBA antigen	Lamina densa-sublamina densa

Because it has intracellular protein features but also manifests collagen components, it is designated as collagen XVII. The extramembranous domain NC16a is the dominant antigenic epitope site for BP and herpes gestationis. The BP180 ectodomain exhibits an extended conformation spanning the lamina lucida and projecting into the lamina densa. The terminal portion of the BP180 ectodomain is in close apposition to the lamina densa and is the autoreactive site for cicatricial pemphigoid.[1]

Antibodies to BPAg1 and BPAg2 are involved in the pathogenesis of BP, with 70% of patients manifesting circulating antibodies against BP230 and 55% having antibodies to BP180. The serum level of anti-BPAg1 autoantibodies inversely correlates with prognosis.[2,3] For BP and herpes gestationis, IgG4 is the predominant IgG anti-BPAg2 subclass.[4] Patients with BP have IgG anti-BP180, which reduces hemidesmosomal BP180, weakening hemidesmosomal attachment to the lamina densa. BP180 immune complex formation induces inflammation and may damage the lamina lucida and explain the BP split at the level of the lamina lucida.[5] High titers of both IgG and IgE anti-NC16a in patients' sera indicate a more severe disease course. Enzyme-linked immunosorbent assay (ELISA) for both IgG and IgE anti-NC16a compared with IgG alone gives better diagnostic and prognostic information.[6,7] High titer of BP180 antibodies correlates with high risk of relapse after cessation of therapy in patients with BP.[3]

Deficiency of BPAg2 and a reduced amount of the corresponding messenger RNA has recently been implicated in generalized atrophic benign epidermolysis bullosa, a form of nonlethal junctional epidermolysis bullosa clinically characterized by generalized blistering after birth, atrophic healing, and alopecia with onset in childhood.[8]

Laminin 5

Laminin 5 is localized in the lamina lucida where it may contribute to the formation of anchoring filaments. It is a high-molecular-weight glycoprotein complex of epithelial basement membranes that is identical to the autoantigen epiligrin and has also been referred to as BM 600, nicein, and kalinin. Autoantibodies directed against laminin 5 are relevant for a certain subtypes of cicatricial pemphigoid referred to as antiepiligrin cicatricial pemphigoid. Mutations in the laminin 5 chain can also be observed in certain forms of junctional epidermolysis bullosa.[1]

Uncein

Uncein is an anchoring filament component that consists of 3 polypeptide chains (100, 135, and 165 kDa) and is related to, but distinct from, laminin 5.

Antibodies to uncein have recently been described in a disease that has overlap features of cicatricial pemphigoid and EBA.[9]

Ladinin

A component of anchoring filaments, ladinin (LAD-1), with a molecular weight of 97 kDa, is a novel secretory protein that has basic properties as a result of enrichment of the N-terminal end with basic amino acids. Immunoelectron microscopy localizes ladinin to the lamina lucida beneath the hemidesmosomes. Ladinin seems to be the autoantigen in most cases of linear IgA disease and in chronic bullous disease of childhood.[1]

EBA antigen

Localized within and subjacent to the lamina densa, the EBA antigen constitutes a fibronectin heterodimer that represents the noncollagenous domain of type VII collagen (145 kDa and 290 kDa). The antibody in bullous SLE manifests similar antigen specificity. Mainly synthesized and secreted by keratinocytes, type VII collagen is found in basement membranes beneath the stratified squamous epithelia of the skin, lip, buccal mucosa, upper esophagus, trachea, vagina, and amnion of mammals; it is not found in birds, reptiles, or fish. It is the constituent molecule of the anchoring fibrils that attach the basement membrane to the underlying dermis.[1]

Salt-Split Skin Assay

Incubating normal skin with a 1-M solution of sodium chloride separates the epidermis from the dermis, whereby the upper lamina lucida and the hemidesmosomes including the BP antigens remain adherent to the epidermis. The other BMZ components, including lower lamina lucida antigenic components such as laminin 5, the lamina densa, and anchoring fibrils, remain with the dermal side after separation.[10–12] This technique enables more precise localization of immunoreactants relative to the lamina lucida, increasing the specificity of DIF. There are certain distinctive vesiculobullous disorders showing localization of immune reactants to the roof of the saline-induced split, namely BP, herpes gestationis, cicatricial pemphigoid (excluding the antiepiligrin variant), and certain cases of linear IgA disease in which the antigenic specificity is to BP antigens. Those diseases showing floor localization include P200 pemphigoid, antiepiligrin pemphigoid, EBA, bullous SLE, and a subset of patients with linear IgA disease.

BP

BP occurs most commonly in the elderly and is associated with intense pruritus, blisters, and frequent truncal localization. Exogenous triggers such as drug therapy or trauma are implicated in some cases.[13,14] BP is attributable to antibodies to BPAg1 or BPAg2, those components of the BMZ that localize above the salt-split skin zone. BPAg2 is a transmembrane protein, although the antigenic target eliciting BP is the extracellular noncollagenous zone. The less common antigenic epitope, BPAg1, localizes to the hemidesmosomes.

Light microscopy

The biopsy shows an eosinophil-rich subepidermal blistering dermatosis. Early phases of the disease may manifest an eosinophilic interface dermatitis with incipient or no cleft formation or, in some cases, urticarial changes (**Fig. 1A, B**). An elderly individual presenting with an intensely pruritic eruption may represent a prebullous lesion of BP.

DIF

The DIF profile shows a homogeneous linear staining of IgG along the dermal-epidermal junction (DEJ) (see **Fig. 1C**). The main immunoglobulin implicated is IgG4.

Salt-split skin

Because of the proximal localization of the BP antigens, the salt-split skin assay shows a dominant localization within the roof of the saline-induced split (see **Fig. 1D**).

Herpes Gestationis

Herpes gestationis is a distinctive blistering dermatosis related to pregnancy, appearing most commonly in the second and third trimester of pregnancy and rarely in the postpartum period. The eruption ranges from an urticarial process to one associated with blister formation (**Fig. 2A**).

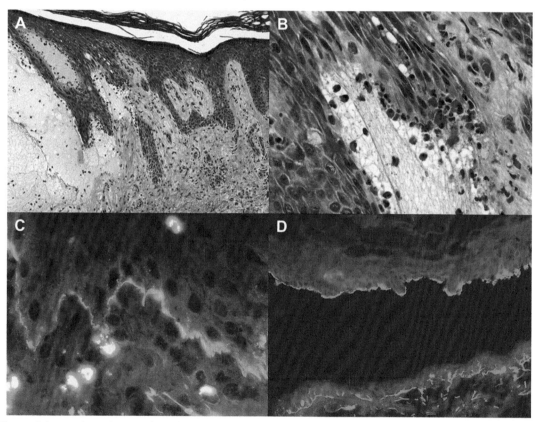

Fig. 1. (*A*) In a classic lesion of BP there is prominent tissue eosinophilia with eosinophils tagging along the dermal-epidermal junction and variable papillary dermal edema with subepidermal blister(s). (*B*) Higher power magnification shows an eosinophilic interface dermatitis. The autoimmune vesiculobullous disorders often manifest a granulocytic interface dermatitis predominated by specific leukocyte subsets such as eosinophils in the setting of pemphigoid or neutrophils in cases of linear IgA disease and DH. (*C*) DIF studies show thin homogeneous linear deposition of IgG along the dermal-epidermal junction (DEJ). Other immunoglobulins of lesser intensity may be observed. There is typically concomitant C3 showing a similar localization pattern. (*D*) The salt-split skin assay shows localization of immunoreactivity to the roof of the saline-induced split.

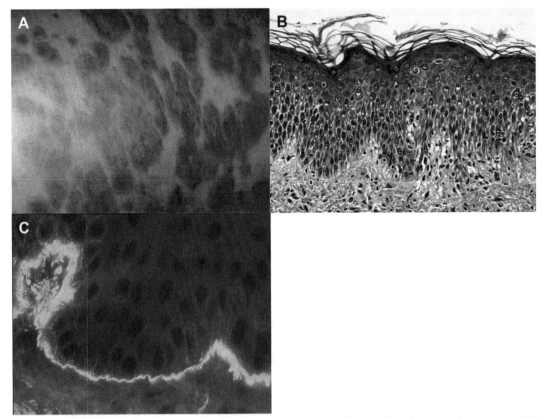

Fig. 2. (*A*) In herpes gestationis, blisters are uncommon. An urticaria-like reaction is more often observed. (*B*) Analogous to the clinical presentation, seeing a bulla on biopsy is not common. Classic light microscopic features include focal eosinophilic interface dermatitis with basilar vacuolar change and dyskeratosis, often accentuated in the suprapapillary plates. (*C*) Direct immunofluorescent studies characteristically show homogeneous linear C3 within the epidermal BMZ in the absence of IgG.

The antibody specificity is to the noncollagenous domain of BPAg2. This antigenic epitope is also found in the placental BMZ; initially antibodies are formed against the placental BMZ and may induce placental insufficiency.

Light microscopy
The papillary dermis is edematous with eosinophil tagging along the DEJ. Dyskeratotic cells predominantly in the basal layer of the epidermis are characteristic and eosinophilic spongiosis may be seen. Frank subepidermal bulla formation is unusual (see **Fig. 2**B).

DIF
C3 is typically observed along the DEJ in the absence of IgG (see **Fig.** 2C). Often accompanying C3 staining is C1q, C4, C5, factor B, and properdin.

IIF
Routine IIF studies are negative. However, complement fixation studies are positive for IgG in the presence of indirect complement-added IF.[15] A complement-binding factor, historically known as herpes gestationis (HG) factor, is often found in patients with HG. This BMZ antibody activates the complement pathway in vivo.

Salt-split skin
In salt-split skin specimens, IgG antibody deposition is observed along the epidermal roof and may persist for up to a year after lesions have cleared. There are cases in which IgG1 and C3 have also been detected in the BMZ.[16]

Anti-p200 Pemphigoid

Anti-P200 pemphigoid is an autoimmune vesiculobullous disorder characterized by a lack of mucosal involvement and the presence of non-scarring urticarial plaques.[17] The implicated antibody in anti-P200 pemphigoid is directed against a noncollagenous glycoprotein in the lower portion of the lamina lucida. The clinical presentation can be heterogeneous, combining cases resembling

BP, DH and/or linear IgA disease. However, the most common presentation is in the context of lesions resembling those of BP. Half of the cases of anti-P200 pemphigoid occur in patients with psoriasis.[18]

The P200 antigen represents laminin $\chi 1$ with localization to dermal extracts. Laminin $\chi 1$ is a 200-kDa end-linked glycoprotein that is part of the cutaneous BMZ and is different from the other laminin heterotrimers contributing to epidermal-dermal adhesion outside the hemidesmosome complex.[19,20] Knockout mice that do not have the laminin $\chi 1$ gene exhibit embryonic demise at day 5 because of the inability to form BMZ in various organ systems.[21]

Light microscopy

Neutrophils are characteristic, reflecting the elaboration of interleukin-8 by keratinocytes stimulated by the anti-P200 antigen-antibody interaction.[22] A rare morphologic expression is similar to that noted in other forms of cicatricial pemphigoid; namely, lymphocytes and plasma cells in the absence of granulocytes. In 1 review, discernible dermal fibrosis was present in only 5 of 15 specimens.

DIF

There is localization of type IV collagen to the floor of the blister, immunoglobulin deposition within the floor of the saline-induced split, and the continued seroreactivity to generic skin devoid in the expression of type VII collagen.[23,24]

Cicatricial Pemphigoid

Cicatricial pemphigoid (CP) is a chronic blistering disease of the elderly involving mainly the oral and ocular mucous membranes, although any mucosal surface can be involved, including those of the nasopharynx, esophagus, larynx, and genitalia (**Fig. 3**A).[25] In the variant of CP called Brunsting-Perry, the scarring blisters occur on the head and neck area; mucosal involvement is rare.[26] Concomitant generalized cutaneous bullous eruptions have been reported in 20% to 33% of patients with CP.

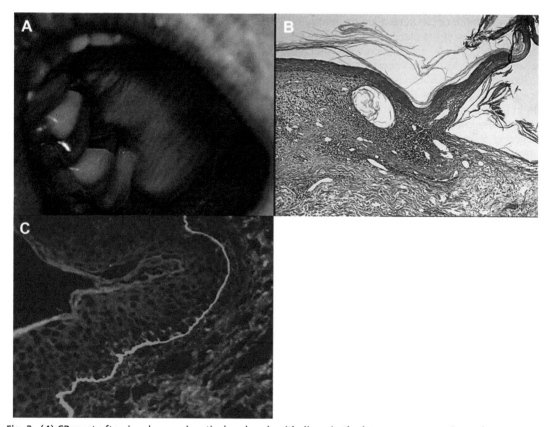

Fig. 3. (A) CP most often involves conjunctival and oral epithelium, in the latter case generating a desquamative gingivitis potentially associated with tooth loss. (B) The histopathology comprises fibrosis with a lymphocytic infiltrate as opposed to what is seen in CP. This photomicrograph shows milia with fibrosis and a patchy lymphocytic infiltrate, a constellation of findings characteristic of cicatricial pemphigoid. (C) DIF of perilesional epithelium in CP shows linear deposits of IgG and complement along the BMZ.

The recently described antiepiligrin variant of CP has been seen in association with malignancy including endometrial, lung, and gastric carcinoma, suggesting that this variant of CP may be a form of paraneoplastic blistering disease.[27–29]

Light microscopy

The light microscopic picture comprises subepithelial blistering with a lymphocytic infiltrate and fibrosis, but a variable infiltrate of neutrophils, eosinophils, and plasma cells can be seen (see **Fig. 3B**).

DIF

Although DIF of perilesional epithelium shows linear deposits of IgG and complement along the BMZ (see **Fig. 3C**), there is a higher incidence of false-negative IF results in CP because of technical problems; if the biopsy is performed on perilesional mucosa, the epithelium may peel off and make interpretation difficult.

Immunoelectron microscopy

In vivo deposits of IgG in fresh nonbullous perilesional skin of patients with noncicatricial BP are located within the upper lamina lucida, mainly on the outer surface of the plasma membrane of the basal keratinocytes in association with hemidesmosomes. This distribution corresponds with the location of the noncollagenous NC16a domain extracellular epitope of BPAg2. In contrast with BP, in patients with CP, the localization of IgG is mainly in the lower lamina lucida associated with anchoring filaments, defining the lamina lucida/lamina densa interface.[30]

IIF

Up to 70% of patients with classic nonscarring BP have circulating antibodies to BMZ material. In contrast, the incidence of circulating antibodies is low in patients with CP. It is suggested that circulating antibodies of IgG and IgA subtype are associated with a more severe course.[31,32] In one study by IIF of salt-split human skin, IgG and IgA of sera reacted with the epidermal side of the split and only rarely with the dermal side. By immunoblotting of epidermal extracts, IgG of sera reacted with BPAg1 and either the carboxy terminus or NC16a domain of BPAg2. The cases that showed dermal reactivity had antibody specificity to epiligrin.

Pathogenesis

Antibodies in most patients with CP recognize an epitope on the BP 180-kDa antigen, which is different from that recognized by patients with HG and BP. The immunolocalization pattern of BP and HG sera is primarily to the upper lamina lucida

region and correlates with the noncollagenous NC16a domain of BP180 immediately subjacent to the hemidesomsome.[33–35] Most CP sera exhibit a lower lamina lucida labeling pattern analogous to the BP180 carboxyl terminal region, associated with anchoring filaments; the antigenic epitope comprises interrupted collagen domains. Nevertheless, the salt-split skin studies show localization of immunoreactivity to the roof of the saline-induced split. A group of patients with classic nonscarring BP recently manifested autoimmunity to the carboxyl terminal region of the BP 180-kDa antigen. Fewer patients with CP have antibodies to the intracellular BPAg1 and to the NC16a domain of BPAg1, hence provoking symptoms indistinguishable from classic nonscarring BP.[36]

A form of severe CP associated with malignancy is anti–laminin 5 pemphigoid.[33–35,37–39] Laminin 5 is known by various terms including laminin 332, epiligrin, calanin, kalinin, and nicien.[33,34] The molecular composition of laminin 5 comprises a heterodimer defined by 3 distinct chains designated $\alpha3$, $\beta3$, and $\Omega2$.[32,40] Most patients who have this form of CP have antibodies against the $\alpha3$ subunit.[36] There are specific criteria for rendering a diagnosis of anti–laminin 5 pemphigoid, including the presence of a subepidermal blister as revealed by routine light microscopy, linear deposits of IgG showing dermal localization within the epidermal BMZ, circulating IgG antibodies reacting with the dermal side of a saline-induced split in skin devoid of collagen VII, and circulating IgG antibodies to laminin 5 detected by immunoblotting or immunoprecipitation.[33,34,41] Nonetheless, these features are not unique to antiepiligrin pemphigoid and can be shared by anti-P200 pemphigoid, at least with respect to the light microscopic and IF profile.[41] The association of antiepiligrin pemphigoid with underlying malignancy may be related to the expression of laminin 5 by certain types of malignancy.[32,42,43] High mortality reflects the underlying cancer and immunosuppressive sequelae of drug therapy. Similar to other forms of CP, the main mucosal sites involved in antiepiligrin pemphigoid are mouth and eye, whereas other mucosal sites can include the nose, larynx, and anogenital regions. Relative to other forms of CP, nasal and laryngeal involvement occur more frequently. Although skin involvement is common, the mucosal disease is the most prominent aspect of the clinical presentation in most cases.

A variant of acquired junctional epidermolysis bullosa associated with IgG autoantibodies to the subunit of laminin 5 has been described. Such cases are impossible to distinguish from antiepiligrin CP, but have a higher incidence of skin involvement. By Western blot, the antibody specificity is to the β subunit of laminin 5 rather than the α subunit. The phenotype is of blisters on normal-appearing skin all over the body with accentuation at sites exposed to trauma such as the elbows and the back of the hands. Erosions can be observed in the conjunctiva, mouth, and larynx. The lesions heal with formation of atrophic scars and milia. There are no mutilating deformities.

Regarding the pathophysiology of the fibrosis in CP, fibrogenic cytokines in the conjunctiva of patients with acute ocular CP have been shown via in situ hybridization. Acute disease showed increased levels of mRNA for transforming growth factor β (TGF-β) 1 and 3, mainly in stromal fibro-blasts and macrophages. In the stroma, there were concordant increases in latent and activated TGF-β1 and TGF-β3 and TGF-β receptor expression by fibroblasts. No cytokines or receptors are significantly increased in chronic disease, indicating that the fibroblasts in ocular CP conjunctiva may remain functionally and morphologically abnormal after the withdrawal of cytokine influences.[44]

Antibodies specific to the β-4 component of the α 6 β 4 integrin have been primarily implicated in oral CP whereas antibodies to the α 6 component of the α 6 β 4 integrin are thought to be pathogenetically important in ocular CP. In addition, a minority of patients with oral CP have antibody specificity to a 168-kDa mucosal antigen, which is different from laminin 5 subunits and shares no epitopes with BPAg1, BPAg2, or the EBA antigen.[10,45–47]

Differential diagnosis of CP

Scarring of the conjunctiva is not unique to CP, occurring in patients with EBA, and a syndrome indistinguishable from CP may occur in 10% to 15% of patients with linear IgA dermatosis.[48] Trauma, especially from alkali burns such as those incurred with exploding airbags and past episodes of erythema multiforme, Stevens Johnson syndrome, or toxic epidermal necrolysis can be associated with conjunctival scarring. The application of ocular agents can be associated with scar formation that is indistinguishable pathologically and clinically from CP. The term drug-induced cicatricial conjunctivitis is used for this severe scarring conjunctival process; patients have auto-antibodies to components of the BMZ like those seen in CP. Glaucoma agents such as pilocarpine and epinephrine are most frequently implicated.[49]

EBA

Although patients with classic EBA typically develop disease in the fourth to sixth decades of life, EBA is described in children as young as 1 year of age. The criteria for diagnosis of EBA are (1) adult onset and a negative family history for epidermolysis bullosa, (2) spontaneous or trauma-induced blisters resembling those of familial dystrophic epidermolysis bullosa, and (3) the exclusion of other blistering diseases.

The classic expression is of a mechanobullous eruption with erosions on a noninflamed base that heal with scarring and milia formation. Scarring alopecia and nail dystrophy can be seen. All patients have skin fragility such that minor trauma induces a blister or erosion. There are 2 other distinctive variants, one resembling BP and another that resembles CP. The latter patients manifest extensive involvement of mucous membranes and can have chronic blisters and erosions in the mouth, upper esophagus, anus, and vagina.

Antiepiligrin CP may be difficult to separate from the mucosal dominant phenotype of EBA. Both exhibit localization of immunoreactivity to the floor of salt-split skin; however, immunogold electron microscopy reveals labeling beneath the lamina densa in EBA versus within the lamina densa and lower portion of the lamina lucida in antiepiligrin CP. Western blotting reveals antibodies directed against 2 discrete proteins weighing 290 kDa and 145 kDa, both directed against type VII collagen in patients with EBA.[38]

There are various diseases associated with EBA, including inflammatory bowel disease (especially Crohn disease), SLE, thyroiditis, amyloidosis, diabetes mellitus, lymphoma, multiple myeloma, hypothyroidism, multiple endocrinopathy syndromes, and autoimmune thrombocytopenia. Patients have a high incidence of HLA type DR2, similar to bullous SLE. EBA is a chronic disease process that rarely remits. Inflammatory EBA seems to be more amenable to treatment with prednisone.

Light microscopy

Biopsies reveal a sparse inflammatory infiltrate in classic noninflammatory EBA (**Fig. 4**A) and, because of the activation of complement, numerous neutrophils in the inflammatory variant.

IIF

Up to 50% of patients with EBA have positive IIF. The circulating IgG autoantibodies are directed against multiple epitopes located in the noncollagenous NC1 domain of collagen VII.

DIF

EBA belongs to the group of disorders that produce a fine, sharp, linear band of deposition of immunoreactants along the DEJ (see **Fig. 4**B). Understanding its pathophysiologic basis, it is possible to differentiate EBA from other subepidermal bullous diseases by sophisticated techniques

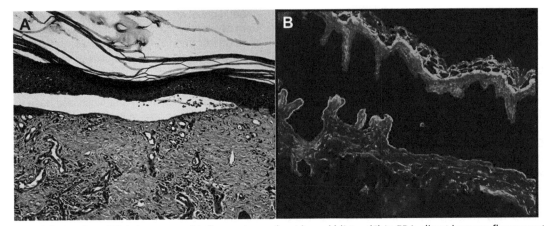

Fig. 4. (*A*) Biopsies of EBA show a pauci-inflammatory subepidermal blister. (*B*) In EBA, direct immunofluorescent studies show homogeneous linear staining along the DEJ. Salt-split skin studies show localization to the floor of the saline-induced split.

such as immunoelectron microscopy, salt-split skin antigen mapping, fluorescence overlay antigen mapping, immunoblot, and ELISA. In studying the DIF patterns in 157 patients with various subepidermal immunobullous diseases, Vodegel and colleagues[50] found 3 distinct linear DIF patterns along the BMZ that they designated as true linear pattern, n-serrated pattern, and u-serrated pattern. The true linear pattern, often seen in conjunction with either the n-serrated or the u-serrated pattern, was found in subepidermal immunobullous disease with linear DIF patterns. In BP, cicatricial pemphigoid, antiepiligrin CP, p200 pemphigoid, and linear IgA disease, the n-serrated pattern was typical (**Fig. 5**). They contend that this pattern correlated with deposition of immunoglobulin in hemidesmosomes, lamina lucida, or lamina densa. However, in EBA and bullous SLE, the u-serrated staining pattern was seen, corresponding with the ultralocalization of type VII collagen in the sublamina densa zone. The investigators confirmed their

findings with immunoelectron microscopy, salt-split skin antigen mapping, fluorescence overlay antigen mapping, or immunoblotting. In our experience, the u-serrated versus n-serrated pattern is difficult to appreciate.

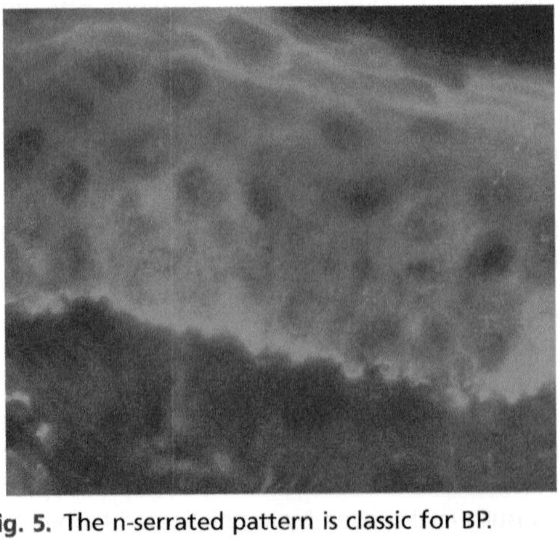

Linear IgA Disease

The eruption in classic linear IgA disease (LAD) (**Fig. 6**A) comprises vesiculobullous skin lesions involving the trunk, inner thigh, and pelvic region that respond to dapsone and may resemble DH and/or BP but never manifest the symmetric distribution of DH. Pruritus is not a consistent finding as it is in DH. Spontaneous resolution occurs in 10% to 33% of cases. There is no well-documented association with gluten-sensitive enteropathy.[48] Mucosal involvement, seen in up to 50% of cases, is usually without scarring, although some cases manifest scarring of the oral, conjunctival, and genital mucosa that resembles CP. In this cicatricial phenotype of LAD, if the antibody specificity is to type VII collagen, some investigators use the designation CP phenotype of IgA EBA.[51,52] A variant of LAD resembling classic cutaneous EBA has also been described, although some children with an otherwise typical LAD clinical phenotype manifest antibody to type VII collagen, which may reflect a poorly recognized form of EBA.[53–55] The diversity of clinical presentation and lack of consensus in eponymy reflects the broad spectrum of implicated BMZ-associated antigens.

There may be a slightly increased risk of malignancy associated with LAD, specifically in regards to lymphoproliferative disease.[48] In a series from the United Kingdom, 7% of patients with LAD had ulcerative colitis, versus a rate of ulcerative colitis in the United Kingdom of 0.05%; abnormal mucosal B cells and IgA1 production are implicated.[56,57]

Fig. 5. The n-serrated pattern is classic for BP.

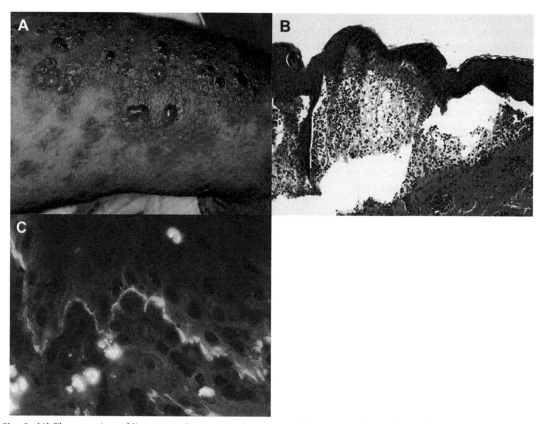

Fig. 6. (*A*) The eruption of linear IgA disease may have a serpiginous annular quality with superimposed vesicles and small bullae likened to a string of pearls. (*B*) The classic light microscopic findings are a subepidermal blistering dermatosis rich in neutrophils. Other neutrophil-rich subepidermal bullous diseases include P200 pemphigoid and bullous SLE. (*C*) Direct immunofluorescent studies show homogeneous linear deposits of IgA along the DEJ. Deposits of other immunoglobulins can be observed but are of lesser intensity.

LAD has been associated with drugs including vancomycin, penicillin, lithium, phenytoin, and diclophenac.[14,58–61] In drug-associated LAD, lesions clear with drug cessation, whereas rechallenge may result in a more severe eruption with a shorter latency period between drug intake and lesional onset.[56,58,60,61] Drug-induced linear IgA lesions range from extreme reactions that, with a single dose, resemble toxic epidermal necrolysis, to few lesions with multiple supratherapeutic doses; the extent and severity of disease is typically not dose dependent.[62]

Chronic bullous disease of childhood closely resembles adult-associated LAD with respect to clinical features, light microscopic findings, and immunopathogenesis; an association with concurrent mucosal infection may exist in some cases.[63]

IgA deposits have a variable location, being found within the lamina lucida, within the hemidesmosomal plaques and adjacent lamina lucida, below the lamina densa, or on both sides of the lamina densa.[64] IgA autoantibodies specifically target the 120-kDa antigen (LAD-1) and 97-kDa antigen

(LABD97) in the ectodomain of collagen XVII.[65,66] A 97-kDa/120-kDa antigen obtained from epidermal extracts and a 285-kDa dermal antigen are the target antigens in linear IgA disease.[67,68] The former is associated with an antibody whose specificity is directed toward anchoring filament protein and is designated as LAD-1. It is synthesized and secreted by epidermal keratinocytes.[69] There seems to be colocalization of LAD-1 and the extracellular portion of BPAg2 in the lamina lucida, possibly forming a complex with the extracellular domain of BPAg2.[70–72] The 285-kDa antigen represents the NC1 domain of collagen type VII, the classic epitope for EBA.[67] IgA antibodies have recently been described, directed to the carboxyl terminus of BPAg2 identical to that seen in IgG-mediated CP, in patients who present with a phenotype indistinguishable from CP. Antibodies to BPAg1 have been identified in a few patients with linear IgA disease. Antibody specificity via an immunoblotting technique to type VII collagen, the LAD-1 antigen, and BPAg1, have recently been shown in cases of drug-associated linear IgA disease, indicating a common pathogenetic basis with idiopathic linear IgA disease.[59] Between 10% and 30% of patients with linear IgA disease have circulating antibodies of IgA type to various components of the BMZ.

Light microscopy

Biopsies show a neutrophil-rich interface dermatitis (see **Fig. 6B**) with effacement of the epidermal architecture and variable tissue eosinophilia. Neutrophils bear IgA receptors; once IgA is bound to specific antigenic components of the BMZ, hemidesmosomes could function as ligands for neutrophil adherence and activation.

DIF

A homogeneous, sharp, thin linear band of staining for IgA is seen along the DEJ (see **Fig. 6C**) in a pattern identical to that observed with EBA and BP. Other immunoglobulins may be seen, such as IgM and IgG, but the intensity of staining is less. The nosology of cases showing linear granular deposits along the DEJ without deposition within the dermal papillae is unclear[48]; the designation linear–granular linear IgA disease has been applied. This variant resembles DH clinically with respect to lesional distribution and morphology and to the high incidence of positive potassium iodide patch testing; however, the incidence of HLA-B8 positivity and gluten-sensitive enteropathy is similar to that of the homogeneous linear subtype of linear IgA disease, being significantly less than is observed with DH.

DH

DH manifests as a symmetric grouped vesicular eruption involving the extensor surfaces of the elbows and knees, posterior scalp, and the buttock area, whereas LAD has a more polymorphic presentation and a more widespread distribution; mucosal involvement may occur in either. Although patients with LAD lack villous atrophy on small bowel biopsy, even in those DH case without symptoms, at least 80% have an abnormal jejunal biopsy with epitheliotropic lymphocytes, degenerative epithelial alterations, and incipient crypt hyperplastic villous atrophy. Other differences include a high incidence of HLAB8, DR3, and Cw7; hypochlorhydria with gastric atrophy; a high incidence of thyroid abnormalities including hyperthyroidism, hypothyroidism, thyroid nodules, and thyroid cancer; insulin-dependent diabetes mellitus; and an increased incidence of gastrointestinal tract lymphoma in patients with DH.[73] Other disease associations that have been identified in patients with DH include sarcoidosis, Sjögren syndrome, pernicious anemia, SLE, and scleroderma. More frequent than overt clinical symptoms are organ-specific autoantibodies, namely anti-thyroid cell antibodies in 39% and antiparietal cell antibodies in 19% of patients with DH.[74,75]

The treatment of choice for DH is dapsone. Sulfapyridine is indicated in those patients intolerant of dapsone. In patients who fail to respond to sulfones, the addition of prednisone in escalating doses is usually sufficient to achieve control.

Light microscopy

The prototype morphology is a focal neutrophil-rich interface dermatitis with subepidermal cleft formation (**Fig. 7A**). Leukocytoclasia is noted and there may be focal red cell extravasation. On occasion, a large blister can be seen, resulting in a condition characterized by a neutrophil-rich subepidermal blistering dermatosis.

DIF

In DH, DIF reveals irregular coarse granular deposits in the dermal papillae with variable granular deposition along the DEJ (see **Fig. 7B**). The deposits are found in perilesional skin; reduced sensitivity is found when biopsies of remote nonlesional or lesional skin are used. Sources of IgA deposition in the skin were formerly thought to reflect circulating mucosal-derived IgA depositing in cutaneous structures for which there was nonimmunologic affinity, circulating immune complexes of gliadin and IgA, or immunologic specificity of the IgA to components in the skin that cross react with gliadin. The antibody specificity has since been shown to be to epidermal transglutaminase.[76] The IgA in DH resembles mucosal IgA because it is polymeric with the presence of J chains.[74] In contrast, patients with LAD have antibody specificity to specific components of the BMZ[74,75]; the IgA is polyclonal and comprises both κ and λ light chains lacking J chain or secretory components.

A subepidermal disease with clinical and histopathologic features of DH and IF characteristics of BP has been described, and is considered a subtype of BP. Salt-split skin studies reveal dominant localization to the base of the blister with only weak staining of the roof. Western blot analysis shows reactivity with a 200-kDa dermal protein but none with the 290-kDa EBA antigen or the recently described 125-kDa and 105-kDa lamina lucida antigens found in some patients with BP. Patient serum does not react significantly with the classic BPAg1 and BPAg2.[77]

BULLOUS DISORDERS UNRELATED TO AN AUTOIMMUNE-BASED CAUSE
Pseudoporphyria and Porphyria

Porphyria is a photoinduced bullous disorder reflecting a hereditary disorder of porphyrin metabolism;

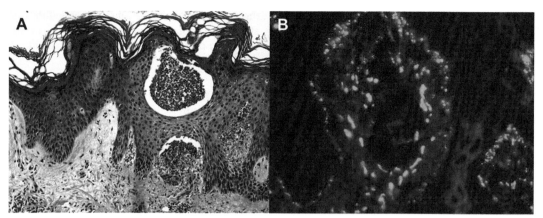

Fig. 7. (A) In classic DH dermal papillae microabscesses are seen. At times, these abscesses coalesce to result in a neutrophilic subepidermal bulla. (B) DIF in DH shows granular deposits of IgA in dermal papillae.

porphyria cutanea tarda (PCT) has also been associated with hepatitis C, including in patients with human immunodeficiency virus (HIV) infection.[78–80] The circulating porphyrins act as endogenous phototoxic agents. The most common clinical manifestations of PCT include vesicles and bullae on sun-exposed skin, sclerodermoid lesions, hyperpigmentation, and malar hypertrichosis.

Pseudo-PCT is a photoinduced bullous disease of the skin clinically and histologically resembling PCT, but in which porphyrin metabolism is normal. The sclerodermoid complications of PCT do not occur in pseudo-PCT. Among the drugs implicated in the evolution of pseudo-PCT are flutamide; the nonsteroidal antiinflammatory agents (NSAIDs) naproxen, ibuprofen, mefenamic acid, and nabumetone; tetracycline; nalidixic acid; isotretinoin; dapsone; chlorthalidone; furosemide; and bumetanide.[81–84] Chronic renal failure and hemodialysis may also produce a condition resembling pseudo-PCT. A precipitating factor in the development of pseudo-PCT is exposure to ultraviolet radiation.

In PCT, photoactivation of the complement system in the presence of uroporphyrin results in activation of dermal mast cells. Disease states like alcoholism, hepatitis C, and HIV infection increase mast cell tryptase and TGF-β elaboration and generate collagen production through the interaction between the activated mast cell and the fibroblast,[85] ultimately generating sclerodermoid alterations in some patients. Other mast cell products implicated in the pathogenesis of PCT include vasoactive agents such as the prostaglandins, the eosinophil chemoattractant histamine, and enzymes such as heparin and chymotrypsinlike proteinase. The proteases evoke vascular injury and dissolve the lamina lucida, resulting in separation of the DEJ. Mast cell tryptase

can damage the BMZ and may contribute to subepidermal cleavage. A similar end point of light-induced complement activation may exist in patients with pseudo-PCT. The mechanism by which NSAIDs are associated with pseudo-PCT may reflect the ability of NSAIDs to inhibit production of cyclic AMP, low levels of which promote mast cell degranulation. Many patients develop pseudo-PCT in the setting of NSAID therapy having serologic or IF features suggesting a preexisting state of endogenous photosensitivity, whereas other patients are on drugs that provoke photosensitivity. The presence of intense granular deposits of C5b-9 within the cutaneous vasculature of either condition corroborates the role of complement activation in the pathogenesis of the vasculopathy of both PCT and pseudo-PCT.[84]

Light microscopy
The prototypic histopathology of PCT and pseudo-PCT comprises a pauci-inflammatory subepidermal blister in concert with homogeneous eosinophilic expansion of the walls and perivascular connective tissue of superficial blood vessels (Fig. 8A), best visualized by a periodic acid-Schiff (PAS) stain. At times, the epidermal BMZ is thickened as well. Caterpillar bodies are elongate, segmented, eosinophilic, and PAS+ globules distributed linearly on the roof of a PCT or erythropoietic porphyria blister.[86] The vasculopathy of PCT and pseudo-PCT may be subtle and only discernible on PAS-stained sections. Because of the activation of the complement system, there is variable tissue neutrophilia.

DIF
DIF reveals broad homogeneous mantles of all classes of immunoglobulin along the DEJ and within the cutaneous vasculature in both PCT and pseudo-PCT. In addition to immunoglobulin

deposition in blood vessels, C3d and C4d immuno-histochemistry shows homogenous staining in the setting of PCT and pseudoporphyria.[87] Homogenous deposition of C5b-9 in vessels is a distinguishing IF pattern of both PCT and bullosis diabeticorum (see **Fig. 8B, C**).[88]

In PCT, C5b-9 deposition reflects complement activation via ultraviolet light (UVL)–activated uroporphyrins. Plasma uroporphyrins become increased in PCT because of an acquired or hereditary defect of uroporphyrinogen decarboxylase. Those at risk for acquired PCT include individuals with hemochromatosis and hepatitis C virus infection. It is thought that the increased hepatic iron found in these conditions leads to free radical formation, which in turn inhibits uroporphyrinogen decarboxylase; exposure to UVL in the 400-nm to 410-nm spectrum activates circulating uroporphyrins. In 1985, Torinuki and colleagues[89,90] irradiated

the sera from 3 patients with established PCT and showed a dose-dependent diminution of total hemolytic complement components including C1, C4, C2, C3, and C5.

Diabetic Microangiopathy/Bullosa Diabeticorum

The IF profile is very similar to the pattern observed in PCT and pseudo-PCT, comprising homogeneous broad mantles of vascular staining of immunoglobulin along with combined homogeneous and granular deposits of complement within the vascular BMZs. In diabetes mellitus, hyperglycemia results in CD59 inactivation. CD59 is a complement regulatory protein, serving to restrict C5b-9 assembly and deposition in vivo. It has been shown that preferential glycosylation near the active site of the molecule results in decreased

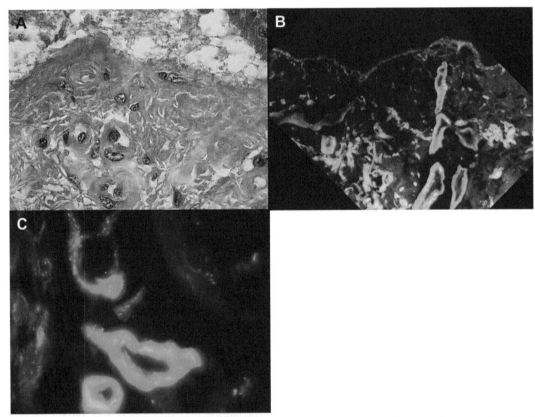

Fig. 8. (A) In PCT, the blood vessels show thickened BMZs reflective of intravascular complement activation by light-irradiated porphyrins passing through the superficial cutaneous vasculature. (B) There is deposition of C5b-9 in vessels resulting in broad mantles of C5b-9 deposited as a combined broad homogeneous and granular pattern. A homogeneous pattern is observed for other immunoglobulins, as opposed to the combined homogeneous and granular pattern typical for C5b-9 and other components of complement activation. (C) Higher power magnification shows C5b-9 deposition in an expanded homogeneous and granular fashion in the blood vessels. The same light microscopic and immunofluorescent profile is observed in bullosa diabeticorum, which, with porphyria, is among the subepidermal blistering dermatoses whose pathogenesis is unassociated with antibodies to the epidermal BMZ.

CD59 activity. Diabetic urine contains glycosylated CD59, whereas the urine of nondiabetics contains little or no glycosylated CD59[91]; the functional deficiency in CD59 is thought to lead to unrepressed C5b-9 deposition. Formed in varying degrees in all humans because of constant exposure to foreign antigen triggering complement activation, C5b-9 results in the formation of transmembrane pores that trigger cytodegenerative change, and allows the release of growth factors from endothelium, perhaps contributing to the neovascularization that defines part of the microvascular changes encountered in diabetes mellitus.[88] It has long been realized that tight control of glycemia delays the onset and progression of microvascular complications; current standards set the ideal hemoglobin A1c, a glycosylated form of hemoglobin, at less than 7%. It is reasonable to assume that glycosylation of hemoglobin A parallels that of CD59. Colocalization of C5b-9 and C1q is described in the blood vessels in brains of patients who died of diabetic ketoacidosis.

AUTOIMMUNE CONDITIONS TARGETING THE COMPONENTS OF THE INTERCELLULAR JUNCTION OF THE EPIDERMIS
Constituents and Antigens of the Desmosome

Pemphigus is a group of autoimmune disorders characterized by the loss of cell-to-cell adhesion between keratinocytes mediated by autoantibodies, most often of IgG isotype, directed against structural epithelial proteins involved in intercellular adhesion. The intercellular junction within stratified epithelium is referred to as the desmosome. The most prominent ultrastructural component of the desmosome is an electron-dense plaque that is in an intracellular location and has 2 components: a submembranous dense portion referred to as plakoglobin with a molecular weight of 83 kDa and an inner, less-dense portion called desmoplakin. Desmoplakin serves as a critical insertion point for the intracellular cytokeratin filaments and is one of the antigenic targets in paraneoplastic pemphigus and, in some cases, of erythema multiforme. Intercellular adhesion is mediated by transmembrane molecules, the desmosomal cadherins, which comprise desmogleins 1, 2, and 3 and desmocollins 1, 2, and 3. These molecules have an intracellular portion and an extracellular portion. The intracellular component extends from the plasma membrane into the outer dense plaque (plakoglobin) whereas the extracellular portion extends into the extracellular gap situated between the 2 juxtaposed keratinocytes. Antibodies to the desmosomal cadherins are associated with pemphigus vulgaris (PV) and pemphigus foliaceus

(PF). Desmoglein 1 has a molecular weight of 160 kDa and is maximally expressed in the upper epidermal layers. Desmoglein 1 is the autoantigen in PF, desmoglein 3 is implicated in PV, and desmocollin 1 is the target in IgA pemphigus.[1]

PF

This disease is characterized by small, flaccid, fragile blisters that yield shallow erosions with crusting and erythema. PF is associated with less morbidity and mortality than PV. Oral lesions are uncommon.

Light microscopy
Loss of cell-to-cell cohesion is mainly restricted to the granular cell layer (**Fig. 9**A, B); the acantholytic granular cell layer merges with a loosely adherent stratum corneum, often with eosinophils, spongiosis, and secondary impetiginization. In bullous impetigo (see **Fig. 9**C, D), the light microscopic findings closely resemble those encountered in PF, including the pattern of superficial acantholysis, attributable in this setting to staphylococcal exotoxin, which cleaves intercellular bridges in the superficial epidermal layers. DIF is negative in bullous impetigo.

Special variants of PF
Pemphigus erythematosus (Senear-Usher disease) PF-like lesions are largely confined to photodistributed areas and are most striking in the facial area. The DIF pattern characteristically manifests a positive lupus band in concert with intercellular deposition of IgG between keratinocytes.

Endemic PF/Brazilian pemphigus This condition is identical to PF but is endemic to Brazil. Fogo selvagem (known as wild fire) in more than 1 family member has been reported, suggesting a hereditary component, but most cases seem to relate to bites from a blackfly of the Simuliidae family, whose saliva may contain antigens that cross react with desmoglein 1. This form of endemic PF mainly affects young persons in rural areas at the base of mountains, with the incidence diminishing at higher altitudes. Patients often share a common immunogenetic background, with specific HLA alleles apparently predisposing to the disease. The most prevalent species is *Simulium nigrimanum*.[92] A group of patients with endemic PF in Colombia showed various histologic patterns compared with past reports of endemic PF, with most showing a PF pattern and other patients having features of SLE or scleroderma with absent appendage structures.[93]

PV

PV typically commences in the oral mucosa and then spreads to involve the head and neck, trunk,

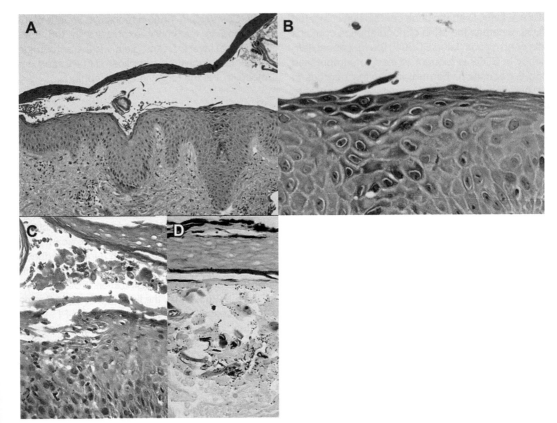

Fig. 9. (*A*) In PF, the pattern of acantholysis is superficial, primarily involving the granular cell layer. (*B*) Higher magnification of the acantholysis within the granular cell layer. (*C*) This is another superficial acantholytic dermatosis that resembles PF, namely bullous impetigo. (*D*) It is important in cases of suspect PF to perform a Gram stain. In this case of bullous impetigo, gram-positive cocci are identified.

and intertriginous areas as multiple small flaccid bullae that break down and coalesce to produce large zones of denudement. Before treatment with prednisone was introduced in the 1950s, the eruption was fatal after 5 years. A variant referred to as pemphigus vegetans encompasses the less common, but more benign, Hallopeau type and the severe Neumann variant, both of which manifest vegetative hypertrophic weeping plaques.

Light microscopy

Dyshesion affects all layers of the epidermis where desmosomal attachments between keratinocytes are lost (**Fig. 10A**), whereas intact hemidesmosomes maintain the attachment of basal layer keratinocytes to the BMZ. As the attachments are lost, the keratin filaments retract from the intracellular component of the desmosome and the keratinocytes assume a rounded appearance with condensed, hypereosinophilic cytoplasm. There is variable dermal and epidermal inflammation, typically comprising eosinophils and neutrophils with foci of eosinophilic microabscess formation.

Pemphigus Herpetiformis

Pemphigus herpetiformis is a distinct variant in which lesions clinically resemble DH. The disease can resemble PV or PF. On histology, the biopsy has some morphologic resemblance to IgA pemphigus with subcorneal acantholysis, vesiculation, and neutrophilic and eosinophilic spongiosis. The DIF studies reveal intercellular staining for IgG. Immunoprecipitation has shown immunoreactivity against the 80-kDa and 45-kDa desmoglein 1 fragments. These desmoglein fragments are recognized by 100% of PF sera and 50% of PV sera. The 80-kDa fragment represents the ectodomain of desmoglein 1 and hence it is assumed that PV autoantibodies may recognize cross-reactive epitopes present in desmoglein 1.[94,95]

Drug-induced Pemphigus

Most cases are clinically similar to PF, with a minority resembling PV. Some do not have evidence of autoantibody production and, in those patients, thiol groups are thought to directly

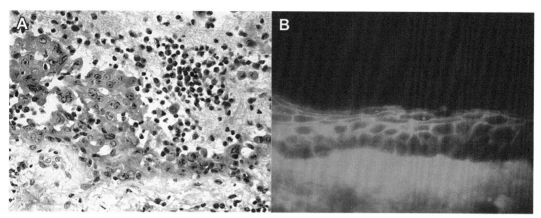

Fig. 10. (A) A classic example of PV. There is striking acantholysis involving much of the epidermis. Basal layer keratinocytes show intercellular dyshesion resulting in a tombstone effect reflective of isolated basal layer keratinocytes detached from one another but linked to the subjacent dermis through intact hemidesmosomes. It is common in PV to see prominent eosinophilic spongiosis as well as spongiform pustulation. (B) The DIF profile is characterized by intercellular deposition of immunoglobulins and complement within the epidermis.

damage the intercellular bridge components. By DIF, complement only is detected in many cases and/or the DIF may be negative, as in the IIF. The main implicated drugs are those with reactive sulfhydryl groups such as D-penicillamine and captopril. The disease typically resolves within 6 months of discontinuing the drug, although some patients develop true autoimmune pemphigus. Patients with penicillamine-induced and other thiol drug–induced pemphigus may recover spontaneously once the drug is discontinued, but those with nonthiol drug–induced pemphigus show clinical, histologic, immunologic, and evolutionary aspects consistent with idiopathic pemphigus. Only 15% of patients with nonthiol-induced pemphigus, such as that caused by ingestion of penicillin and its synthetic derivatives, can be expected to recover. Nonthiol-induced pemphigus resembles idiopathic PV, and it is possible that bacterial, viral, or endogenous peptides bind to drug hapten inducing an autoantibody with intercellular substance specificity. In contrast, the thiol drugs induce acantholysis absent an immunogenic event; a similar phenomenon occurs with drugs such as penicillins or cephalosporins that undergo metabolic change to a thiol-containing drug, and, in both cases, presentation is as the PV variant, often with negative IF. Drug-induced pemphigus can generate antibodies to desmoglein 1 and/or 3 with a positive IF profile.[96,97] Because the histology may not deviate from idiopathic pemphigus, exclusion of a drug-based cause might be suggested for all newly diagnosed pemphigus cases.

Paraneoplastic Pemphigus

Apart from thymomas and retroperitoneal sarcomas, most cases of paraneoplastic pemphigus occur in the setting of hematologic malignancies including chronic lymphocytic leukemia and Castleman disease. Oral lesions are prominent and the tracheobronchial tree may be involved. The cutaneous eruption is polymorphous with episodes of blistering and healing.[98] Paraneoplastic pemphigus is associated with considerable morbidity and mortality. The presentations are varied and include cases resembling classic BP, CP, lichen planus, erythema multiforme, toxic epidermal necrolysis, and graft-versus-host disease.

Light microscopy
There is suprabasilar acantholysis similar to PV in concert with an erythema multiforme–like interface or lichenoid dermatitis.[99]

IgA Pemphigus

The term was first introduced in 1982. There are 2 variants: an intraepidermal neutrophilic dermatosis in which the blisters occur in the lower epidermis, and subcorneal pustular dermatosis, in which the acantholysis occurs in the upper epidermis and the clinical presentation is as Sneddon-Wilkinson disease. There is in vivo bound IgA in concert with circulating IgA antibodies that target the epidermal cell surface component. It is not clear why some people develop IgA rather than IgG autoantibodies against the same target antigen. The generation of antibodies is a complex immunologic process involving both T and B lymphocytes.[100]

DIF Testing for Pemphigus

The standard IF pattern in all forms of pemphigus is of intracellular staining in the epidermis (see Fig. 10B). Intercellular staining may be combined with a homogeneous linear pemphigoidlike pattern along the DEJ in paraneoplastic pemphigus. There may be enhanced decoration of the more superficial keratinocytes in PF. False-negative or false-positive results can occur in the setting of an active epidermal inflammatory process because inflammatory cells may digest immunoglobulin; in contrast, epithelial injury may expose novel antigenic epitopes, thereby evoking antibody formation as an epiphenomenon, but the antibodies may not be of pathogenetic significance. Antibodies to select blood group antigens A and B may exhibit a positive IF mimicking pemphigus, although this can be eliminated using a mixture of soluble A and B antigens in solution.[101]

Antigen Specificity in PV Versus PF Versus Paraneoplastic Pemphigus

The sera from patients with PV immunoprecipitate a 130-kDa glycoprotein called the pemphigus vulgaris antigen, identified as desmoglein 3, in all patients and manifests 65% homology with sequenced human desmoglein 1, which is the PF antigen. Desmoglein 3 is present only in the lowermost epidermal cell layers. Antibodies are directed primarily to the N-terminal region of the extracellular portion of the molecules. Desmoglein 1 is a 160-kDa transmembrane glycoprotein that is critical to cell-to-cell adhesion and is found in PF sera. Desmoglein 1 is a transmembrane protein that belongs to the superantigen family of cadherins; it has an intracellular component that traverses through plakoglobin and an extracellular component. Desmoglein 1 is present on the surface of all cells, but its maximal expression is within the superficial layers of the epidermis.[102] Most PF autoantibodies are directed against epitopes on the in vivo accessible extracellular domain of desmoglein 1 and some are conformational and calcium dependent. Because the granular cell layer is poorly formed in the mucous membranes, desmoglein 1 may not be as critical for cell adhesion in the oral mucosa, accounting for the low incidence of oral lesions in PF. Antibodies to desmoglein 1 have also been shown in patients with pemphigus erythematosus (Senear-Usher syndrome). Antibody specificity to a 190-kDa antigen located on a desmosomal plaque and the intracellular portion of the hemidesmosomes has been shown in patients with PF; this is different from BPAG2 and is similar to that described in patients with paraneoplastic pemphigus.[103]

In the subcorneal variant of IgA pemphigus, desmocollin 1, a desmosomal component located primarily in the upper epidermis has recently been identified as a target antigen. The target antigen in the intraepidermal variant is desmoglein 3, the identical antigenic target in classic IgG-mediated PV. The ability of IgA autoantibodies to bind neutrophils may explain tissue neutrophilia; the specific binding site for the monocyte/granulocyte IgA-Fc (fragment crystallizable) receptor has been localized to the constant domain of human IgA distal to the hinge region, an arrangement that may lead to resistance to protease digestion, promoting efficient binding of neutrophils.[104,105]

Antibodies to a 170-kDa transmembrane antigen with an extracellular domain associated with atypical clinical and immunologic features of paraneoplastic pemphigus are described. Antibodies to desmoplakins I and II have been identified in a subset of patients with erythema multiforme major, some of whom had been exposed to NSAIDs and herpes simplex labialis[106]; histology mimics paraneoplastic pemphigus. Patients with PF by clinical, histologic, and IF criteria recently had antibody specificity to antigens implicated in paraneoplastic pemphigus; these antibodies had specificity to desmoplakin I and II in 1 patient and antibodies to desmoplakin I in another.[107] Neither patient had evidence of cancer during a follow-up period.

Autoantibodies in paraneoplastic pemphigus are primarily targeted against cytoplasmic proteins of the plakin family (desmoplakin 1, 2, BPAG1, envoplakin, periplakin, and plectin). Desmoplakins are intracellular cytoplasmic proteins common to desmosomes that serve as an attachment site for keratin filaments and are common to all epithelial structures. Potential targets therefore include respiratory, gut, bladder and oral mucosae, skin and myocardium, explaining the often widespread multiorgan involvement.[98,108–111] ELISA detection of periplakin and envoplakin antibodies is highly sensitive and specific.[112] Cell surface target antigens have recently been identified, including desmoglein 3 and 1, the autoantigens of PV and PF respectively.[102,108,109] In particular, antibodies to desmoglein 1 and 3 may be involved in the early stages of disease.[99] Anti–desmoglein 3 antibodies purified from patients with paraneoplastic pemphigus induce blisters in neonatal mice, indicating that anti–desmoglein 3 and possibly anti-desmoglein 1 play a pathogenic role. The sera may also have specificity for the 230-kDa BPAg. In our experience, and based on this pathophysiology, paraneoplastic pemphigus may manifest perplexing fluctuations of DIF findings over time.

IIF in Pemphigus

IIF is a more sensitive assay than immunoblotting for the detection of circulating antibodies in patients with pemphigus, particularly the foliaceus variant.

There is also a strong correlation between substrate specificity of intercellular antibodies, the type of pemphigus, and the presence of antibodies against either the 130-kDa PV or the160-kDa PF antigen. There is a higher degree of immunoreactivity when using monkey versus guinea pig esophagus in sera from patients with PF. Because the converse is true in patients with PV, substrate specificity can help to define the type of pemphigus, reflecting differential expression of desmoglein 1 and desmoglein 3 in monkey and guinea pig esophagus. By IIF using urothelium as substrate, intercellular staining is observed with paraneoplastic pemphigus serum, a finding not observed in routine pemphigus states.

Mechanisms of Acantholysis in Pemphigus

Pemphigus sera can fix C1q, C3, and C4. Complement is demonstrable in lesional skin but absent in nonlesional skin. Complement likely causes the inflammatory cell infiltrate seen in lesions of pemphigus and may augment acantholysis. The critical event is the binding of antibody to the epidermis. In typical pemphigus, IgG binds to the surface of the epidermal cells, leading to increased plasminogen activator activity that produces localized increases in levels of epidermal plasmin, which cleaves cell-to-cell adhesion molecules.[113]

IF IN DIAGNOSIS OF COLLAGEN VASCULAR DISEASE

The lupus band test (LBT) and the deposition pattern of the supramolecular membrane attack complex of complement C_{5B-9} are valuable in establishing the presence of autoimmune CTD, and for further precise classification of the diseases. In our view, DIF performed in conjunction with conventional histology boosts sensitivity and specificity of diagnosis.[114]

LBT

The LBT was introduced in 1963 by Burnham and colleagues,[115] who referred to the deposition of IgG, IgA, and IgM along the DEJ in lesional skin. The definition has since expanded to encompass lesional and nonlesional skin in sun-exposed and sun-protected sites.[116–121]

The most frequent immunoglobulin isotype deposited is IgM, and the least frequently deposited is IgA. In discoid lupus erythematosus (DLE) lesions, the frequency of IgG deposition is low compared with that of IgM, which is seen in 90% of lesional skin biopsies. In clinically normal deltoid region skin from patients with SLE and other rheumatic diseases in 1 study, DEJ deposition of immunoglobulin was seen in 73% of patients with SLE (**Fig. 11**A) and in 36% of other patients, yielding a specificity of 64% and a predictive value of 57%. The predictive value for SLE was greater with C4 (100%), properdin (91.3%), and IgA (86.2%) than with IgM (59%). The specificity and predictive value increases with the number of immunoreactants detected at the DEJ.[115–122] The pattern of deposition is typically as granules or closely spaced vertically oriented fibrils, or occasionally as a thick, homogeneous band. We do not designate as a positive LBT a sharply defined thin linear band of decoration similar to that seen

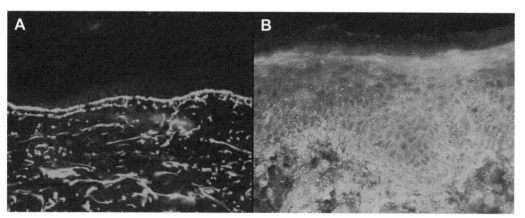

Fig. 11. (A) An example of a positive LBT. There is a continuous band of granular deposition within the epidermal BMZ. The IgM variant of a positive LBT is the least specific for underlying lupus erythematosus. In classic lupus erythematosus, all immunoglobulin isotypes are observed within the epidermal BMZ. The specificity of a positive LBT for lupus erythematosus increases as more classes of immunoglobulin are deposited within the epidermal BMZ. (B) Epidermal deposition of IgG in keratinocyte nuclei in a granular fashion. This finding correlates strongly with antibodies to an extractable nuclear antigen such as Ro, La, Smith, and/or RNP. Hence this staining pattern can be observed in subacute cutaneous lupus erythematosus, anti-Ro–associated SLE, and mixed connective tissue disease.

in BP. Globular deposits positive for complement and/or immunoglobulins that correlate with colloid bodies in dermal papillae, although indicating antecedent keratinocyte injury, are not specific as to cause. The degree of deposition that warrants designation as a positive LBT is controversial; differences in criteria partly explain the disparity of results in various series. We consider the deposition of IgM in sun-exposed skin in a continuous band of least moderate intensity over at least 50% of the width of the biopsy specimen to be a positive LBT.[121] Weak IgM decoration along the DEJ is common in sun-exposed skin of patients who do not have lupus erythematosus (LE), such as in lesions of actinic keratosis and rosacea, and in 20% of normal skin specimens from healthy young adults[123,124]; deposition of IgG, IgA, and C3 is seen in less than 5% of such individuals. One of us (ANC) has seen a fibrillar band of IgG deposition in a young woman with pyoderma faciale, a form of rosacea, in the absence of associated signs of a systemic CTD. In comparing the IF profile of dermatomyositis with LE, we found weak discontinuous DEJ deposition of IgM on sun-exposed lesional skin in more than 50% of dermatomyositis patients, but never of sufficient intensity to warrant designation as a positive LBT using the strict criteria outlined earlier.[125] Up to 13.5% of patients with systemic scleroderma manifest a positive LBT, a finding that seems to herald a more aggressive course.[126,127] Biopsied lesions of cutaneous vasculitis, irrespective of cause, may also exhibit a positive LBT.

In sun-protected skin, an interrupted band of IgM of at least moderate intensity is sufficient for designation as a positive LBT, assuming that the biopsy is not a lesion of lichen planus, in which granular deposition of IgM as an interrupted band along the DEJ is seen at sites of colloid body deposition. The deposition of IgG is usually less intense than that of IgM and false-positive results are rare, so it is therefore likely adequate to see an interrupted weak band of IgG deposition, even in sun-exposed skin.[121,128] The concomitant deposition of IgA enhances the specificity of the assay. We have seen many examples of positive LBTs composed of fine granules of IgM isotype unaccompanied by the deposition of any additional immunoglobulins in patients with other forms of autoimmune disease such as alopecia areata, a subgroup of patients with female pattern hair loss, idiopathic and autoimmune-associated small fiber neuropathy, and in the setting of apparent drug hypersensitivity. In patients with LE, all classes of immunoglobulin are characteristically observed, as opposed to isolated immunoglobulin isotypes within the epidermal BMZ. The

clinician must be alert to the relative lack of specificity of the IgM variant of the positive LBT.

Our view is that sun-exposed lesional skin should be used to substantiate an initial diagnosis of LE so as to avoid the problem of false-negative results caused by reduced sensitivity in sun-protected skin. After the diagnosis of LE is made, a biopsy of nonlesional skin may be performed to further assist in subclassification and prognostication.

LBT in subtypes of lupus erythematosus

In sun-exposed nonlesional skin, the LBT is positive in 70% to 80% of patients with SLE, whereas it is negative in patients with DLE and subacute cutaneous LE (SCLE). A positive LBT in sun-protected nonlesional skin of patients with SLE, seen in roughly 55% of cases, correlates with severe extracutaneous disease, particularly of renal origin, and with antibodies to double-stranded DNA.[121,129,130] Most patients with DLE have a positive LBT in lesional skin. Only 50% of patients with SCLE show a positive LBT. In most patients in whom the LBT is positive, all classes of immunoglobulin are deposited along the DEJ. A negative LBT is common if there is a prior and/or concurrent history of topical and/or systemic steroid use.

Pathogenesis of the LBT

In biopsies of sun-exposed forearm skin, early studies showed a positive LBT in 77% of cases, versus 33% of non–sun-exposed buttock skin.[131] It was therefore postulated that UVL plays a role in the denaturing of keratinocyte DNA, which then diffuses across the BMZ and becomes trapped because of the natural avidity of native DNA for type IV collagen. This DNA then binds with anti-nuclear antibodies (ANAs), being visualized as the granular deposits that constitute the positive LBT. Another source of immunoreactivity is circulating immune complexes comprising DNA and antibodies to DNA. Antibodies directed against BMZ components do not play a significant role in the genesis of a positive LBT.[121,131]

Relationship of LBT to disease severity in SLE

The relationship between a positive LBT and the severity of renal disease in SLE is controversial. Some investigators suggest a significant relationship between a positive LBT in nonlesional sun-protected skin and renal disorders, with 70% of such patients having active nephritis, and with serious renal disease being 3 times more common. The deposition of IgG in nonlesional sun-protected skin correlates with anti–nuclear DNA (anti-nDNA) antibodies and with a higher incidence of renal disease.[118,119,129,130] However, a negative LBT does not exclude active renal disease. Patients with pure IgM deposition in clinically normal skin have anti-nDNA antibodies restricted to the IgM class and tend to have a more benign course.[129] Several studies have correlated a positive LBT on buttock skin with active systemic disease. Because C1q avidly binds to DNA, C1q deposition along the DEJ in the skin of patients with SLE may reflect the presence of DNA at the DEJ; such patients have a higher index of disease activity.[129,130]

Biopsy site for LBT

The recommended site for a sun-exposed nonlesional skin biopsy to establish an initial diagnosis of SLE is the shoulder. The upper arm and the extensor aspect of the forearm are positive in 67% of cases. The volar aspect of the forearm or the upper third of the extensor aspect of the forearm are the typical sites chosen to represent sun-protected nonlesional skin; the volar aspect of the forearm is positive in 50% of cases. Buttock skin generates a positive LBT in 35% to 40% of patients with active SLE.[120]

C_{5B-9} in Subclassification of LE and Other Forms of CTD

The C_{5b-9} assay is a useful adjunct in the subclassification of CTD.[132,133] Dako anti-C_{5b-9} aE11 is a monoclonal mouse antihuman antibody targeting the neoepitope resident on activated C9 of the terminal complement complex comprising complement fractions C5b, C6, C7, C8, and C9. The supramolecular structure C_{5b-9} forms following activation of the classic or alternate pathways, and induces plasmalemmal pores that lead to cell injury and permit access of other antibodies to the cytosol and to the nucleus of keratinocytes and endothelia.[125,134] The method used is a sandwich technique that, by definition, is an IIF method even though patient skin is used as the substrate.[121]

SLE

Lesional skin Intense granular deposition of C_{5b-9} along the DEJ is seen in 80% of cases.[128] Granular nuclear and cytoplasmic deposits of IgG and C_{5b-9} are also observed in keratinocytes in patients with antibodies to one of the extractable nuclear antigens (ENAs): Ro, La, Sm, or U1RNP (see **Fig. 11B**).

Nonlesional skin In patients with SLE with an antibody to an ENA, immunoreactivity for C_{5b-9} and IgG within keratinocytes is common.[128] C_{5b-9} deposits are also seen in the cutaneous vasculature of lesional and nonlesional skin in patients with anti-Ro–associated SLE.[135,136]

SCLE

Deposition of C_{5b-9} along the DEJ is observed in 66% of patients with SCLE. A more specific finding

is the presence of granular nuclear and or cytoplasmic epidermal decoration for IgG[136] and C_{5b-9},[125,128] an IF profile independent of serologic findings observed in patients with and without antibodies to Ro.[125] There is usually absent vascular decoration except in patients who have drug-associated SCLE.[137] In vivo keratinocyte fluorescence seen using reagents is associated with ANA by serologic testing in 70% of patients; the positive predictive value of an in vivo ANA for systemic CTD is 75%.[138] Twenty of 28 patients with positive keratinocyte fluorescence for IgG, IgA, or IgM, or C3 had autoantibodies and 17 had an antibody to an ENA. Nine of these 17 patients were proved to have SLE, 3 had MCTD, 3 had an overlap syndrome, and 1 each had Sjögren disease or CREST (calcinosis, Raynaud syndrome, esophageal dysmotility, sclerodactyly, telangiectasia) syndrome.[138] C_{5b-9} in keratinocytes is more specific than IgG decoration of keratinocytes. In our experience, IgG expression in keratinocytes without C_{5b-9} is not associated with antibodies to an ENA but may indicate a positive ANA.

DLE

Intense granular decoration for C_{5b-9} along the DEJ is seen in most cases. Decoration of epidermal keratinocytes or endothelia for either IgG or C_{5b-9} is typically absent, although there may be some granular staining within the vessel wall.

MCTD

Granular nuclear and cytoplasmic keratinocyte deposition of C_{5b-9} and IgG is seen in 100% of cases, corresponding to antibodies to ribonucleoprotein (RNP), which are a defining feature of this disease process. Intense granular deposits are seen along the DEJ in almost all cases, usually in concert with granular vascular decoration.[139] The IF profile is virtually indistinguishable from that of anti-Ro/SSA–positive SLE.[135]

Dermatomyositis

The typical finding in dermatomyositis (DM) is C_{5b-9} deposition as a continuous granular band along the DEJ of lesional sun-exposed and sun-protected skin (**Fig. 12A, B**). In more than 90% of cases, there is granular vascular staining that is most conspicuous in dermal papillae capillaries. Granular keratinocyte nuclear staining for C_{5b-9} or IgG is observed in only those patients in whom there is a positive ANA.[128,134]

In the appropriate clinical setting, the constellation of a negative LBT, C_{5b-9} deposition along the DEJ and within blood vessels, with variable keratinocyte decoration for C_{5b-9} and IgG, in the absence of antibodies to Ro/SSA or RNP, strongly suggests DM.

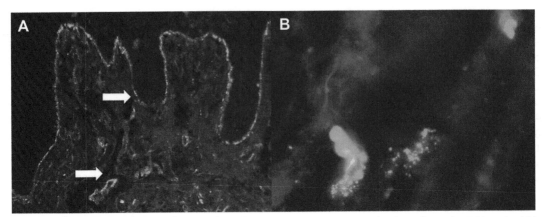

Fig. 12. (*A*) In dermatomyositis, the typical pattern is prominent deposits of C5b-9 along the DEJ and within blood vessels (*arrows*). (*B*) This is a high magnification of C5b-9 within blood vessels; C5b-9 is the likely effector of microvascular injury triggered by antiendothelial cell antibodies.

Pathogenesis of C5b-9 decoration

In the setting of LE or MCTD, DEJ deposition of C_{5b-9} may reflect activation within the BMZ of the complement pathway caused by the deposition of immune complexes or by passively absorbed keratinocyte-derived DNA complexed with an ANA. In the setting of DM, we have postulated that the mechanism of deposition may relate to nonspecific trapping of C_{5b-9} passing across damaged dermal papillae capillaries.[125,134] Once deposited, C_{5b-9} may contribute to epidermal injury.[125,134] The epidermal deposition of C_{5b-9} in SCLE, anti-Ro/SSA–positive SLE, MCTD, and ANA-positive DM correlates strongly with an antibody to an ENA.[125,134,135,139] Antibodies to ENAs in DM include those that are directed against histidyl-transfer RNA synthetase, and 4 other aminoacyl transfer RNA synthetases, namely threonine, glycine, isoleucine, and alanine.[140–143] Relocation of nuclear and cytoplasmic Ro/SSA antigens to the cell surface has been implicated as a key event that allows the binding of autoantibodies. Ultraviolet light exposure, viral infection, and estrogen treatment of cultured keratinocytes have been shown to displace Ro antigen to the cell membrane.[140–143] A similar mechanism of surface displacement has been shown for RNP and may also occur with DM-associated ENAs.[125,134] The presence of C_{5b-9} in keratinocytes suggests a role for complement-induced pores in the propagation of keratinocyte injury. Most studies indicate that C_{5b-9} binding to keratinocytes is not cytotoxic and that the principal mechanism of injury is antibody-dependent cellular immunity. However, it is possible that C_{5b-9} may be capable of lysing cells whose repair mechanisms have been previously or concurrently suppressed.[144,145] The pores may also allow circulating antibodies access to the cytoplasmic and nuclear antigens of the Ro/SSA, RNP, and histidyl-transfer RNA synthetase complexes seen in SCLE and anti-Ro/SSA–associated SLE, MCTD, and anti-Jo1–associated DM, respectively. Intracellular decoration may reflect an in vivo phenomenon initiated by complement-mediated pore formation.[128,134,137,139] Deposition of C_{5b-9} in dermal blood vessels in anti-Ro/SSA–associated SLE, DM, and MCTD suggests that endothelium is a prime antigenic target in these CTDs.[128,134,135,139]

One of the authors (CMM) has published on the usefulness of C3d and C4d in CTD evaluation via an immunohistochemical methodology. Intense C3d deposition along the DEJ without C4d is typical of DLE, combined C3d and C4d is characteristic of SLE, and C4d in vessels in the absence of C4d along the DEJ is characteristic of DM. Although C4d may decorate the nuclei of keratinocytes in cases of SCLE, this pattern is difficult to interpret; under oil-immersion magnification, a distinct fine granular appearance is noted within nuclei.

UNCOMMON SUBTYPES OF LUPUS ERYTHEMATOSUS
Anti-Ro/SSA–Associated SLE

Anti-Ro/SSA–positive patients with SLE have variable clinical manifestations including an SCLE-like rash, malar erythema, a DM-like rash, and vascular disease involving the skin, heart, pulmonary system, and nervous system.[135] The sequela of vasculopathy in the lungs is hypovascularity of the interalveolar septal capillary bed, whereas microvascular injury in skeletal muscle produces a muscle injury pattern similar to that of DM.[135,146] In vitro studies showing endothelial localization of the Ro/SSA antigen,[142] and the correlation of serum

C_{5b-9} levels with evidence of active central nervous system disease,[136,147] suggest that humoral injury mediated by anti-Ro/SSA antibody bound to endothelial Ro antigen may be operative. In patients with Sjögren syndrome, but seemingly not in a cohort of patients with SLE, the degree of skin disease activity seems to correlate with the levels of antibodies to Ro/SSA.[148]

Bullous SLE

Bullous SLE is a distinctive cutaneous manifestation of SLE. It has been encountered as a presenting manifestation of SLE[149] but patients typically have 1 or more features of SLE preceding the eruption by 8 months to 6 years. Bullae on an urticarial base resemble BP or linear IgA disease, whereas grouped vesicular lesions may mimic DH,[150,151] sometimes preceded by diffuse erythema. The eruption is generalized, with a propensity to involve the trunk and flexural surfaces. A bullous eruption confined to the face has been described, which some investigators think is not bullous SLE but rather an unrelated, poorly defined form of cutaneous SLE.

Proposed criteria for a diagnosis of bullous SLE are (1) a diagnosis of SLE by criteria of the American College of Rheumatology, (2) a widespread, nonscarring, vesiculobullous eruption, (3) subepidermal blisters with dermal inflammation characterized by neutrophilic papillary microabscesses similar to those of DH, and (4) DIF of lesional or nonlesional skin showing linear or granular IgG and/or IgM. The newly revised criteria do not require salt-split skin dermal binding of immunoreactants or antibodies to type VII collagen.[152] Although in most patients antigenicity lies in the noncollagenous domain of type VII collagen, some patients have antigen specificity to other components of the BMZ.[153]

Light microscopy

Skin biopsies show a neutrophilic interface dermatitis with dermal papillae microabscess formation reminiscent of DH. The interface inflammation may be broad and associated with effacement of the rete ridge architecture, recapitulating a morphology that closely resembles linear IgA disease. Histiocytes containing engulfed nuclear fragments of disintegrating neutrophils may be observed. Tissue eosinophilia may be prominent. Vacuolar interface dermatitis with concomitant mesenchymal mucinosis often completes the picture.[151,152]

DIF

DIF of lesional skin reveals a continuous band of IgG deposition along the DEJ, which may appear homogeneous with a $400\times$ objective but, at $1000\times$, oil-immersion microscopy reveals a superimposed coarse and fine granular band of deposition (CMM, personal observation, 2012). The band is wider than the sharp, thin, linear band seen with BP and EBA. There is also codominant expression of other isotypes of immunoglobulin, specifically IgA and IgM, with an increased incidence of IgA deposition in bullous SLE versus nonbullous SLE (76% vs 17%). Although IgA or IgM along the DEJ can be observed in BP and EBA, it is of lesser staining intensity than the dominant, intense pattern of IgG decoration in either disorder.[151–153] Salt-split skin studies reveal localization of immunoreactivity to the floor consistent with antigenic localization to the sublamina densa region, similar to that of EBA, and unlike BP, in which immunoreactivity localizes to the roof.

IIF

Substrates used are either normal skin or salt-split skin, the latter enhancing sensitivity of the assay for circulating antibodies. The hallmark is a linear pattern of deposition along the DEJ with localization to the floor in those cases in which salt-split skin is the substrate.

Immunoelectron microscopy

Immunogold electron microscopy performed on perilesional skin shows localization of immunoreactants to the sublamina densa region.[151–153]

Immunoblot analysis

Immunoblot analysis reveals IgG binding to 2 distinct protein bands with molecular weights of 290 and 145 kDa, which migrate with bands previously reported for EBA and have specificity for type VII collagen.[11,12,154–156] It has recently been suggested that there is immunogenic heterogeneity in bullous SLE, whereby some patients lack antibodies to type VII collagen and manifest epidermal staining with salt-split skin. In contrast, not all patients with SLE who have antibodies to components of the BMZ have bullous eruptions. Patients with nonbullous LE are described who had antibodies to BPAg2 and BPAg1 without correlation between immunoblotting studies and the IF findings of lesional skin, the latter being typical of LE and not of a vesiculobullous disorder.[157]

Immunomapping

IIF mapping uses antibodies to 3 known components of the BMZ of human skin: (1) BP antigen, (2) laminin, and (3) type IV collagen. In bullous SLE, the BMZ components reside in the roof of the vesicle, designating the level of the cleavage plane to be beneath the lamina densa, hence defining a dermolytic process. There are some reports of the cleavage point in lesions of bullous

SLE being within the lamina lucida; rather than reflecting a different antigenic target, this finding likely reflects the lamina lucida being the weakest part of the BMZ (locus minoris resistensiae). There may alternatively be a preferential localization of proteolytic enzymes to the lamina lucida in such cases.

Pathogenesis

Antibodies to the noncollagenous component of type VII collagen are the pathogenic basis of bullous SLE; activating the complement cascade sequence results in acute inflammation caused by the generation of C5a, a major neutrophil chemoattractant and leukocyte-activating complement peptide.

Treatment

Patients often, but not always, respond to dapsone therapy. High-dose prednisone may be the only option for control of the disease.[153]

Differential diagnosis

The main differential diagnosis, EBA, can coexist with SLE. Concomitant cell-poor vacuolar interface dermatitis and mesenchymal mucinosis, and the demonstration by DIF of a broader band with codominant localization with IgA and superimposed granular decoration of the DEJ, would support a diagnosis of bullous SLE rather than EBA.[151]

Sclerodermatomyositis

Sclerodermatomyositis is a distinctive CTD that combines overlapping features of DM and scleroderma, characteristically without the same severity of systemic involvement. The patients have pinched facies similar to that encountered in scleroderma, roughened cuticles, and the so-called mechanics hand similar that seen in any of the antisynthetase syndromes. There may be Gottron papules analogous to those seen in patients with DM. The patients have antibodies to Pm Scl and Ku, both of which are nucleolar-based antigens resulting in a distinctive nucleolar staining pattern in keratinocytes by DIF (**Fig. 13**).[158–160]

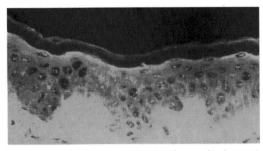

Fig. 13. In sclerodermatomyositis, the antibody specificity is to nucleolar antigens, therefore keratinocyte nucleolar decoration is characteristic.

LINEAR IGM DEPOSITION ALONG THE DEJ

A sharp linear band of IgM along the DEJ in isolation from other immunoreactants may occasionally be seen in a variety of disorders including urticaria, paraneoplastic pemphigus, Grover disease, pigmented purpuric dermatosis, leukocytoclastic vasculitis, folliculitis, and so-called hypersensitivity dermatitis.[161,162] Described in a pregnant patient with a pruritic follicular-based eruption was an entity designated as linear IgM disease of pregnancy.[163] Subsequent studies revealed that 9% of patients with polymorphous eruption of pregnancy had deposits of IgM along the DEJ, suggesting that IgM may be found in various eruptions of pregnancy and not in just a specific IgM dermatitis.

Certain immune complex–mediated diseases may be associated with a narrow fibrillar band of IgM deposition mimicking the sharp linear pattern of deposition seen in conditions with antibody specificity to components of the BMZ. Only 1 patient to date with linear IgM deposition has had evidence of circulating IgM antibodies to BMZ components; the patient had atypical BP with serum IgM BMZ antibodies detected by IIF in the setting of an underlying IgM paraproteinemia.[164] The presumed basis was IgM κ protein affinity to an epitope within the lamina lucida.

Ultrastructural localization of linear IgM immunoreactants is to the sublamina densa consistent with nonspecific immune complex deposition. A frequent histologic finding is marked papillary dermal edema, which may be a sign of exudation and subsequent filtration of immune complexes at the BMZ.

We consider linear IgM deposition to represent an epiphenomenon reflecting nonspecific trapping of immune complexes along the DEJ; hence its association with vasculitis, urticaria, drug reactions, and CTD.

IF IN DIAGNOSIS OF VASCULOPATHIC CONDITIONS

The vasculitic or vasculopathic conditions in which IF may be of help include IgA-associated vasculitis, non-IgA leukocytoclastic vasculitis (LCV) attributable to cryoprecipitates, urticarial vasculitis, the antineutrophil cytoplasmic antibody (ANCA)–mediated vasculitic syndromes, and pauci-inflammatory thrombogenic vasculopathy syndromes, including antiphospholipid antibody syndrome. In addition, in vascular injury syndromes attributable to antiendothelial cell antibodies and/or in which such antibodies may be important in mediating some component of microvascular injury, an IIF assay to assess for the presence of antiendothelial cell antibodies can be of help diagnostically. Independent of the vasculitic lesion biopsied, it has been our experience that DIF should be performed on lesional skin to enhance sensitivity.[165]

IgA Vasculitis

Henoch-Schönlein purpura (HSP) is the most common morphologic expression of IgA vasculitis in the context of a neutrophil-rich LCV linked with an infectious trigger.[166] There is a minor subset of IgA-mediated vascular injury syndromes in which the dominant inflammatory cell infiltrate is lymphocytic.[166] The older criteria set forth by the American College of Rheumatology for HSP did not include an IF profile of dominant IgA deposits within the microvasculature; these have since been revised such that dominant deposits of IgA in the vasculature are a requisite (Fig. 14). The old, obsolete criteria for HSP could also apply to other vasculitic syndromes such as mixed cryoglobulinemia, Wegener granulomatosis, CTD, hypocomplementemic vasculitis, and microscopic polyarteritis nodosa,[167] all of which can present with palpable purpura and abdominal symptoms caused by small vessel vasculitis. Other common features seen in HSP, such as glomerulonephritis and arthritis, can also be seen in these systemic vasculitides. HSP typically occurs in childhood, is triggered by antecedent infection, and is associated with IgA deposits in the skin, intestine, and kidney. In adult patients with HSP, IgA anticardiolipin antibodies have significant correlation with early disease activity, arthralgia, and proteinuria.[168,169] However, there are many reported cases of cutaneous IgA-associated vasculitis that lack the extracutaneous manifestations of HSP. The DIF criterion that we use to suggest a diagnosis of IgA vasculitis is prominent vascular deposition of IgA that is dominant with respect to IgG and IgM.

Although HSP is a form of IgA vasculitis, the designation is only applied to those cases accompanied by arthritis, abdominal pain, and/or evidence of glomerulonephritis. A variety of microbial pathogens acting as antigenic triggers are associated with HSP; 18% to 29% of patients have evidence of group A or C streptococcal infections. Mycoplasma pneumoniae, Yersinia, Salmonella hirshfeldii, hepatitis A or C, Parvovirus B 19, and denatured microbial pathogens are also implicated, as is the use of streptokinase following myocardial infarction. The rash of HSP prototypically involves the upper and lower extremities, buttocks, and abdomen.[166]

Vascular IgA deposition is not unique to HSP or even to vasculitis per se, because it is seen in non-lesional skin of patients with IgA nephropathy, alcoholism, and DH,[170] and in vasculitic lesions in patients with inflammatory bowel disease, ankylosing spondylitis, SLE with anti-Ro antibodies, rheumatoid arthritis, prostatic and bronchogenic neoplasms, hypersensitivity reactions to drugs including carbamazepine, and IgA paraproteinemia.[166]

In our series, 1 of the 7 patients with IgA vasculitis without infection, had one of these associations established either before or after the biopsy. One additional patient developed IgA vasculitis in the setting of lymphoma, an association that was then novel to our experience. IgA-associated vasculitis occurs as a paraneoplastic phenomenon in adult patients in whom a microbial trigger may not be isolated.[171,172]

Non-IgA Vasculitis

Any vascular injury syndrome can exhibit IgM deposition within blood vessel walls accompanied by components of complement. In exuberant delayed-type hypersensitivity reactions without any apparent immune complex deposits, it is common to see deposits of IgM and C5b-9 within the vessel walls; hence, interpreting vascular immunoglobulin and complement deposits requires correlation with the clinical presentation and the light microscopic findings. In a classic necrotizing vasculitis that is not mediated by IgA, the most common vascular immunoglobulin deposited is IgM, along with components of the classic complement cascade sequence. It is unusual to see IgG deposition within the vessel wall except in the setting of mixed cryoglobulinemic vasculitis and certain cases of SLE in which palpable purpura develops. Fibrinogen is invariably present in an endovascular, perivascular, and/or

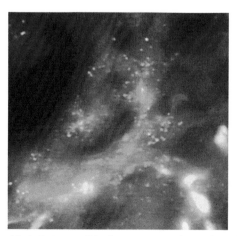

Fig. 14. In IgA vasculitis, there are prominent deposits of IgA within the cutaneous vasculature. The IgA deposits are dominant over other immunoglobulins.

interstitial distribution, but fibrinogen deposition in the skin is common and does not always correlate with discernible fibrin by routine light microscopy.

In mixed cryoglobulinemic vasculitis, prominent deposits of immunoglobulin are seen in the vascular lumen and within the vessel walls; IgG is most frequent. The immunoglobulin isotype is important in elucidating the nature of the immune complex. Illustrated is a case of type II mixed cryoglobulinemia comprising a monoclonal rheumatoid factor of IgA isotype complexed to polyclonal IgG (**Fig. 15**).

ANCA-Positive Vasculitic Syndromes

The ANCA-positive vasculitic syndromes are categorized as pauci-immune despite the presence of antibodies with neutrophilic cytoplasmic granule specificity being causally important. Designation as pauci-immune emphasizes a minimal role for immune complex deposition in the pathogenesis of the vascular injury in these distinctive vasculitic syndromes. As with any vascular injury syndrome independent of immune complex deposition, the observation of IgM and complement may be seen. The complement cascade seems to be activated in the ANCA-positive vasculitic syndromes, including in the context of membranolytic attack complex deposition.[173]

Urticarial Vasculitis

In urticarial vasculitis associated with hypocomplementemia, the LBT is characteristically positive and all immunoglobulin isotypes are observed along the DEJ, producing a pattern analogous to SLE. A significant percentage of patients with hypocomplementemic vasculitis in whom this profile is observed develop SLE.

Hemorrhagic Edema of Infancy

Acute hemorrhagic edema of infancy (AHEI), also known as Finklestein disease, Seidlmayer syndrome, and postinfectious cockade purpura, is an LCV seen in infants that has been considered to represent a variant of HSP that is self-limiting and usually resolves without treatment. Affected patients are usually infants aged 2 months to 3 years with a high male/female ratio of 4.64 to 1.[174]

Fever, edema, and purpura characterize AHEI and typically occur 2 days to 1 month after exposure to the causative agent, sometimes a drug. Some cases show no signs of fever. Nonpitting edema often affects the face, extremities, ears, eyelids, lips, penis, and/or scrotum. The most consistent manifestation is purpura, presenting initially as an erythematous macule, papule, or urticarial plaque(s) that quickly develops into annular, cockade, or rounded purpuric lesion(s) that is often symmetric. Extracutaneous symptoms are rare.[174,175]

Although the features of AHEI sometimes overlap with those of HSP, IF studies suggest that they are separate entities. IF studies of AHEI show deposition of fibrinogen, IgG, IgM, IgA, IgE, C3, and C1q in vessel walls (**Fig. 16**). Although HSP also shows reactivity with fibrinogen, C3, and IgM, C1q is not commonly observed.[176] IgA deposition is seen in patients with AHEI but it is not dominant over other immunoglobulins, specifically in regards to IgM.[175,177]

Antiphospholipid Antibody Syndrome

Autoimmune antiphospholipid antibodies (APLA) are a heterogeneous group of autoantibodies. The first APLA to be described was in the context of the Venereal Disease Research Laboratory

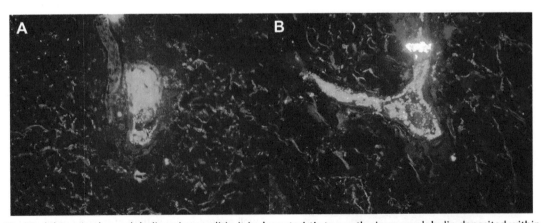

Fig. 15. (*A*) In mixed cryoglobulinemic vasculitis, it is characteristic to see the immunoglobulin deposited within vascular lumina. In this image there are prominent deposits of IgG. (*B*) This case shows prominent deposits of IgA within the vascular lumina in a patient with hepatitis C virus infection–associated mixed cryoglobulinemia with a monoclonal IgA rheumatoid factor.

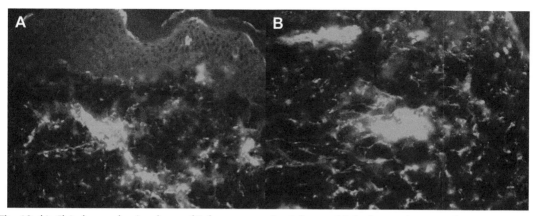

Fig. 16. (A, B) In hemorrhagic edema of infancy, approximately one-third of cases show IgA deposition. In our experience, it is apparent but not as prominent as other immunoglobulins, such as IgM.

(VDRL) test. It has long been known that patients with SLE have a higher frequency of false-positive VDRL and that this correlates with vascular events including migraines, livedo reticularis, and clotting events. The syphilis antigen is embedded in cardiolipin and thus sera that contains anticardiolipin antibodies may react to the embedded cardiolipin, producing the false-positive result. The VDRL test has low sensitivity and low specificity and should not be used as a screening test for APLA. Many APLA have been shown to target complexes of protein bound to phospholipid rather than phospholipid or protein alone. Phospholipid in isolation is not immunogenic, but is rendered immunogenic after the binding of certain proteins to it. These proteins have been erroneously referred to as cofactors because APLA could not be detected in their absence. The 2 proteins that were discovered first and studied most were B2-glycoprotein I and human thrombin. In some instances, the only APLA that is detectable is antiphosphatidyletha-nolamine. The IgG isotype of this unique APLA requires a cofactor, specifically a kinogen of low or high molecular weight. When the lupus anticoagulant assay is positive, there is a greater likelihood that the APLA present is associated with a thrombophilic tendency. The essence of the positive lupus anticoagulant assay is the blockage via the endogenous antibody of the in vitro assembly of the prothrombinase complex, resulting in a prolongation of certain in vitro clotting assays such as activated partial thromboplastin time, the dilute Russell viper venom time, the kaolin clotting time, and (rarely) the prothrombin time. These abnormalities are not reversed when the patient's plasma is diluted 1:1 with normal platelet-free plasma, a procedure that corrects clotting disorders caused by deficient clotting factors. Although the lupus anticoagulant would logically be expected to provoke a bleeding diathesis, the converse is true with arterial and venous thrombosis occurring in 25% to 50% of patients in whom the assay is positive.

Patients with APLA are divided into 6 clinical types: deep vein thrombosis and pulmonary embolus (type I), coronary or peripheral artery thrombosis (type II), cerebrovascular/retinal vessel thrombosis (type III), and the occasional patient who presents with mixtures of the foregoing (type IV). Type V patients are those with APLA and fetal wastage. It is unclear how many seemingly normal individuals who may never develop manifestations of APLA syndrome (type VI) harbor APLA.

Occlusive arterial and venous thrombi are found throughout the dermis and subcutis. An accompanying intramural lymphocytic infiltrate may be present. There is endothelial cell injury, but vessel wall necrosis is usually not present unless the patient has underlying collagen vascular disease.

DIF

Immunofluorescent testing has revealed granular deposits of C5b-9 within the cutaneous vasculature (**Fig. 17**), suggesting a role for humorally mediated vascular injury in the pathogenesis of the cutaneous lesions. C5b-9 may be a critical effector mechanism contributing to vascular thrombosis, which has led to an important therapeutic endeavor: the administration of eculizumab in cases of catastrophic APLA syndrome.[178]

Pathogenesis

Antiphospholipid antibodies are of IgG, IgA, and/or IgM isotypes. Mechanisms of thrombosis include complement-mediated injury via APLA binding to complexes comprising a protein cofactor (ie, β2

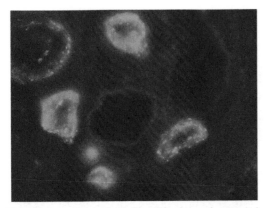

Fig. 17. In antiphospholipid antibody syndrome, it is characteristic to see extensive deposits of C5b-9 within the microvasculature. C5b-9 is likely an effector molecule in propagating vascular thrombosis. Eculizumab has been used to treat catastrophic antiphospholipid antibody syndrome.

glycoprotein, kininogen, and thrombin) and surface (ie, endothelial cell and platelet) phospholipids, leading to platelet aggregation and endothelial dysfunction respectively. Damaged endothelium leads to hidden antigen exposure, leading to a type II immune-based vascular injury syndrome.

IF Detection of Antiendothelial Cell Antibodies

Antibodies with endothelial cell specificity are thought to cause pathologic conditions in the context of APLA, HSP, and CTDs, including scleroderma, DM, MCTD, Behçet disease, and SLE; where they are detected in most patients.[179] Studies have shown that IgG or IgM from patients positive for antiendothelial cell antibodies were capable of causing antibody-dependent cellular cytotoxicity of human umbilical vein endothelial cells.[180–183] Clinical studies have established a link between the antiendothelial cell antibodies in sera and the severity of disease activity in various CTDs.[184]

Potential targeted antigens suggested in other studies focusing on antiendothelial cell antibodies include cytoskeletal proteins (β-actin, α-tubulin, and vimentin), glycolytic enzymes (glucose-3-phosphate-deshydrogenase and α-enolase), and prolyl-4-hydroxylase β subunit, a member of the disulfide isomerase family.[146,185,186]

The typical biopsy finding in those vascular injury syndromes attributed to antiendothelial cell antibodies is of endothelial cell necrosis and denudement, fibrin deposition, and vascular BMZ reduplication.

The frequency of positivity of the antiendothelial cell antibody assay in the setting of DM makes this IIF assay an important adjunct in the evaluation of patients in whom DM is suspected clinically. We typically conduct the assay on a single serum separator tube of blood and send the rest of the sample for the comprehensive myositis panel to the University of Oklahoma's research center. In any cutaneous thrombotic condition, this assay is part of the screening tool in elucidating the underlying cause of the vascular thrombosis. If the process reflects a defect in anticoagulation, such as in the setting of factor V Leiden, the assay is characteristically negative. However, if the process reflects an underlying systemic autoimmune diathesis and/or is attributable to APLA, the assay is strongly positive (Fig. 18).

IMMUNOFLUORESCENT MAPPING
Congenital Epidermolysis Bullosa

Epidermolysis bullosa can be broadly categorized into 4 variants. EBA is an autoimmune dermatosis caused by autoantibodies against the terminus of the noncollagenous α chain of type VII collagen, manifesting a conventional DIF profile indistinguishable from BP. However, salt-split skin studies are discriminatory by virtue of floor localization of immunoreactivity in EBA versus roof localization in BP. In EBA, autoantibodies directed against the terminus of the noncollagenous α chain of type VII collagen cause decreased anchoring in the lamina densa, and yield skin fragility and trauma-induced blisters. For the other forms of epidermolysis bullosa, a technique termed immunofluorescent mapping is used to identify the deficient components of the DEJ on a microanatomic basis.

Patients with congenital epidermolysis bullosa experience skin fragility and blisters that reflect

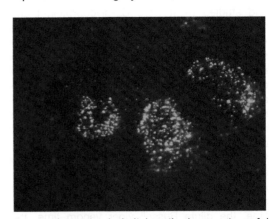

Fig. 18. The antiendothelial antibody assay is useful in certain clinical settings. This patient's serum has been incubated with generic endothelial cells. This granular nuclear pattern is a positive antiendothelial cell antibody assay. This patient had underlying dermatomyositis.

a genetic deficiency of critical BMZ proteins.[187–190] A specialized form of DIF assessment for endogenous BMZ components has emerged as an important diagnostic test in this particular clinical setting. A biopsy is obtained after provoking a blister by rotating a small spherical eraser over an area of skin on which there are no lesions until the epidermis separates from the dermis.

Cases of congenital epidermolysis bullosa are subclassified as 1 of 3 groups: (1) epidermolytic-epidermolysis bullosa simplex (EBS); (2) junctional epidermolysis bullosa (JEB); and (3) dermolytic-dystrophic epidermolysis bullosa (DEB). These categories are based on ultrastructural analysis of where the cleavage occurs, reflecting a congenital deficiency in the genes that encode specific proteins intrinsic to the epidermal BMZ. The nature of the deficient protein determines the subtype of epidermolysis bullosa. Immunofluorescent mapping using monoclonal antibodies directed at the specific epidermal BMZ human proteins defines a critical diagnostic adjunct in the evaluation of such cases and has largely replaced electron microscopy. The antibodies used are directed against human cytokeratin 5, cytokeratin 14, laminin 332, and type VII collagen, and have largely been developed in mice. In the setting of EBS, the deficiency in cytokeratins 5 and/or 14 is manifested by diminished and/or absent staining for these proteins. Minimal or absent staining for type XVII collagen and laminin 332 supports a diagnosis of JEB. DEB would be supported by an absence of, or markedly diminished, staining of antibodies directed against type VII collagen.

Alport Syndrome

In 1927, Cecil A. Alport described a hereditary nephritic disease characterized by progressive impairment of both aural and renal function. Some cases have eye defects as an additional symptom.[191] About 80% of patients inherit Alport syndrome as an X-linked trait, with mutations affecting the α5 chain of type IV collagen, resulting in end-stage renal disease.[192] Less commonly, the disease is inherited as an autosomal recessive or autosomal dominant trait.[193] Although Alport syndrome has been diagnosed primarily through electron microscopy, typically by examining the thinness of the glomerular basement membrane, the addition of IF studies can significantly increase the accuracy of diagnosis. For X-linked Alport syndrome, α5(IV) can be a useful diagnostic marker because it is present in both the glomerular basement membrane as well as the epidermis, whereas the α3(IV) and α4(IV) chains are not present in the skin. IF stains for α5(IV) in a normal skin sample show linear staining of the epidermal BMZ (**Fig. 19**). However, in those with X-linked Alport syndrome, the discontinuity of α5(IV) becomes more distinct compared with the normal linear staining and can even be completely absent.[193] In comparison, patients who inherited Alport syndrome through autosomal recessive or autosomal dominant traits show mutations at the α3(IV) and α4(IV) rather than at the α5(IV) chain, making the IF studies ineffective.

NONSPECIFIC IMMUNOFLUORESCENT PROFILES

It is important not to overinterpret immunoreactant deposition in the skin. Examining IF studies in a clinical vacuum can lead to misinterpretation, primarily overinterpretation of patterns that may not be pathogenically significant. However, several nonspecific patterns could potentially corroborate a particular clinical impression, and a negative test is also informative.

In the setting of eczema or psoriasis, the IF profile is similar even though the conditions are pathogenically distinct; there is nonspecific

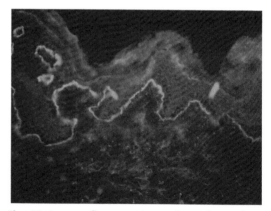

Fig. 19. Immunofluorescent mapping refers to incubating a patient's skin biopsy material with antibodies to components normally present in the skin to assess for a genetic deficiency of such components. This methodology is used in establishing a diagnosis of congenital epidermolysis bullosa or of Alport syndrome. This patient's skin biopsy has been incubated with antibodies to the α5 chain of type IV collagen. A strongly positive reaction is noted, therefore this patient dose not have deficient α5(IV) as seen in X-linked Alport syndrome. However, this does not exclude the possibility of the autosomal recessive or autosomal dominant forms of Alport syndrome caused by mutations of the α3 or α4 chains of type IV collagen. Because these chains of type IV collagen are normally not present in skin, Alport syndrome in which mutations in the α3 or α4 chains are pathogenetically significant cannot be diagnosed on a skin biopsy.

entrapment of immunoglobulin and complement within the stratum corneum and it is common to see some degree of C3, C3d, C4d, and/or C5b-9 within the epidermal BMZ and in blood vessels.

In the setting of type IV cytotoxic interface injury, IgM deposition in a granular fashion is observed along the DEJ in concert with a similar pattern of epidermal BMZ localization of components of complement and highlighting of colloid bodies. A distinctive feature is observed in those interface dermatitis syndromes in which the keratinocyte is rendered antigenic and evokes a memory T cell clonal response characterized by decoration of occasional spinous layer necrotic/apoptotic keratinocytes in a granular fashion by immunoglobulin and complement. The pattern differs from the more uniform pattern of granular cytoplasmic and nuclear staining affecting most keratinocytes in the setting of antibodies to an ENA (ie, SCLE or MCTD). In lichen planus, all of the findings discussed earlier are seen and there is a broad, homogeneous, intense band of staining for fibrinogen along the DEJ.

In hypersensitivity reactions in general, including those that are primarily dermal based, such as a persistent arthropod reaction, epidermal BMZ complement deposition including C5b-9 is common with variable deposition of IgM and complement including C5b-9 within the cutaneous vasculature. The staining can be extensive and, if there are supervening eczematous changes, entrapment of immunoglobulin and serum in the stratum corneum is common.

In many instances, the extent of IgM deposition along the DEJ is equivalent to a positive LBT in the context of a hypersensitivity reaction or androgenetic alopecia. Complement deposition within the follicular BMZ of involuting hairs is common.

In any patient with glucose intolerance, regardless of the rash biopsied, broad mantles of immunoglobulin and complement can be seen in the vessels. The specimen should not be misinterpreted as indicating PCT, pseudo-PCT, or bullosa diabeticorum.

Prominent deposits of C5b-9 and immunoglobulin within the BMZ of the eccrine coil is a common finding in all skin biopsies and should be discounted.

REFERENCES

1. Moll R, Moll I. Epidermal adhesion molecules and basement membrane components as target structures of autoimmunity. Virchows Arch 1998;432:487–504.

2. Bernard P, Bedane C, Bonnetblanc JM. Anti-BP 180 autoantibodies as a marker of poor prognosis in bullous pemphigoid: a cohort analysis of 94 elderly patients. Br J Dermatol 1997;136:694–6.

3. Bernard P, Reguiai Z, Tancrède-Bohin E, et al. Risk factors for relapse in patients with bullous pemphigoid in clinical remission: a multicenter, prospective, cohort study. Arch Dermatol 2009;145:537–42.

4. Patton T, Plunckett RW, Beutner EH, et al. IgG4 as the predominant IgG subclass in pemphigus gestationis. J Cutan Pathol 2006;33:299–302.

5. Iwata H, Kamio N, Aoyama Y, et al. IgG from patients with bullous pemphigoid depletes cultured keratinocytes of the 180-kDa bullous pemphigoid antigen (type XVII collagen) and weakens cell attachment. J Invest Dermatol 2009;129:919–26.

6. Iwata Y, Komura K, Kodera M, et al. Correlation of IgE autoantibody to BP180 with sever form of bullous pemphigoid. Arch Dermatol 2008;144:41–8.

7. Messingham KA, Noe MH, Chapman MA, et al. A novel ELISA reveals high frequencies of BP180-specific IgE production in bullous pemphigoid. J Immunol Methods 2009;346:18–25.

8. Jonkman M, De Jong M, Heeres K, et al. Generalized atrophic benign epidermolysis bullosa. Arch Dermatol 1996;132:145–50.

9. Horiguchi Y, Ueda M, Shimizu H, et al. An acquired bullous dermatosis due to an autoimmune reaction against uncein. Br J Dermatol 1996;134:934–8.

10. Ghohestani RF, Nicolas JF, Rousselle P, et al. Diagnostic value of indirect immunofluorescence on sodium chloride-split skin in differential diagnosis of subepidermal autoimmune bullous dermatoses. Arch Dermatol 1997;133:1102–7.

11. Gammon WR, Briggaman RA, Imman AO III, et al. Differentiating anti-lamina lucida and anti-sublamina densa anti-BMZ antibodies by indirect immunofluorescence on 1.0 M sodium chloride-separated skin. J Invest Dermatol 1984;82:139–44.

12. Gammon WR, Woodley DT, Dole KC, et al. Evidence that the anti-basement membrane zone antibodies in bullous eruption of systemic lupus erythematosus recognize epidermolysis bullosa acquisita autoantigen. J Invest Dermatol 1985;84:472–6.

13. Bernard P, Charneux J. Bullous pemphigoid: a review. Ann Dermatol Venereol 2011;138(3):173–81.

14. Crowson AN, Brown TJ, Magro CM. Progress in the understanding of the pathology and pathogenesis of cutaneous drug eruptions: implications for management. Am J Clin Dermatol 2003;4:407–42.

15. Jordon RE, Heine KG, Tappeiner G, et al. The immunopathology of herpes gestationis. immunofluorescence studies and characterization of "HG factor". J Clin Invest 1976;57(6):1426–31.

16. Bedocs PM, Kumar V, Mahon MJ. Pemphigoid gestationis: a rare case and review. Arch Gynecol Obstet 2009;279(2):235–8.

17. Egan CA, Yee C, Zillikens D, et al. Anti-p200 pemphigoid: diagnosis and treatment of a case presenting as an inflammatory subepidermal

blistering disease. J Am Acad Dermatol 2002;46(5): 786–9.

18. Miyakura T, Yamamoto T, Tashiro A, et al. Anti-p200 pemphigoid associated with annular pustular psoriasis. Eur J Dermatol 2008;18(4):481–2.

19. Zillikens D, Ishiko A, Jonkman MF, et al. Autoantibodies in anti-p200 pemphigoid stain skin lacking laminin 5 and type VII collagen. Br J Dermatol 2000;143:1043–9.

20. Verdolini R, Cerio R. Autoimmune subepidermal bullous skin diseases: the impact of recent findings for the dermatopathologist. Virchows Arch 2003; 443(2):184–93.

21. Smyth N, Vatansever HS, Meyer M, et al. The targeted deletion of the LAMC1 gene. Ann N Y Acad Sci 1998;857:283–6.

22. Dilling A, Rose C, Hashimoto T, et al. Anti-p200 pemphigoid: a novel autoimmune subepidermal blistering disease. J Dermatol 2007;34:1–8.

23. Rose C, Schmidt E, Kerstan A, et al. Histopathology of anti-laminin 5 mucous membrane pemphigoid. J Am Acad Dermatol 2009;61(3):433–40.

24. Jonkman MF, Schuur J, Dijk F, et al. Inflammatory variant of epidermolysis bullosa acquisita with IgG autoantibodies against type VII collagen and laminin alpha3. Arch Dermatol 2000;136:227–31.

25. Taniuchi K, Inaoki M, Nishimura Y, et al. Nonscarring inflammatory epidermolysis bullosa acquisita with esophageal involvement and linear IgG deposits. J Am Acad Dermatol 1997;36:320–2.

26. Hanno R, Foster DR, Bean SF. Brunsting-Perry cicatricial pemphigoid associated with bullous pemphigoid. J Am Acad Dermatol 1980;3(5):470–3.

27. Lenz P, Hsu R, Yee C, et al. Cicatricial pemphigoid with autoantibodies to laminin 5 (epiligrin) in a patient with metastatic endometrial carcinoma. Hautarzt 1998;49:31–5.

28. Gibson GE, Daoud MS, Pittelkow MR. Anti-epiligrin (laminin 5) cicatricial pemphigoid and lung carcinoma: coincidence or association? Br J Dermatol 1997;137:780–2.

29. Fujimoto W, Ishida-Yamamoto A, Hsu R, et al. Anti-epiligrin cicatricial pemphigoid: a case associated with gastric carcinoma and features resembling epidermolysis bullosa acquisita. Br J Dermatol 1998;139:682–7.

30. Robin H, Hoang-Xuan T, Prisant O, et al. Immunoelectron microscopic study of the conjunctiva in cicatricial pemphigoid. Graefes Arch Clin Exp Ophthalmol 1999;237(1):39–44.

31. Setterfield J, Shirlaw PJ, Kerr-Muir M, et al. Mucous membrane pemphigoid: a dual circulating antibody response with IgG and IgA signifies a more severe and persistent disease. Br J Dermatol 1998;138(4):602–10.

32. Murakami H, Nishioka S, Setterfield J, et al. Analysis of antigens targeted by circulating IgG and IgA autoantibodies in 50 patients with cicatricial pemphigoid. J Dermatol Sci 1998;17(1):39–44.

33. Balding SD, Prost C, Diaz LA, et al. Cicatricial pemphigoid autoantibodies react with multiple sites on the BP180 extracellular domain. J Invest Dermatol 1996;106:141–6.

34. Balding SD, Giudice GJ, Diaz LA, et al. Analysis of antigens targeted by circulating IgG and IgA autoantibodies in 50 patients with cicatricial pemphigoid. J Dermatol Sci 1998;17:39–44.

35. Bédane C, McMillan JR, Balding SD, et al. Bullous pemphigoid and cicatricial pemphigoid autoantibodies react with ultrastructurally separable epitopes on the BP180 ectodomain: evidence that BP180 spans the lamina lucida. J Invest Dermatol 1997;108:901–7.

36. Nakatani C, Muramatsu T, Shirai T. Immunoreactivity of bullous pemphigoid (BP) autoantibodies against the NC16A and C-terminal domains of the 180 kDa BP antigen (BP180): immunoblot analysis and enzyme-linked immunosorbent assay using BP180 recombinant proteins. Br J Dermatol 1998; 139:365–70.

37. Albrittion JL, Nousari HC, Anhalt G. Anti-epiligrin (laminin 5) cicatricial pemphigoid. Br J Dermatol 1997;137:992–6.

38. Chan L, Majmudar A, Tran H, et al. Laminin-6 and laminin-5 are recognized by autoantibodies in a subset of cicatricial pemphigoid. J Invest Dermatol 1997;108:848–53.

39. Lazarova Z, Hsu R, Yee C, et al. Antiepiligrin cicatricial pemphigoid represents an autoimmune response to subunits present in laminin 5. Br J Dermatol 1998;139:791–7.

40. Leverkus M, Bhol K, Hirako Y, et al. Cicatricial pemphigoid with circulating autoantibodies to beta4 integrin, bullous pemphigoid 180 and bullous pemphigoid 230. Br J Dermatol 2001;145: 998–1004.

41. Rashid KA, Gürcan HM, Ahmed AR. Antigen specificity in subsets of mucous membrane pemphigoid. J Invest Dermatol 2006;126:2631–6.

42. Leverkus M, Schmidt E, Lazarova Z, et al. Antiepiligrin cicatricial pemphigoid: an underdiagnosed entity within the spectrum of scarring autoimmune subepidermal bullous diseases? Arch Dermatol 1999;135(9):1091–8.

43. Umemoto N, Demitsu T, Toda S, et al. A case of anti-p200 pemphigoid clinically mimicking inflammatory epidermolysis bullosa acquisita. Br J Dermatol 2003;148(5):1058–60.

44. Elder MJ, Dart JK, Lightman S. Conjunctival fibrosis in ocular cicatricial pemphigoid–the role of cytokines. Exp Eye Res 1997;65:165–76.

45. Chang JH, McCluskey PJ. Ocular cicatricial pemphigoid: manifestations and management. Curr Allergy Asthma Rep 2005;5:333–8.

46. Foster CS, Sainz De La Maza M. Ocular cicatricial pemphigoid review. Curr Opin Allergy Clin Immunol 2004;4:435–9.

47. Ahmed M, Zein G, Khawaja F, et al. Ocular cicatricial pemphigoid: pathogenesis, diagnosis and treatment. Prog Retin Eye Res 2004;23:579–92.

48. Leonard J, Haffenden GP, Ring NP, et al. Linear IgA disease in adults. Br J Dermatol 1982;107:301–16.

49. Liesegang TJ. Conjunctival changes associated with glaucoma therapy: implications for the external disease consultant and the treatment of glaucoma. Cornea 1998;17:574–83.

50. Vodegel RM, Jonkman MF, Pas HH, et al. U-serrated immunodeposition pattern differentiates type VII collagen targeting bullous diseases from other forms of subepidermal bullous autoimmune diseases. Br J Dermatol 2004;151(1):112–8.

51. Nie Z, Hashimoto K. IgA antibodies of cicatricial pemphigoid sera specifically react with C-terminus of BP180. J Invest Dermatol 1999;112:254–5.

52. Kirtschig G, Mengel R, Mittag H, et al. Desquamative gingivitis and balanitis–linear IgA disease or cicatricial pemphigoid? Clin Exp Dermatol 1998; 23:173–7.

53. Caux F, Kirtschig G, Lemarchand-Venencie F, et al. IgA-epidermolysis bullosa acquisita in a child resulting in blindness. Br J Dermatol 1997;137:270–5.

54. Callot-Mellot C, Bodemer C, Caux F, et al. Epidermolysis bullosa acquisita in childhood. Arch Dermatol 1997;133:1122–6.

55. Hashimoto T, Ishiko A, Shimizu H, et al. A case of linear IgA bullous dermatosis with IgA anti-type VII collagen autoantibodies. Br J Dermatol 1996; 134:336–9.

56. Paige DG, Leonard JN, Wojnarowska F, et al. Linear IgA disease and ulcerative colitis. Br J Dermatol 1997;136:779–82.

57. De Simone C, Guerriero C, Pellicano R. Linear IgA disease and ulcerative colitis. Eur J Dermatol 1998; 8:48–50.

58. Nousari HC, Kimyai-Asadi A, Caeiro JP, et al. Clinical, demographic, and immunohistologic features of vancomycin-induced linear IgA bullous disease of the skin. Report of 2 cases and review of the literature. Medicine (Baltimore) 1999;78:1–8.

59. Paul C, Wolkenstein P, Prost C, et al. Drug-induced linear IgA disease: target antigens are heterogeneous. Br J Dermatol 1997;136:406–11.

60. Wakelin SH, Allen J, Zhou S, et al. Drug-induced linear IgA disease with antibodies to collagen VII. Br J Dermatol 1998;138:310–4.

61. Acostamadiedo JM, Perniciaro C, Rogers RS 3rd. Phenytoin-induced linear IgA bullous disease. J Am Acad Dermatol 1998;38:352–6.

62. Neughebauer BI, Negron G, Pelton S, et al. Bullous skin disease: an unusual allergic reaction to vancomycin. Am J Med Sci 2002;323(5):273–8.

63. Sillevis Smitt JH, Leusen JH, Stas HG, et al. Chronic bullous disease of childhood and a paecilomyces lung infection in chronic granulomatous disease. Arch Dis Child 1997;77:150–2.

64. Zhou S, Ferguson DJ, Allen J, et al. The localization of target antigens and autoantibodies in linear IgA disease is variable: correlation of immunogold electron microscopy and immunoblotting. J Br Dermatol 1998;139:591–7.

65. Schumann H, Baetge J, Tasanen K, et al. The shed ectodomain of collagen XVII/BP180 is targeted by autoantibodies in different blistering skin diseases. Am J Pathol 2000;156:685–95.

66. Egan CA, Reddy D, Nie Z, et al. IgG anti-LABD97 antibodies in bullous pemphigoid patients' sera react with the mid-portion of the BPAg2 ectodomain. J Invest Dermatol 2001;116:348–50.

67. Allen J, Zhou S, Wakelin SH, et al. Linear IgA disease: a report of two dermal binding sera which recognize a pepsin-sensitive epitope (?NC-1 domain) of collagen type VII. Br J Dermatol 1997;137:526–33.

68. Wojnarowska F, Whitehead P, Leigh IM, et al. Identification of the target antigen in chronic bullous disease of childhood and linear IgA disease of adults. Br J Dermatol 1991;124:157–62.

69. Marinkovich MP, Taylor TB, Keene DR, et al. LAD-1, the linear IgA bullous dermatosis autoantigen is a novel 120-kDa anchoring filament protein synthesized by epidermal cells. J Invest Dermatol 1996; 106:734–8.

70. Ishiko A, Shimizu H, Masunaga T, et al. 97 kDa linear IgA bullous dermatosis antigen localizes in the lamina lucida between the NC16A and carboxyl terminal domains of the 180 kDa bullous pemphigoid antigen. J Invest Dermatol 1998;111:93–6.

71. Ghohestani R, Nicolas JF, Kanitakis J, et al. Linear IgA bullous dermatosis with IgA antibodies exclusively directed against the 180- or 230 kDa epidermal antigens. J Invest Dermatol 1997;108:854–8.

72. Zone JJ, Taylor TB, Meyer LJ, et al. The 97 kDa linear IgA bullous disease antigen is identical to a portion of the extracellular domain of the 180 kDa bullous pemphigoid antigen, BPAg2. J Invest Dermatol 1998;110:207–10.

73. Collier PM, Wojnarowska F, Welsh K, et al. Adult linear IgA disease and chronic bullous disease of childhood: the association with human lymphocyte antigens Cw7, B8, DR3 and tumour necrosis factor influences disease expression. Br J Dermatol 1999; 141:867–75.

74. Hall RP. Dermatitis herpetiformis. J Invest Dermatol 1992;99:873–81.

75. Reunala T, Collins P. Diseases associated with dermatitis herpetiformis. Br J Dermatol 1997;136: 315–8.

76. Asano Y, Makino T, Ishida W, et al. Detection of antibodies to epidermal transglutaminase but not

tissue transglutaminase in Japanese patients with dermatitis herpetiformis. Br J Dermatol 2011; 164(4):883–4.

77. Salmhofer W, Kawahara Y, Soyer H. A subepidermal blistering disease with histopathological features of dermatitis herpetiformis and immunofluorescence characteristics of bullous pemphigoid: a novel subepidermal blistering disease or a variant of bullous pemphigoid? Br J Dermatol 1997;137: 599–604.

78. Jackson JM, Callen JP. Scarring alopecia and sclerodermatous changes of the scalp in a patient with hepatitis C infection. J Am Acad Dermatol 1998;39: 824–6.

79. O'Connor WJ, Badley AD, Dicken CH, et al. Porphyria cutanea tarda and human immunodeficiency virus: two cases associated with hepatitis C. Mayo Clin Proc 1998;73:895–7.

80. Rivera D, Lilli D, Griso D, et al. Hepatitis C virus in patients with porphyria cutanea tarda: relationship to HCV-genotypes. New Microbiol 1998;21:329–34.

81. Borroni G, Brazzelli V, Baldini F, et al. Flutamide-induced pseudoporphyria. Br J Dermatol 1998; 138:711–2.

82. O'Hagan AH, Irvine AD, Allen GE, et al. Pseudoporphyria induced by mefenamic acid. J Dermatol 1998;139:1131–2.

83. Varma S, Lanigan SW. Pseudoporphyria caused by nabumetone. Br J Dermatol 1998;138:549–50.

84. Magro CM, Crowson AN. Pseudo-porphyria cutanea tarda associated with nabumetone (Relafen) therapy. J Cutan Pathol 1999;26:42–7.

85. Lanconi G, Ravinal RC, Costa RS, et al. Mast cells and transforming growth factor-β expression: a possible relationship in the development of porphyria cutanea tarda skin lesions. Int J Dermatol 2008;47:575–81.

86. Fung MA, Murphy MJ, Hoss DM, et al. The sensitivity and specificity of "caterpillar bodies" in the differential diagnosis of subepidermal blistering disorders. Am J Dermatopathol 2003;25(4): 287–90.

87. Magro CM, Dyrsen ME. The use of C3d and C4d immunohistochemistry on formalin-fixed tissue as a diagnostic adjunct in the assessment of inflammatory skin disease. J Am Acad Dermatol 2008; 59(5):822–33.

88. Vasil KE, Magro CM. Cutaneous vascular deposition of C5B-9 and its role as a diagnostic adjunct in the setting of diabetes mellitus and porphyria cutanea tarda. J Am Acad Dermatol 2007;56:96–104.

89. Torinuki W, Miura T, Tagami H. Activation of complement by 405-nm light in serum from porphyria cutanea tarda. Arch Dermatol Res 1985;277(3):174–8.

90. Torinuki W, Miura T, Tagami H. Activation of the alternative complement pathway by 405 nm light

in serum from porphyric rat. Acta Derm Venereol 1984;64(5):367–72.

91. Qin X, Goldfine A, Krumrei N, et al. Glycation inactivation of the complement regulatory protein CD59: a possible role in the pathogenesis of the vascular complications of human diabetes. Diabetes 2004;53(10):2653–61.

92. Eaton DP, Diaz LA, Hans-Filho G, et al. Comparison of black fly species (Diptera: Simuliidae) on an Amerindian reservation with a high prevalence of fogo selvagem to neighboring disease-free sites in the State of Mato Grosso do Sul, Brazil. The Cooperative Group on Fogo Selvagem Research. J Med Entomol 1998;35:120–31.

93. Howard MS, Yepes MM, Maldonado-Estrada JG, et al. Broad histopathologic patterns of nonglabrous skin and glabrous skin from patients with a new variant of endemic pemphigus foliaceus-part 1. J Cutan Pathol 2010;37(2):222–30.

94. Santi C, Maruta C, Aoki V, et al. Pemphigus herpetiformis is a rare clinical expression of nonendemic pemphigus foliaceus, fogo selvagem, and pemphigus vulgaris. J Am Acad Dermatol 1996;34:40–6.

95. Kubo A, Amagai M, Hashimoto T, et al. Herpetiform pemphigus showing reactivity with pemphigus vulgaris antigen (desmoglein 3). Br J Dermatol 1997; 137:109–13.

96. Brenner S, Golan AB, Anhalt G. Recognition of pemphigus antigens in drug-induced pemphigus vulgaris and pemphigus foliaceus. J Am Acad Dermatol 1997;36:919–23.

97. Brenner S, Ruocco VD. Penicillamine-induced pemphigus foliaceus with autoantibodies to desmoglein-1. J Am Acad Dermatol 1998;39:137–8.

98. Sklavounou A, Laskaris G. Paraneoplastic pemphigus: a review. Oral Oncol 1998;34:437–40.

99. Sehgal VN, Srivastava G. Paraneoplastic pemphigus/paraneoplastic autoimmune multiorgan syndrome. Int J Dermatol 2009;48:162–9.

100. Wang J, Kwon J, Ding X, et al. Nonsecretory IgA1 autoantibodies targeting desmosomal component desmoglein 3 in intraepidermal neutrophilic IgA dermatosis. Am J Pathol 1997;150(6):1901–7.

101. Lee FJ, Silvestrini R, Fulcher DA. False-positive intercellular cement substance antibodies due to group A/B red cell antibodies: frequency and approach. Pathology 2010;42(6):574–7.

102. Shirakata Y, Amagai M, Hanakawa Y, et al. Lack of mucosal involvement in pemphigus foliaceus may be due to low expression of desmoglein 1. J Invest Dermatol 1998;110(1):76–8.

103. Jiao D, Bystryn JC. Antibodies to desmoplakin in a patient with pemphigus foliaceous. J Eur Acad Dermatol Venereol 1998;11:169–72.

104. Hashimoto T, Ebihara T, Dmochowski M, et al. IgA antikeratinocyte surface autoantibodies from two types of intercellular IgA vesiculopustular

dermatosis recognize distinct isoforms of desmocollin. Arch Dermatol Res 1996;288:447–52.

105. Hashimoto T, Kiyokawa C, Mori O, et al. Human desmocollin 1 (Dsc1) is an autoantigen for the subcorneal pustular dermatosis type of IgA pemphigus. J Invest Dermatol 1997;109:127–31.

106. Foedinger D, Sterniczky B, Elbe A, et al. Autoantibodies against desmoplakin I and II define a subset of patients with erythema multiforme major. J Invest Dermatol 1996;106:1012–6.

107. Ghohestani R, Joly P, Gilbert D, et al. Autoantibody formation against a 190-kDa antigen of the desmosomal plaque in pemphigus foliaceus. Br J Dermatol 1997;137(5):774–9.

108. Amagai M, Nishikawa T, Nousari HC, et al. Antibodies against desmoglein 3 (pemphigus vulgaris antigen) are present in sera from patients with paraneoplastic pemphigus and cause acantholysis in vivo in neonatal mice. J Clin Invest 1998;102:775–82.

109. Amagai M, Tsunoda K, Zillikens D, et al. The clinical phenotype of pemphigus is defined by the anti-desmoglein autoantibody profile. J Am Acad Dermatol 1999;40(2 Pt 1):167–70.

110. Mahoney MG, Aho S, Uitto J, et al. The members of the plakin family of proteins recognized by paraneoplastic pemphigus antibodies include periplakin. J Invest Dermatol 1998;111:308–13.

111. Chorxelski TP, Hashimoto T, Jablonska S. Paraneoplastic pemphigus. Are autoantibodies pathogenic or an epiphenomenon? A reply. Eur J Dermatol 1996;2:152–3.

112. Huang Y, Li J, Zhu X. Detection of anti-envoplakin and anti-periplakin autoantibodies by ELISA in patients with paraneoplastic pemphigus. Arch Dermatol Res 2009;301:703–9.

113. Mascaro JM Jr, España A, Liu Z, et al. Mechanisms of acantholysis in pemphigus vulgaris: role of IgG valence. Clin Immunol Immunopathol 1997;85(1):90–6.

114. Al-Suwaid AR, Venkataram MN, Bhushnurmath SR. Cutaneous lupus erythematosus: comparison of direct immunofluorescence findings with histopathology. Int J Dermatol 1995;34:480–2.

115. Burnham TK, Neblett TR, Fine G. Immunofluorescent "band" test for lupus erythematosus. II. Employing skin lesions. Arch Dermatol 1970;102:42–50.

116. Harrist TJ, Mihm MC Jr. Cutaneous immunopathology. The diagnostic use of direct and indirect immunofluorescence techniques in dermatologic disease. Hum Pathol 1979;10:625–53.

117. Harrist TJ, Mihm MC Jr. The specificity and clinical usefulness of the lupus band test. Arthritis Rheum 1980;23:479–90.

118. Provost TT. Lupus band test. Int J Dermatol 1981; 20:475–81.

119. Smith CD, Marino C, Rothfield NF. The clinical utility of the lupus band test. Arthritis Rheum 1984;27:382–7.

120. Jordon RE. Lupus band test: clinical applications. Clin Dermatol 1985;3:113–22.

121. Magro CM, Crowson AN. The application of immunofluorescence testing in diagnostic dermatopathology. In: Cockerell CJ, editor. Advances in dermatology. St Louis (MO): Mosby; 1999. p. 441–86.

122. Cardinali C, Caproni M, Fabbri P. The utility of the lupus band test on sun-protected non-lesional skin for the diagnosis of systemic lupus erythematosus. Clin Exp Rheumatol 1999;17:427–32.

123. Leibold AM, Bennion S, David-Bajar K, et al. Occurrence of positive immunofluorescence in the dermoepidermal junction of sun-exposed skin of normal adults. J Cutan Pathol 1994;21:200–6.

124. Weigand DA. Lupus band test: anatomic regional variations in discoid lupus erythematosus. J Am Acad Dermatol 1986;14:426–8.

125. Magro CM, Crowson AN. The immunofluorescent profile of dermatomyositis. A comparative study with lupus erythematosus. J Cutan Pathol 1997; 24:543–52.

126. Kondo S, Tone M, Teramoto N, et al. Clinical studies of 15 cases of progressive systemic sclerosis (PSS) associated with positive proteinuria and membranous glomerulonephritis. Nippon Hifuka Gakkai Zasshi 1989;99:1105–10 [in Japanese].

127. Shibeshi D, Blaszczyk M, Jarzabek-Chorzelska M, et al. Immunopathologic findings in systemic sclerosis patients: clinical and immunopathologic relationships. Int J Dermatol 1989;28:650–6.

128. Magro CM, Crowson AN, Harrist TJ. The use of antibody to C5b-9 in the subclassification of lupus erythematosus. Br J Dermatol 1996;134:855–62.

129. Provost TT, Andres G, Maddison PJ, et al. Lupus band test in untreated SLE patients: correlation of immunoglobulin deposition in the skin of the extensor forearm with clinical renal disease and serological abnormalities. J Invest Dermatol 1980; 74:407–12.

130. Liu T, Liu FR. Prognostic value of lupus band test in unexposed normal skin of patients with systemic lupus erythematosus. Chin Med J 1989;102:620–4.

131. Gilliam JN. The significance of cutaneous immunoglobulin deposits in lupus erythematosus and NZB/NZW F1 hybrid mice. J Invest Dermatol 1975;65: 154–61.

132. Helm KF, Peters MS. Deposition of membrane attack complex in cutaneous lesions of lupus erythematosus. J Am Acad Dermatol 1993;28:687–91.

133. Crowson AN, Magro CM. C5b-9 deposition at the dermoepidermal junction in lupus erythematosus. J Am Acad Dermatol 1994;31:515–6.

134. Crowson AN, Magro CM. The role of microvascular injury in the pathogenesis of cutaneous lesion of dermatomyositis. Hum Pathol 1996;26:14–9.

135. Magro CM, Crowson AN. The cutaneous pathology associated with seropositivity for antibodies to Ro:

a clinicopathological study of 23 adult patients without subacute cutaneous lupus erythematosus. Am J Dermatopathol 1999;21:129–37.

136. Provost TT, Talal N, Harley JB, et al. The relationship between anti-Ro(SS-A) antibody-positive Sjogren's syndrome and anti-Ro(SS-A) antibody-positive lupus erythematosus. Arch Dermatol 1988;124:63–71.

137. Crowson AN, Magro CM. Subacute cutaneous lupus erythematosus arising in the setting of calcium channel blocker therapy. Hum Pathol 1997;28:67–73.

138. Sousa JX Jr, Miyamoto D, Zimbres JM, et al. Clinicopathological evaluation of in vivo epidermal nuclear fluorescence. Clin Exp Dermatol 2009; 34(3):314–8.

139. Magro CM, Crowson AN, Regauer S. Mixed connective tissue disease. A clinical, histologic, and immunofluorescence study of eight cases. Am J Dermatopathol 1997;19:206–13.

140. Furukawa F, Lyons MB, Lee LA, et al. Estradiol enhances binding to cultured human keratinocytes of antibodies specific for SS-A/Ro and SS-B/La. Another possible mechanism for estradiol influence of lupus erythematosus. J Immunol 1988;141:1480–8.

141. Furukawa F, Kahihara-Sawami M, Lyons MB, et al. Binding of antibodies to ENA SS-A/Ro and SS-B/La is induced on the surface of human keratinocytes by UVL: implications for the pathogenesis of photosensitive cutaneous lupus. J Invest Dermatol 1990;94:77–85.

142. Lanto B, Bohm F, Meffert H, et al. The cytotoxic effect of anti-Ro- (SS-A) antibodies and UVA light on human endothelial cells in vitro. Dermatol Monatsschr 1990;176:305–11 [in German].

143. Ben-Chetrit E. The molecular basis of the SSA/Ro antigens and the clinical significance of their autoantibodies. Br J Rheumatol 1993;32:396–402.

144. Norris DA, Lee LA. Antibody-dependent cellular cytotoxicity and skin disease. J Invest Dermatol 1985;85(Suppl 1):165S–75S.

145. Norris DA. Pathomechanisms of photosensitive lupus erythematosus. J Invest Dermatol 1993;100: 58S–68S.

146. Magro CM, Ross P, Marsh CB, et al. The role of anti-endothelial cell antibody-mediated microvascular injury in the evolution of pulmonary fibrosis in the setting of collagen vascular disease. Am J Clin Pathol 2007;127(2):237–47.

147. Alexander E, Provost T, Sanders M, et al. Serum complement activation in central nervous system disease in Sjogren's syndrome. Am J Med 1988; 85:513–8.

148. Prapotnik S, Bozic B, Kveder T, et al. Fluctuation of anti-Ro/SS-A antibody levels in patients with systemic lupus erythematosus and Sjogren's syndrome: a prospective study. Clin Exp Rheumatol 1999;17:63–8.

149. LaFleur L, Kuykendall T, Crowson AN, et al. Vesiculo-bullous systemic lupus erythematosus in a 4 year old girl presenting as mixed bullous dermatosis of childhood. J Am Acad Dermatol 2006; 54(3):AB139.

150. Burrows NP, Bhogal BS, Black MM, et al. Bullous eruption of systemic lupus erythematosus: a clinicopathological study of four cases. Br J Dermatol 1993;128:332.

151. Rappersberger K, Tschachler E, Tani M, et al. Bullous disease in systemic lupus erythematosus. J Am Acad Dermatol 1989;21:745.

152. Yell JA, Allen J, Wojnarowska F, et al. Bullous systemic lupus erythematosus: revised criteria for diagnosis. Br J Dermatol 1995;132:921.

153. Borradori L, Hohl D, Monteil M, et al. Bullous systemic lupus erythematosus. Dermatology 1993;187:306.

154. Barton DD, Fine JD, Gammon WR, et al. Bullous systemic lupus erythematosus: an unusual clinical course and detectable circulating autoantibodies to the epidermolysis bullosa acquisita antigen. J Am Acad Dermatol 1986;15(2 Pt 2):369–73.

155. Jones DA, Hunt SW 3rd, Prisayanh PS, et al. Immunodominant autoepitopes of type VII collagen are short, paired peptide sequences within the fibronectin type III homology region of the noncollagenous (NC1) domain. J Invest Dermatol 1995;104:231–5.

156. Shirahama S, Furukawa F, Yagi H, et al. Bullous systemic lupus erythematosus: detection of antibodies against noncollagenous domain of type VII collagen. J Am Acad Dermatol 1998;38:844–8.

157. Ishikawa O, Zaw K, Miyachi Y, et al. The presence of anti-basement zone antibodies in the sera of patients with non-bullous lupus erythematosus. Br J Dermatol 1997;136:222–6.

158. Vandergheynst F, Ocmant A, Sordet C, et al. Anti-pm/scl antibodies in connective tissue disease: clinical and biological assessment of 14 patients. Clin Exp Rheumatol 2006;24(2):129–33.

159. Toll A, Monfort J, Benito P, et al. Sclerodermatomyositis associated with severe arthritis. Dermatol Online J 2004;10(2):18.

160. García-Patos V, Bartralot R, Fonollosa V, et al. Childhood sclerodermatomyositis: report of a case with the anti-PM/Scl antibody and mechanic's hands. Br J Dermatol 1996;135(4):613–6.

161. Helm T, Valenzuela R. Continuous dermoepidermal junction IgM detected by direct immunofluorescence: a report of nine cases. J Am Acad Dermatol 1992;26:203–6.

162. Velthuis PJ, Jong MCJM, Kruis MH. Is there a linear IgM dermatosis? Significance of linear IgM junctional staining in cutaneous immunopathology. Acta Derm Venereol (Stockh) 1988;68:8–14.

163. Acalay J, Ingber A, David M, et al. Linear IgM dermatosis of pregnancy. J Am Acad Dermatol 1988;18:412–5.

164. Whittaker SJ, Bhogal BS, Black MM. Acquired immunobullous disease: a cutaneous manifestation of IgM macroglobulinaemia. Br J Dermatol 1996; 135:283–6.

165. Barnadas MA, Pérez E, Gich I, et al. Diagnostic, prognostic and pathogenic value of the direct immunofluorescence test in cutaneous leukocytoclastic vasculitis. Int J Dermatol 2004;43(1):19–26.

166. Magro CM, Crowson AN. A clinical and histologic study of 37 cases of immunoglobulin A associated vasculitis. Am J Dermatopathol 1999;21(3):234–40.

167. Mills JA, Michel BA, Bloch DA, et al. The American College of Rheumatology 1990 criteria for the classification of Henoch-Schönlein purpura. Arthritis Rheum 1990;33(8):1114–21.

168. Kawakami T, Watabe H, Mizoguchi M, et al. Elevated serum IgA anticardiolipin antibody levels in adult Henoch-Schönlein purpura. Br J Dermatol 2006;154:983–7.

169. Cioc AM, Sedmak DD, Nuovo GJ, et al. Parvovirus B19 associated adult Henoch Schönlein purpura. J Cutan Pathol 2002;29(10):602–7.

170. Crowson AN, Usmani A, Magro CM, et al. Immunoglobulin-A associated lymphocytic vasculopathy: a clinical and pathological entity resembling pigmentary purpura. J Cutan Pathol 2002;29:596–601.

171. Greer JM, Longley S, Edwards NL, et al. Vasculitis associated with malignancy. Experience with 13 patients and literature review. Medicine (Baltimore) 1988;67(4):220–30.

172. Pertuiset E, Lioté F, Launay-Russ E, et al. Adult Henoch-Schönlein purpura associated with malignancy. Semin Arthritis Rheum 2000;29(6):360–7.

173. Timmeren MM, Chen M, Heeringa P. Review article: pathogenic role of complement activation in anti-neutrophil cytoplasmic auto-antibody-associated vasculitis. Nephrology (Carlton) 2009;14(1):16–25.

174. AlSufyani MA. Acute hemorrhagic edema of infancy: unusual scarring and review of the English language literature. Int J Dermatol 2009;48(6):617–22.

175. Karremann M, Jordan AJ, Bell N, et al. Acute hemorrhagic edema of infancy: report of 4 cases and review of the current literature. Clin Pediatr (Phila) 2009;48(3):323–6.

176. da Silva Manzoni AP, Viecili JB, de Andrade CB, et al. Acute hemorrhagic edema of infancy: a case report. Int J Dermatol 2004;43(1):48–51.

177. Lai-Cheong JE, Banerjee P, Hill V, et al. Bullous acute haemorrhagic oedema of skin in infancy. Clin Exp Dermatol 2007;32(4):467–8.

178. Lonze BE, Singer AL, Montgomery RA. Eculizumab and renal transplantation in a patient with CAPS. N Engl J Med 2010;362(18):1744–5.

179. Shingu M, Hurd ER. Sera from patients with systemic lupus erythematosus reactive with human endothelial cells. J Rheumatol 1981;8(4):581–6.

180. Tripathy NK, Upadhyaya S, Sinha N, et al. Complement and cell mediated cytotoxicity by antiendothelial cell antibodies in Takayasu's arteritis. J Rheumatol 2001;28:805–8.

181. Kaneko K, Savage CO, Pottinger BE, et al. Antiendothelial cell antibodies can be cytotoxic to endothelial cells without cytokine pre-stimulation and correlate with ELISA antibody measurement in Kawasaki disease. Clin Exp Immunol 1994;98:264–9.

182. del Papa N, Meroni PL, Barcellini W, et al. Antibodies to endothelial cells in primary vasculitides mediate in vitro endothelial cytotoxicity in the presence of normal peripheral blood mononuclear cells. Clin Immunol Immunopathol 1992;63:267–74.

183. Negi VS, Tripathy NK, Misra R, et al. Antiendothelial cell antibodies in scleroderma correlate with severe digital ischemia and pulmonary arterial hypertension. J Rheumatol 1998;25:462–6.

184. Magro CM, Pope Harman A, Klinger D, et al. Use of C4d as a diagnostic adjunct in lung allograft biopsies. Am J Transplant 2003;3:1143–54.

185. Ationu A. Identification of endothelial antigens relevant to transplant coronary artery disease from a human endothelial cell cDNA expression library. Int J Mol Med 1998;1(6):1007–10.

186. Alvarez-Marquez A, Aguilera I, Blanco RM, et al. Positive association of anticytoskeletal endothelial cell antibodies and cardiac allograft rejection. Hum Immunol 2008;69(3):143–8.

187. Cepeda-Valdes R, Pohla-Gubo G, Borbolla-Escoboza JR, et al. Immunofluorescence mapping for diagnosis of congenital epidermolysis bullosa. Actas Dermosifiliogr 2010;101(8):673–82 [in Spanish].

188. Abrams ML, Smidt A, Benjamin L, et al. Congenital epidermolysis bullosa acquisita: vertical transfer of maternal autoantibody from mother to infant. Arch Dermatol 2011;147(3):337–41.

189. Hintner H, Stingl G, Schuler G, et al. Immunofluorescence mapping of antigenic determinants within the dermal-epidermal junction in the mechanobullous diseases. J Invest Dermatol 1981;76(2):113–8.

190. Heagerty AH, Kennedy AR, Leigh IM, et al. Identification of an epidermal basement membrane defect in recessive forms of dystrophic epidermolysis bullosa by LH 7:2 monoclonal antibody: use in diagnosis. Br J Dermatol 1986;115(2):125–31.

191. Van Agtmael T, Bruckner-Tuderman L. Basement membranes and human disease. Cell Tissue Res 2010;339(1):167–88.

192. Lagona E, Tsartsali L, Kostaridou S, et al. Skin biopsy for the diagnosis of Alport syndrome. Hippokratia 2008;12(2):116–8.

193. Haas M. Alport syndrome and thin glomerular basement membrane nephropathy: a practical approach to diagnosis. Arch Pathol Lab Med 2009;133(2):224–32.

New Directions in Dermatopathology
In Vivo Confocal Microscopy in Clinical Practice

Caterina Longo, MD[a], Iris Zalaudek, MD[b],
Giuseppe Argenziano, MD[a], Giovanni Pellacani, MD[c],*

KEYWORDS

- In vivo confocal microscopy • Skin tumors • Inflammatory diseases • Infectious diseases

KEY POINTS

- Reflectance confocal microscopy (RCM) is a novel noninvasive imaging technique that enables the identification of cells and tissues with nearly histologic resolution.
- In the epidermis, keratinocytes are clearly visualized as small polygonal nucleated structures, and epidermal alterations, such as acanthosis, hyperkeratosis, exocytosis, and spongiosis, and others can be easily identified.
- RCM also enables the visualization of dermal structures up to the papillary dermis.
- In melanocytic and epithelial skin tumors, cytologic atypia as well as architectural disarrangement can be visualized, helping in the achievement of a more accurate diagnosis.
- The application in inflammatory and infectious skin diseases showed good correlation with microscopic findings, although inflammatory cell subpopulations cannot be distinguished.

INTRODUCTION

Reflectance confocal microscopy (RCM) represents a new imaging tool that enables the identification of cells and tissues with nearly histologic resolution.[1–3] Although several noninvasive tools have been explored to test their potential application in the clinical field, RCM has emerged as a unique instrument because it can visualize the skin tissue with a resolution that is comparable with conventional histopathology. It allows a horizontal scanning of the imaged tissue, with the advantage of exploring a larger field of view compared with vertical sectioning. Moreover, the horizontal plane offers a perfect correlation with clinical and dermoscopic aspects, which is crucial when dealing with skin tumor diagnosis. In this article, we present the main confocal findings and their correlations with histopathology along with a brief description of confocal applications in the clinic arena.

INSTRUMENTS

The commercially available confocal microscope (VivaScope 1500, Lucid, Rochester, NY) contains a probe (the head of the microscope), which is attached to the skin by using a disposable plastic window, which is in turn taped to a metal ring. A confocal microscope consists of a point source of light, condenser, objective lenses, and a point detector.[1,2] The pinhole collects light emanating only from the in focus plane. The mechanism of bright contrast in RCM is backscattering. In grayscale confocal images, structures that appear bright (white) have components with high refractive

No conflict of interest to disclose.

[a] Dermatology and Skin Care Unit, Arcispedale Santa Maria Nuova-IRCCS, Viale Risorgimento 80, 42100 Reggio Emilia, Italy; [b] Department of Dermatology, University of Graz, Austria; [c] Dermatology Unit, University of Modena and Reggio Emilia, via del Pozzo 71, 41124 Modena, Italy
* Corresponding author.
E-mail address: pellacani.giovanni@gmail.com

index compared with their surroundings and are similar in size to the wavelength of light. Backscattering is primarily governed by the refractive index of the structure compared with surrounding medium. Highly reflective skin components include melanin, collagen, and keratin. The confocal scanning produces high-resolution black-and-white horizontal images (0.5 × 0.5 mm) with a lateral resolution of 1.0 μm and axial resolution of 3 to 5 μm. A sequence of full-resolution individual images at a given depth is acquired and stitched together to create a mosaic ranging in size from 2 × 2 mm to 8 × 8 mm. For inflammatory or physiologic skin conditions, a 3 × 3 mm VivaCube (Lucid, Rochester, NY) composed of 4 mosaics with a 25-μm step is usually acquired, whereas for skin tumor examination, the imaging should include the entire lesion. Besides the horizontal mosaic, a vertical VivaStack can be imaged. It consists of single high-resolution images acquired from the top skin surface up to 200 μm, corresponding to the papillary dermis, to obtain a sort of optic biopsy. The VivaStack (Lucid, Rochester, NY) modality is useful for the assessment of the epidermal thickness either in physiologic condition or in the presence of dysfunctional epidermis.

Recently, a handheld RCM has been introduced on the market (VivaScope 3000). This version is a smaller, flexible device, which is useful in areas that are difficult to access (eg, skin folds, ears). Unlike the 1500 version, it has an on-instrument control for laser power, imaging depth, and capture but it does not allow scanning of a large field of view, which is needed, for example, in some tumors to obtain an overview of the architecture. However, it is a promising tool, which can be used for surgical premapping or when multiple site imaging is requested.

MAIN HISTOPATHOLOGIC CORRELATES OF CONFOCAL CRITERIA
Epidermis

The epidermis can be affected by several injuries that lead to different morphologic changes involving the keratinocytes (KCs) or other cells of the epidermis, such as melanocytes.

The epidermal changes are described as phenomenon per se regardless of their relationship with either inflammatory or skin tumors.

In healthy young skin, the epidermis appears as a multilayer tissue with paradigmatic confocal aspects depending on the skin level.[4,5] The stratum corneum appears as a highly refractive surface surrounded by visible skin furrows. At this level, the corneocytes are large, ranging from 10 to 30 μm, polygonal, and without a visible nucleus. Skin furrows appear as dark folds between islands of KCs. In young people, the skin furrows are arranged in a rhomboidal pattern formed by intersecting skin furrows. However, the shape and arrangement of the skin folds strongly depends on the body site (being almost absent on the forehead and well represented on the abdomen) and the individual's age. The stratum granulosum is composed of polygonal KCs presenting a bright and grainy cytoplasm because of the presence of organelles. The KCs cohesively assemble, forming a structure that gives rise to a honeycombed pattern.[5] The contour of the cell is usually brighter than the cytoplasm and perfectly outlined. Pigmented KCs are usually bright cells, small in size and always polygonal, separated by a darker contour (cobblestone pattern), resembling the negative of the honeycombed pattern. In the honeycombed pattern, the KCs appear black with bright contour, whereas in the cobblestone pattern, these cells show a bright cytoplasm because of the high melanin content (ie, brightness) (**Fig. 1**). On the face, a peculiar pattern is caused by the presence of numerous hair follicles that appear as dark round areas (donutlike appearance, H Rabinovitz, personal observation). At the stratum spinosum level, the size of KCs tends to decrease but the cells still have a polygonal shape. The honeycombed pattern is easily observable.

Acanthosis is one of the most frequent findings and it can be observed in several conditions. Histopathologically, acanthosis is defined as diffuse epidermal hyperplasia caused by the increased thickness of the stratum spinosum constituted by the prickle cells.

Because of the horizontal sectioning, only an indirect correlate with acanthosis is feasible on RCM. The granulosum and spinosum layers of an acanthotic epidermis consist of islands of KCs with broadened greyish outlines (**Fig. 2**). Moreover, when using the VivaStack modality, an increased thickness of the stratum granulosum/spinosum can be detected and measured by counting the layers.

Dermoepidermal Junction

Below the spinous layer, there is a single layer of basal cells at the dermoepidermal junction (DEJ).[4] Basal cells are uniform in size and shape but are smaller and more refractive than spinous KCs because of the melanin caps forming bright disks on top of the nuclei. The brightness of KCs is strongly dependent on the skin phototype. Dark skin phototypes show basal KCs that are bright round cells with highly refractive cytoplasm forming a cobblestone pattern at the epidermal level and

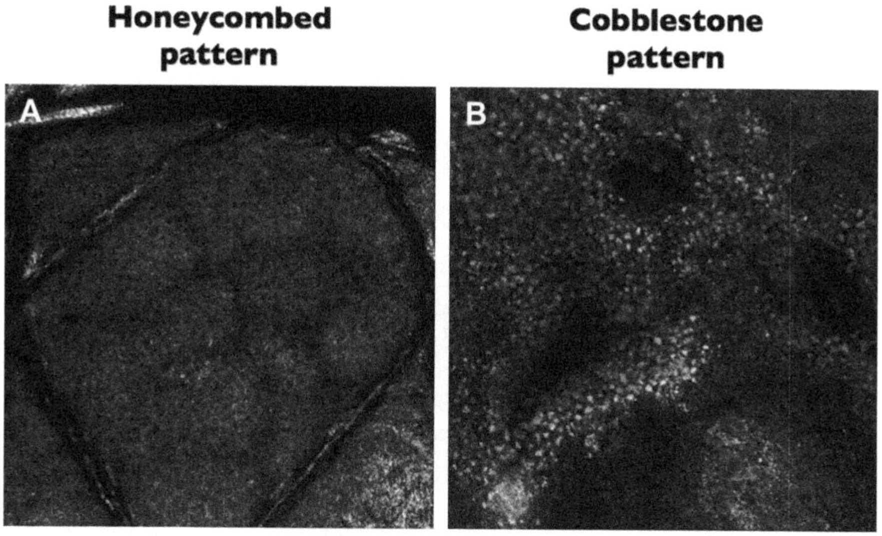

Honeycombed pattern

Cobblestone pattern

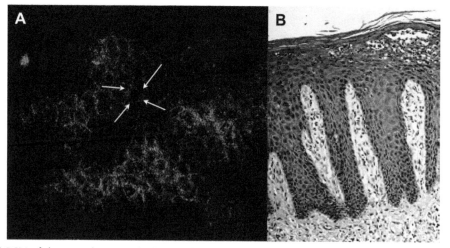

Fig. 1. (*A*) The honeycombed pattern is constituted by polygonal KCs, which appear black with bright contour with RCM, whereas in the cobblestone pattern (*B*), these cells show a bright cytoplasm caused by the high melanin content and are separated by a darker contour.

bright rings at the dermoepidermal junction level. On the other hand, skin phototype I-II are characterized by basal KCs with low refractivity that constitute barely visible dermal papillae (**Fig. 3**). At the dermoepidermal level, in the presence of regular rete-ridges, basal cells form round or oval rings of bright cells (KCs) surrounding dark dermal papillae. Within the dark dermal papillae, it is possible to visualize tiny canalicular blood vessels.

In solar lentigos and in seborrheic keratosis, the DEJ reveals small bud-acanthotic proliferations, often anastomosing, and hyperpigmentation of the basal layer. This histologic finding translates into polycyclic bright contours or bulbous projections caused by the anastomosing elongated structures, separated by dark areas (**Fig. 4**), on horizontal plane RCM.[6]

In skin cancer and in melanocytic proliferations, the DEJ is often distorted and occupied by tumor proliferations. In nevi, junctional nests can be seen as compact, well-outlined, roundish-to-oval structures, sometimes connected with the epidermis.[7,8] In some instances, a few atypical large and bright cells can occasionally be found in nevi.

Acanthosis

Fig. 2. (*A*) RCM of the granulosum and spinosum layers of an acanthotic epidermis consist of islands of KCs with broadened greyish outlines (*arrows*). (*B*) The histopathologic correlate is psoriasis.

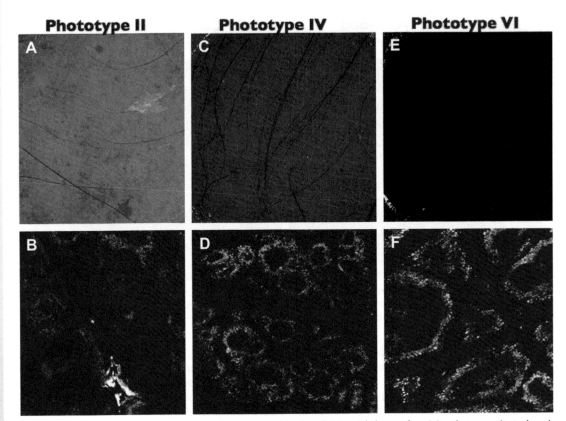

Phototype II   **Phototype IV**   **Phototype VI**

Fig. 3. (*A*) Light skin phototypes (I-II) are characterized by basal KCs with low refractivity that constitute barely visible dermal papillae on RCM (*B*). (*C, E*) Darker skin phototypes (IV-VI) show basal KCs that are bright cells with highly refractive cytoplasm forming bright rings at the DEJ level on RCM (*D, F*).

Many junctional nests form the so-called meshwork pattern (**Fig. 5**). This pattern is made by the enlargement of the interpapillary spaces formed by aggregated cells or clusters bulging within the dermal papilla in contiguity with the basal layer. When several nests are located within the dermal papillae, the general architecture is called clod pattern and corresponds to the presence of dermal

Solar lentigo

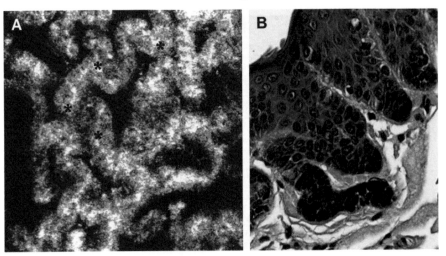

Fig. 4. (*A*) In solar lentigo, there are polycyclic bright contours or bulbous projections (*asterisks*) on RCM, corresponding to the anastomosing rete-ridge on histopathology (*B*).

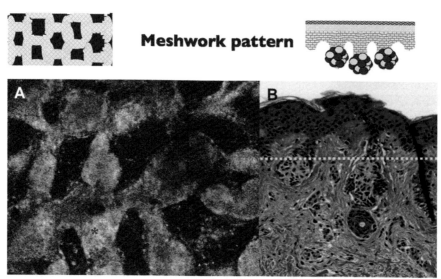

Fig. 5. (*A*) On RCM, the meshwork pattern is made by the enlargement of the interpapillary spaces formed by junctional nests bulging within the dermal papilla in contiguity with the basal layer. The junctional nests can be seen as compact, well-outlined, roundish-to-oval structures, sometimes connected with the epidermis (*asterisks*). (*B*) The histopathologic correlate is nevus with compact junctional nests at the tips of the cristae (*dashed line* corresponds to the level of RCM imaging). **Figs. 5–9** show the horizontal view (*left corner*) and vertical view (*right corner*).

nests seen in the superficial dermis in compound nevi (**Fig. 6**). In malignant melanoma, the DEJ can show areas of flattening and disarrangement of the architecture, responsible for fuzzy and not well-defined papillary contours (so-called non-edged papillae),[9] alternating with single-cell proliferations or nests of large pleomorphic atypical cells (aspecific pattern, **Fig. 7**).

Papillary Dermis

In the papillary dermis, the main findings that can be evaluated with high resolution using RCM are the inflammatory infiltrate, the regression phenomenon, and solar elastosis. The tumoral proliferation of the dermal compartment is reported in a specific section.

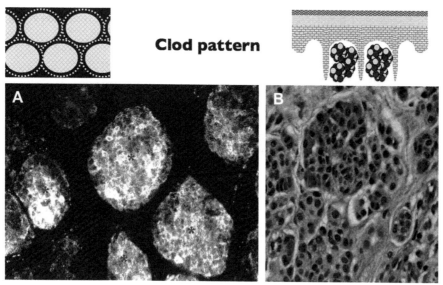

Fig. 6. (*A*) The clod pattern on RCM is formed by dermal nests (*asterisks*) seen in the superficial dermis of compound nevi. (*B*) The histopathologic correlate is a compound nevus with regular nests.

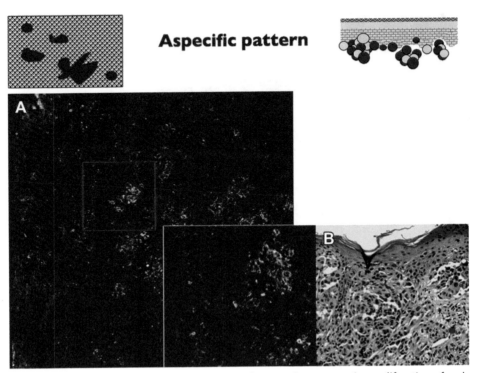

Fig. 7. (*A*) The aspecific pattern on RCM in an invasive melanoma shows a massive proliferation of melanocytes loosely arranged in nests (*red square*), correlating with the atypical nests seen on histopathology (*B*).

The inflammatory infiltrate is constituted by distinct cell types. On RCM, we can readily detect melanophages and lymphocytes. Melanophages appear as plump, large, bright cells with ill-defined borders and no visible nucleus.[10,11] These cells are usually seen within the dermal papillae or in the dermis and are often clustered (**Fig. 8**). In the regression phenomenon, melanophages are seen admixed with coarse and bright collagen fibers corresponding to a fibrotic response. Occasionally, a few melanocytes can be found, but their distinction from the inflammatory infiltrate is not always feasible in regressive areas (**Fig. 9**). Lymphocytes show up as small bright triangular structures, which can be focal or widespread. In aged skin or heavily sun-damaged skin, it is possible to detect the presence of curled bright fibers[12,13] that correspond to fragmented elastic fibers on histochemistry.

MAIN CLINICAL APPLICATIONS OF IN VIVO CONFOCAL MICROSCOPY
Skin Tumors

In skin oncology, the goal is to make an early diagnosis and reduce the number of unnecessary biopsies. Because the skin is easy to access, several instruments have been applied in oncology, although the gold standard in clinical practice is considered the combination of clinical inspection and dermoscopy. Dermoscopy is a noninvasive and cheap technique, which has proved to be an essential tool in skin oncology[14,15] and general dermatology.[16] RCM represents a second-level examination in clinical practice, which found its application in challenging cases or in special instances. In addition to dermoscopy, RCM is capable of delivering single-cell resolution in a few minutes at the patient's bedside.[17–20]

Melanocytic Tumors

In common nevi, RCM reveals a symmetric architecture that is characterized by junctional nests (meshwork pattern, see **Fig. 5**) or dermal nests (clod pattern, see **Fig. 6**) with little or no cytologic atypia.[21–26] When dealing with the so-called gray zone constituted by atypical or dysplastic nevi, a puzzling picture is shared by both RCM and histopathology. On RCM, it is possible to detect some morphologic aspects such as bridging of the nests or the presence of atypical cells, but it is not always feasible to draw a line between a severe dysplastic nevus and an incipient melanoma.[27] This challenge relies on the clinician's ability to read the confocal image or on their belief in the existence of a precursor lesion. The same scenario is present also in dermatopathology and accounts for the

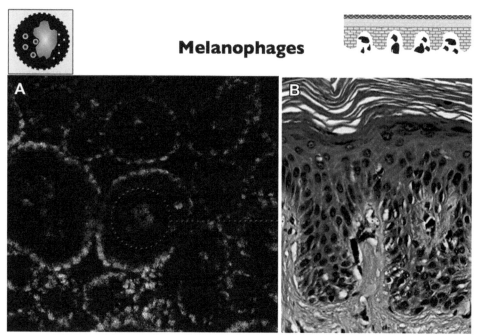

Fig. 8. (*A*) Melanophages appear as plump, large, bright cells with ill-defined borders and no visible nucleus (*circle*) on RCM. These cells are usually seen within the dermal papillae or in the dermis and are often clustered. (*B*) Histopathology shows the presence of melanin-laden melanophages within the dermal papillae.

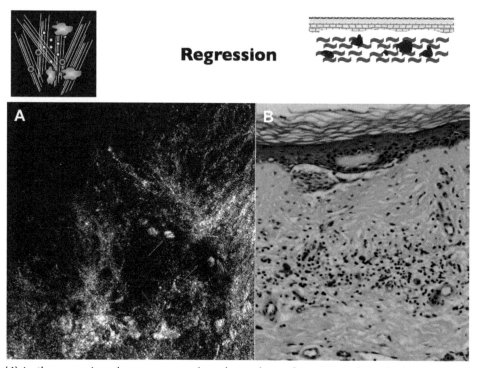

Fig. 9. (*A*) In the regression phenomenon, melanophages (*arrows*) are seen admixed with coarse and bright collagen fibers corresponding to a fibrotic response on RCM. Occasionally, a few melanocytes can be found, but their distinction from the inflammatory infiltrate is not always feasible in regressive areas. (*B*) Hematoxylin-eosin sections show a regressive area in a melanoma for comparison.

low interobserver agreement found when analyzing these kinds of pigmented lesions.[28,29] Spitzoid lesions represent another challenging situation in clinical practice. Although the confocal features of Spitz nevi are partially characteristic, they remain in most cases indistinguishable from melanoma. A good correlation was found for some histopathologic aspects and RCM features, some of which are considered characteristic of Spitz nevi, such as sharp lateral demarcation and presence of spindled cells. Other correlates that are not specific include pagetoid infiltration, junctional and dermal nests, parakeratosis, transepidermal melanin elimination, and inflammatory infiltrate rich in melanophages.[30,31] However, no correlate was found for other characteristic histologic aspects, such as Kamino bodies and maturation with depth. The frequent presence of features suggestive of malignancy in Spitz nevi, such as pagetoid infiltration (Fig. 10) and atypical cells, nonedged papillae, dishomogeneous nests, and the impossibility to explore the deeper parts of a given lesion, hamper a reliable diagnosis with RCM.

Melanoma comprises several subtypes with distinct morphologic and biologic aspects.[32–35] RCM diagnosis is based on major and minor criteria that have been extensively identified and tested for diagnostic accuracy.[17,18,36] Among them, the presence of pagetoid spread is one of the most striking criteria.[37–40] This term refers to the presence of melanocytes singly or in small nests, within the epidermis. Pagetoid spread is present in superficial spreading melanomas and in lentigo maligna type.[20,41] Conversely, in pure nodular melanoma, pagetoid cells are rare, whereas ulceration is a common finding at the epidermal level.[34]

RCM highlights different shapes of melanocytes scattered throughout the epidermis at various levels in melanoma.[35] Pagetoid cells usually have a round shape with bright granular cytoplasm and hyporefractive nucleus but can have a dendritic shape with a barely visible body and variably long branching terminal structures (see Fig. 10E). A clear-cut distinction between dendritic-shaped melanocytes and Langherans cells has not yet been established.[40] However, our personal experience is that the latter always has a triangular body with long and thin dendrites, in contrast to the true pagetoid cells characterized by thick and short dendrites with a more bizarre-shaped body. It is possible to analyze the pagetoid cell distribution (focal, widespread, patchy) and the cell density by counting the cells within the imaged field of view.[37] The possibility of exploring the entire epidermis in a horizontal plane is crucial to establishing if pagetoid cells are located in the center

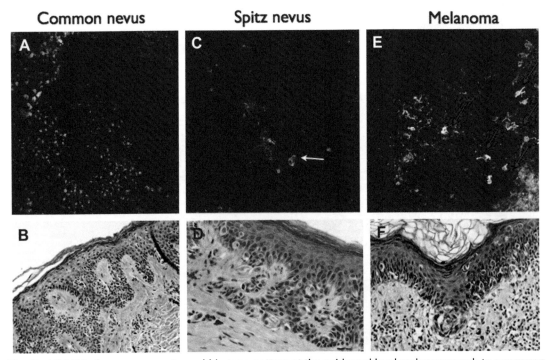

Fig. 10. (A) RCM of a nevus presents a cobblestone pattern at the epidermal level and corresponds to a common nevus on histopathology (B). (C). RCM of a Spitz nevus reveals a few pagetoid cells (arrow), which corresponds with the histopathology (D). (E) Multiple bright pagetoid cells with dendrites (arrows) located in the upper layers of the epidermis on RCM correspond to the pagetoid infiltration on histopathology in a melanoma (F).

of the lesion (a common phenomenon in congenital nevi, Spitz/Reed or traumatized nevi), or through the whole lesion.

In melanomas, the DEJ is characterized by ringed or meshwork architecture with large and bright pleomorphic (atypical) cells in early melanomas.[17] The cells can show the tendency to form nests that can still be compact or can be loosely arranged, depending on tumor progression. In early lesions, it is a common finding to observe alteration or abrupt interruption of the normal DEJ architecture caused by flattening of rete-ridges, resulting in irregularly shaped and not well-defined papillae (nonedged papillae)[9] or disappearance of dermal papillae substituted by strands of atypical cells. In advanced stage, the massive tumor proliferation occupies the entire junction and can push up into the epidermal layers as loose aggregates of bright, large, and pleomorphic melanocytes.

In nodular melanomas, RCM shows the presence of so-called cerebriform nests,[21,22] which consist of small and hyporefractive cells forming a large tumor mass separated by dark thin fissures and bright collagen septae.

Besides its diagnostic application, RCM is useful in large lesions suspicious for lentigo maligna of the face that present a challenge because of sampling error when partial biopsies are performed.[42] Because RCM scans the skin horizontally, it allows for the ability to scan the entire area of the lesion to direct the biopsies. RCM may be also used to guide gross pathologic sectioning of melanomas arising in nevi. In addition, RCM is useful in recurrent lesions in which repigmentation within a scar is present and the nature of the pigmentation is unknown.[43,44] Lesions with regression represent an important indication for RCM. More specifically, areas with bluish to greyish granules represent a common challenge among clinicians and can represent either a lichenoid keratosis or a regressive melanoma. RCM is able to discriminate between the former, showing only a florid inflammatory infiltrate, and the latter, constituted by atypical melanocytes admixed with inflammatory infiltrate.[5,45]

NONMELANOMA SKIN TUMORS

Nonmelanocytic tumors include basal cell carcinoma (BCC), actinic keratosis (AK) and squamous cell carcinoma (SCC), to name the most common tumors (**Fig. 11**). Confocal features of BCC consist of tightly packed aggregates with peripheral palisading and lobulated shape.[46–49] These aggregates are outlined by a dark space (corresponding to mucin) (see **Fig. 11A**) and are often surrounded by a prominent vascularity. Histopathologically,

the aggregates correspond to the basaloid islands. RCM highlights the presence of dendritic melanocytes entrapped within the basaloid islands observable in heavily pigmented BCC.[50,51]

AK and SCC show the presence of variable KC atypia. At the stratum corneum level, superficial disruption with single detached KCs seen as bright, polygonal cells of high reflectance can be observed.[52–57] Furthermore, nucleated, highly reflective cells with dark center and sharp demarcation appear within the stratum corneum, corresponding to parakeratosis. Atypical honeycombed pattern and architectural disarray of variable degree are seen at the level of the stratum granulosum and stratum spinosum, corresponding to different degrees of KC dysplasia on histopathologic examination.[58] Although different degrees of KC atypia can be detected, it is not possible to have a reliable diagnostic cutoff between severely atypical AKs and in situ SCCs. Round blood vessels traversing through the dermal papillae perpendicular to the skin surface and scale crust appearing as brightly reflective amorphous islands on the surface of the skin are common findings in SCC.[58] In cases with marked hyperkeratosis or abundant scale covering the entire lesion, in-depth imaging is limited by the keratin scattering, limiting exploration of the DEJ, which is fundamental for diagnosis.

Another potential use of RCM is presurgical assessment of margins. This approach is better performed by using the handheld device (VivaScope 3000), which allows faster and easier scanning of large areas.

Inflammatory Skin Diseases (Spongiotic, Psoriasiform, Interface, and Pigmentary)

The role of RCM has also been explored in inflammatory skin diseases, and the main confocal findings have been correlated with histopathology, although no systematic studies are available. After the histopathologic traditional classification, inflammatory skin diseases can be roughly grouped into 4 categories: (1) spongiotic dermatitis (ie, allergic and irritant contact dermatitis), (2) psoriasiform diseases (ie, psoriasis), (3) diseases with interface involvement (eg, lupus erythematosus, lichen planus, dermatomyositis), (4) pigmentary nontumoral skin disorders (ie, vitiligo, melasma) (**Fig. 12**).

The main feature of spongiotic dermatitis on RCM is the presence of intercellular or intracellular spongiosis. This feature corresponds to an increased intercellular brightness caused by intercellular or intracellular fluid accumulation, which leads to the appearance of a regular honeycombed morphology.[59–64] When spongiosis is more pronounced, it is possible to detect vesicle

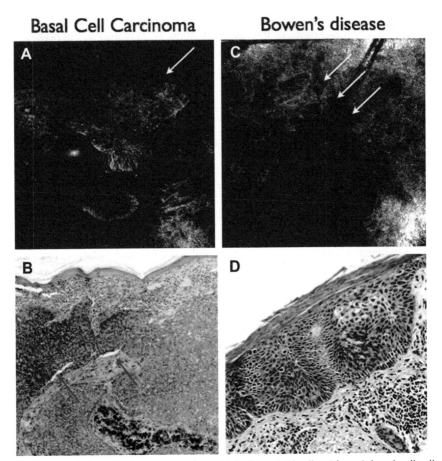

Fig. 11. (*A*) RCM shows tightly packed aggregates (*asterisks*) of basaloid cells with peripheral palisading outlined by a dark space (*arrow*). (*B*) Basaloid islands by light microscopy in a nodular BCC with surrounding cleftlike spaces (*arrows*) correspond to the dark outline seen on RCM, representing mucin. (*C*) RCM reveals the presence of irregularly shaped KCs with prominent black nuclei (*arrows*) in Bowen disease. (*D*) Hematoxylin-eosin sections of Bowen disease are characterized by full-thickness atypia.

formation, which appears as well-demarcated, dark hollow spaces (see **Fig. 12**A) between granular and spinous layer KCs. Commonly, exocytosis is associated with spongiosis, whereby the inflammatory cells are seen on RCM as bright, round highly refractive structures of about 8 to 10 μm, interspersed between KCs. Inflammatory cells may also be observed to various extents in a perifollicular, perivascular, or interstitial dermal distribution.

Psoriasiform disease is distinctive in the presence of nonrimmed papillae at the DEJ, resulting in a junctional profile similar to the normal skin but with papillae surrounded by faint rings of basal KCs, instead of the typical bright rings (see **Fig. 12**C).[65,66] Further confocal findings include epidermal thickening, up-located papillae (sometimes visible in the most superficial layers immediately below a thickened corneum), and several, sometimes tortuous, vessels within the nonrimmed papillae.

The hallmark in interface dermatitis is the inflammatory involvement of the DEJ. The inflammatory cells tend to obscure the junction profile and the dermal papillae, with a more diffuse involvement in lichen planus and a focal distribution in lupus erythematosus.[67,68] In the latter, the presence of inflammatory infiltrate can be seen close to the adnexa, which usually appear dilated (larger than 80–100 mm) and filled by highly refractive material in the lumen (hyperkeratotic infundibula).

Among the acquired pigmented disorders, vitiligo has been analyzed by RCM. Vitiligo lesional skin shows disappearance of the normal brightness at the DEJ, where the edged papillae appear as a remnant of the preexisting papillary ring.[69] In addition, the KCs, usually seen in normal skin as bright polygonal cells, are generally hyporeflecting in vitiligo lesions because of the lack of melanin. In nonlesional skin in vitiligo, an abnormal distribution pattern of brightness (ie, pigment) at the DEJ is

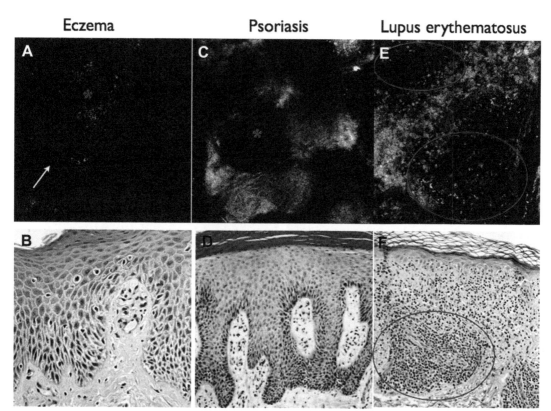

Fig. 12. (*A*) RCM shows the presence of a spongiotic vesicle (*arrow*), which appears as a well-demarcated, dark hollow space containing mildly refractive particles corresponding to leukocytes and debris (*asterisk*). (*B*) Hematoxylin-eosin sections are characterized by spongiotic dermatitis. (*C*) The RCM image of psoriasis displays non-rimmed papillae at the DEJ (*asterisk*), resulting in a junctional profile similar to the normal skin but with papillae surrounded by faint rings of basal KCs, instead of the typical bright rings. (*D*) The histopathology of psoriasis shows acanthosis, parakeratosis, and orthokeratosis. (*E*) RCM showing the presence of the inflammatory involvement (*circles*) of the DEJ corresponds well to the ones (*circle*) seen on histopathology (*F*) in lupus erythematosus.

seen. The characteristic ring structures are barely observable and they show up as half-ring bright structures outlining only a part of the dermal papilla (scalloped papillae). After ultraviolet B-narrow band treatment, activated melanocytes located at the DEJ can be detected by RCM even when there is not yet any clinical evidence of repigmentation. Characteristically, melanocytes appear as bipolar or stellate dendritic structures, with a predominant perifollicular distribution.

Infectious Diseases (Scabies, Mycosis, Demodex, Syphilis)

RCM has been applied in some infectious diseases, although its value in clinical practice needs to be tested on a larger scale. Superficial mycosis can be easily detected by RCM because it has a high-level resolution for the upper epidermis. Dermatophyte hyphae appear as bright linear branching structures within the epidermis, with an excellent correlation with the ones seen on light microscopy.[70] With the same high resolution, it is possible to detect the presence of *Demodex folliculorum* within the hair follicles.[71,72] *Demodex* usually show up as multiple, roundish, well-outlined structures corresponding to the head-down mites living in the hair follicles (**Fig. 13**). The possibility to readily detect these mites in a few minutes can be useful in treatment monitoring in *Demodex*-related skin diseases. *Sarcoptes scabiei* is seen well on RCM (see **Fig. 13**), as well as its feces and eggs within the burrow.[73]

Some investigators report the potential use of RCM in secondary syphilis, in which RCM displays the *Treponema pallidum* as elongate, spiral bright particles.[74]

Monitoring of Nonsurgical Therapies

Because of its noninvasiveness and high resolution, RCM is a suitable candidate for treatment monitoring. Its role has been investigated for monitoring treatment efficacy of imiquimod in AK.[75] RCM was able to visualize the inflammatory response induced by imiquimod in clinically visible

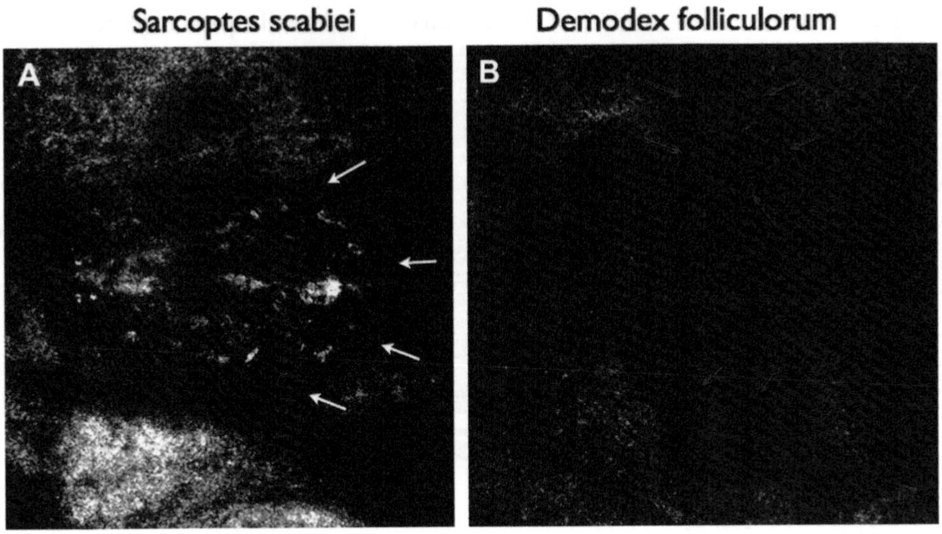

Sarcoptes scabiei   Demodex folliculorum

Fig. 13. (A) The head of the *Sarcoptes scabiei* mite is outlined by arrows on RCM. (B) Multiple *Demodex folliculorum* (*arrows*) are located within the hair follicles on RCM.

as well as in subclinical lesions within the cancerization field. Moreover, RCM offered in vivo insight into immune-modulatory effects of imiquimod by visualizing the inflammatory cells, especially Langerhans cells, followed by apoptosis of atypical KCs. At 4-week follow-up, RCN detected the replacement of KC atypia with a regular honeycombed pattern and the detection of residual disease after treatment in a few cases. Another study evaluated the efficacy of cryotherapy for superficial BCC,[76] showing early cell necrosis at the basal layer and within the superficial dermis 5 hours after application of liquid nitrogen, indicating effective cryotherapy. In this regard, RCM may allow the immediate evaluation of treatment efficacy after cryotherapy and may indicate if a second cryotherapy session is needed. RCM has also been used in lentigo maligna treated with imiquimod.[77] In this situation, the presence of dendritic-shaped Langerhans cells could represent a potential pitfall in the evaluation of treatment efficacy because these cells may resemble residual dendritic atypical melanocytes. However, these activated Langerhans cells usually completely disappear within 1 to 3 months after treatment ends. RCM has also found application for the efficacy assessment of laser therapy for solar lentigines,[78] vascular lesions,[79] skin rejuvenation,[80] and acne scars,[80] showing the skin changes occurring after treatment and in long-term follow-up. The possibility to closely monitor the morphologic changes over time and gain new insight into the mechanism of action of laser devices could be useful in understanding side effects.

SUMMARY

In Vivo Dermatopathology: Light and Dark

The development of RCM for in vivo examination of the epidermis, papillary, and superficial dermis at a resolution approaching histologic detail has significant implications for clinical care. The possibility of near-histologic resolution at the patient's bedside is fundamental in skin oncology not only for diagnostic purposes but also for nevi follow-up to better understand the dynamic process of growth. In addition, RCM provides an excellent assessment of skin changes after treatment, with the main advantage that it is painless, not scarring, and repeatable over time. RCM requires clinicians to become familiar with the histopathology and how essential it is for the correct interpretation of horizontal confocal images. This requirement is even more important for young residents and fellows, who may not have adequate teaching of this matter in their residency programs.

The potential of in vivo RCM to aid clinical dermatology looks promising but instrumentation advances and clinical research must occur before these technologies can be applied in routine clinical practice. In this regard, the first-generation confocal microscopes (VivaScope 1000) were time-consuming to use and not able to provide an overview of the skin area but only a snapshot of a limited field. The next generation (VivaScope 1500) moved the technology from the bench to the bedside, reducing the time for imaging a lesion from almost 30 minutes to approximately 5 minutes, and enabling the high-resolution exploration of a wide field of view (up to 8 × 8 mm).

However, it has a complex configuration that cannot be conveniently placed on certain anatomic areas such as the ear, medial canthus, or on intertriginous areas because of the need to stitch a metal ring onto the area of interest. As with other imaging technologies, fast improvement of the technology has led to a handheld device (VivaScope 3000), which allows simpler and faster delivery of images for as many body sites as preferred, but does not allow a wide-field examination of the lesion. So far, mainly referral centers and academic institutes are using these devices for research or clinical applications. In the future, more widespread knowledge and capability of interpreting difficult images, along with better cost-effective packages, will allow spread of this technology into dermatology practice. Along with technical improvements, there is an urgent need for courses teaching use of the instrument but, even more important, correct interpretation of the confocal images and their correlates in the clinical context. Face-to-face lessons and Web-based courses are already available or will be in the near future. Moreover, a teleconsult (VivaNet) is going to be available soon to increase the scientific exchange and to offer a teaching outlet. The images will be safely stored in a root server, which provides a permanent and secure medical archive. Confocal microscopy holds the unique possibility to move the art of histology closer to the bedside for diagnostic purposes and also for treatment monitoring or for the understanding of the biologic processes underlying the morphologic aspects.

REFERENCES

1. Rajadhyaksha M, Grossman M, Esterowitz D, et al. In vivo confocal scanning laser microscopy of human skin: melanin provides strong contrast. J Invest Dermatol 1995;104:946–52.
2. Rajadhyaksha M, Gonzalez S, Zavislan JM, et al. In vivo confocal laser microscopy of human skin II: advances in instrumentation and comparison with histology. J Invest Dermatol 1999;113:293–303.
3. Gonzalez S, Sackstein R, Anderson RR, et al. Real-time evidence of in vivo leukocyte trafficking in human skin by reflectance confocal microscopy. J Invest Dermatol 2001;117:384–6.
4. Huzaira M, Rius F, Rajadhyaksha M, et al. Topographic variations in normal skin, as viewed by in vivo reflectance confocal microscopy. J Invest Dermatol 2001;116(6):846–52.
5. Scope A, Benvenuto-Andrade C, Agero AL, et al. In vivo reflectance confocal microscopy imaging of melanocytic skin lesions: consensus terminology glossary and illustrative images. J Am Acad Dermatol 2007;57:644–58.
6. Langley RG, Burton E, Walsh N, et al. In vivo confocal scanning laser microscopy of benign lentigines: comparison to conventional histology and in vivo characteristics of lentigo maligna. J Am Acad Dermatol 2006;55:88–97.
7. Ahlgrimm-Siess V, Massone C, Koller S, et al. In vivo confocal scanning laser microscopy of common naevi with globular, homogeneous and reticular pattern in dermoscopy. Br J Dermatol 2008;158(5):1000–7.
8. Pellacani G, Scope A, Ferrari B, et al. New insights into nevogenesis: in vivo characterization and follow-up of melanocytic nevi by reflectance confocal microscopy. J Am Acad Dermatol 2009;61(6):1001–13.
9. Pellacani G, Cesinaro AM, Longo C, et al. Microscopic in vivo description of cellular architecture of dermoscopic pigment network in nevi and melanomas. Arch Dermatol 2005;141:147–54.
10. Busam KJ, Charles C, Lee G, et al. Morphologic features of melanocytes, pigmented keratinocytes, and melanophages by in vivo confocal scanning laser microscopy. Mod Pathol 2001;14:862–8.
11. Guitera P, Li LX, Scolyer RA, et al. Morphologic features of melanophages under in vivo reflectance confocal microscopy. Arch Dermatol 2010;146(5):492–8.
12. Sauermann K, Clemann S, Jaspers S, et al. Age related changes of human skin investigated with histometric measurements by confocal laser scanning microscopy in vivo. Skin Res Technol 2002;8(1):52–6.
13. Longo C, Casari A, Beretti F, et al. Skin aging: in vivo microscopic assessment of epidermal and dermal changes by means of confocal microscopy. J Am Acad Dermatol 2011 Oct 13. [Epub ahead of print].
14. Argenziano G, Puig S, Zalaudek I, et al. Dermoscopy improves accuracy of primary care physicians to triage lesions suggestive of skin cancer. J Clin Oncol 2006;24(12):1877–82.
15. Argenziano G, Cerroni L, Zalaudek I, et al. Accuracy in melanoma detection: a 10-year multicenter survey. J Am Acad Dermatol 2012;67(1):54–9.
16. Zalaudek I, Argenziano G, Di Stefani A, et al. Dermoscopy in general dermatology. Dermatology 2006;212(1):7–18.
17. Pellacani G, Cesinaro AM, Seidenari S. Reflectance-mode confocal microscopy of pigmented skin lesions–improvement in melanoma diagnostic specificity. J Am Acad Dermatol 2005;53:979–85.
18. Gerger A, Koller S, Weger W, et al. Sensitivity and specificity of confocal laser-scanning microscopy for in vivo diagnosis of malignant skin tumors. Cancer 2006;107:193–200.
19. Pellacani G, Guitera P, Longo C, et al. The impact of in vivo reflectance confocal microscopy for the diagnostic accuracy of melanoma and equivocal melanocytic lesions. J Invest Dermatol 2007;127:2759–65.

20. Guitera P, Pellacani G, Crotty KA, et al. The impact of in vivo reflectance confocal microscopy on the diagnostic accuracy of lentigo maligna and equivocal pigmented and nonpigmented macules of the face. J Invest Dermatol 2010;130(8):2080–91.

21. Pellacani G, Cesinaro AM, Seidenari S. In vivo confocal reflectance microscopy for the characterization of melanocytic nests and correlation with dermoscopy and histology. Br J Dermatol 2005;152:384–6.

22. Pellacani G, Cesinaro AM, Seidenari S. In vivo assessment of melanocytic nests in nevi and melanomas by reflectance confocal microscopy. Mod Pathol 2005;18:469–74.

23. Pellacani G, Bassoli S, Longo C, et al. Diving into the blue: in vivo microscopic characterization of the dermoscopic blue hue. J Am Acad Dermatol 2007;57:96–104.

24. Scope A, Benvenuto-Andrade C, Agero AL, et al. Correlation of dermoscopic structures of melanocytic lesions to reflectance confocal microscopy. Arch Dermatol 2007;143:176–85.

25. Scope A, Gill M, Benveuto-Andrade C, et al. Correlation of dermoscopy with in vivo reflectance confocal microscopy of streaks in melanocytic lesions. Arch Dermatol 2007;143:727–34.

26. Pellacani G, Longo C, Malvehy J, et al. In vivo confocal microscopic and histopathologic correlations of dermoscopic features in 202 melanocytic lesions. Arch Dermatol 2008;144(12):1597–608.

27. Pellacani G, Farnetani F, Gonzalez S, et al. In vivo confocal microscopy for detection and grading of dysplastic nevi: a pilot study. J Am Acad Dermatol 2012;66(3):e109–21.

28. Shoo BA, Sagebiel RW, Kashani-Sabet M. Discordance in the histopathologic diagnosis of melanoma at a melanoma referral center. J Am Acad Dermatol 2010;62(5):751–6.

29. Weyers W. The 'epidemic' of melanoma between under- and overdiagnosis. J Cutan Pathol 2012;39(1):9–16.

30. Pellacani G, Cesinaro AM, Grana C, et al. In-vivo confocal scanning laser microscopy of pigmented Spitz nevi. Comparison of in-vivo confocal images with dermoscopy and routine histopathology. J Am Acad Dermatol 2004;51:371–6.

31. Pellacani G, Longo C, Ferrara G, et al. Spitz nevi: in vivo confocal microscopic features, dermatoscopic aspects, histopathologic correlates, and diagnostic significance. J Am Acad Dermatol 2009;60(2):236–47.

32. Langley RGB, Rajadhyaksha M, Dwyer PJ, et al. Confocal scanning laser microscopy of benign and malignant melanocytic skin lesions in vivo. J Am Acad Dermatol 2001;45:365–76.

33. Zalaudek I, Marghoob AA, Scope A, et al. Three roots of melanoma. Arch Dermatol 2008;144(10):1375–9.

34. Segura S, Pellacani G, Puig S, et al. In vivo microscopic features of nodular melanomas: dermoscopy, confocal microscopy, and histopathologic correlates. Arch Dermatol 2008;144(10):1311–20.

35. Longo C, Rito C, Beretti F, et al. De novo melanoma and melanoma arising from pre-existing nevus: in vivo morphologic differences as evaluated by confocal microscopy. J Am Acad Dermatol 2011;65(3):604–14.

36. Segura S, Puig S, Carrera C, et al. Development of a two-step method for the diagnosis of melanoma by reflectance confocal microscopy. J Am Acad Dermatol 2009;61(2):216–29.

37. Pellacani G, Cesinaro AM, Seidenari S. Reflectance-mode confocal microscopy for the in vivo characterization of pagetoid melanocytosis in melanomas and nevi. J Invest Dermatol 2005;125:532–7.

38. Longo C, Fantini F, Cesinaro AM, et al. Pigmented mammary Paget disease: dermoscopic, in vivo reflectance-mode confocal microscopic, and immunohistochemical study of a case. Arch Dermatol 2007;143(6):752–4.

39. Guitera P, Scolyer RA, Gill M, et al. Reflectance confocal microscopy for diagnosis of mammary and extramammary Paget's disease. J Eur Acad Dermatol Venereol 2012 Jan 3. http://dx.doi.org/10.1111/j.1468-3083.2011.04423.x. [Epub ahead of print].

40. Hashemi P, Pulitzer MP, Scope A, et al. Langerhans cells and melanocytes share similar morphologic features under in vivo reflectance confocal microscopy: a challenge for melanoma diagnosis. J Am Acad Dermatol 2012;66(3):452–62.

41. Tannous ZS, Mihm MC, Flotte TJ, et al. In vivo examination of lentigo maligna and malignant melanoma in situ, lentigo maligna type by near-infrared reflectance confocal microscopy: comparison of in vivo confocal images with histologic sections. J Am Acad Dermatol 2002;46:260–3.

42. Chen CS, Elias M, Busam K, et al. Multimodal in vivo optical imaging, including confocal microscopy, facilitates presurgical margin mapping for clinically complex lentigo maligna melanoma. Br J Dermatol 2005;153:1031–6.

43. Longo C, Moscarella E, Pepe P, et al. Confocal microscopy of recurrent naevi and recurrent melanomas: a retrospective morphological study. Br J Dermatol 2011;165(1):61–8.

44. Moscarella E, Zalaudek I, Pellacani G, et al. Lichenoid keratosis-like melanomas. J Am Acad Dermatol 2011;65(3):e85–7.

45. Bassoli S, Rabinovitz HS, Pellacani G, et al. Reflectance confocal microscopy criteria of lichen planus-like keratosis. J Eur Acad Dermatol Venereol 2012;26(5):578–90.

46. González S, Tannous Z. Real-time, in vivo confocal reflectance microscopy of basal cell carcinoma. J Am Acad Dermatol 2002;47:869–74.

47. Ulrich M, Roewert-Huber J, González S, et al. Peritumoral clefting in basal cell carcinoma: correlation of in vivo reflectance confocal microscopy and routine histology. J Cutan Pathol 2011;38(2):190–5.

48. Nori S, Rius-Díaz F, Cuevas J, et al. Sensitivity and specificity of reflectance-mode confocal microscopy for in vivo diagnosis of basal cell carcinoma: a multicenter study. J Am Acad Dermatol 2004;51:923–30.

49. Agero AL, Busam KJ, Benvenuto-Andrade C, et al. Reflectance confocal microscopy of pigmented basal cell carcinoma. J Am Acad Dermatol 2006; 54:638–43.

50. Segura S, Puig S, Carrera C, et al. Dendritic cells in pigmented basal cell carcinoma: a relevant finding by reflectance-mode confocal microscopy. Arch Dermatol 2007;143:883–6.

51. Casari A, Pellacani G, Seidenari S, et al. Pigmented nodular basal cell carcinomas in differential diagnosis with nodular melanomas: confocal microscopy as a reliable tool for in vivo histologic diagnosis. J Skin Cancer 2011;2011:406859.

52. Aghassi D, Anderson R, Gonzalez S. Confocal laser microscopic imaging of actinic keratosis in vivo: a preliminary report. J Am Acad Dermatol 2000;43: 42–8.

53. Ulrich M, González S, Lange-Asschenfeldt B, et al. Non-invasive diagnosis and monitoring of actinic cheilitis with reflectance confocal microscopy. J Eur Acad Dermatol Venereol 2011;25(3):276–84.

54. Ulrich M, Maltusch A, Rius-Diaz F, et al. Clinical applicability of in vivo reflectance confocal microscopy for the diagnosis of actinic keratoses. Dermatol Surg 2008;34(5):610–9.

55. Ulrich M, Stockfleth E, Roewert-Huber J, et al. Noninvasive diagnostic tools for nonmelanoma skin cancer. Br J Dermatol 2007;157(Suppl 2):56–8.

56. Ulrich M, Forschner T, Röwert-Huber J, et al. Differentiation between actinic keratoses and disseminated superficial actinic porokeratoses with reflectance confocal microscopy. Br J Dermatol 2007;156(Suppl 3): 47–52.

57. Ulrich M, Maltusch A, Röwert-Huber J, et al. Actinic keratoses: non-invasive diagnosis for field cancerisation. Br J Dermatol 2007;156(Suppl 3):13–7.

58. Rishpon A, Kim N, Scope A, et al. Reflectance confocal microscopy criteria for squamous cell carcinomas and actinic keratoses. Arch Dermatol 2009;145(7):766–72.

59. González S, González E, White WM, et al. Allergic contact dermatitis: correlation of in vivo confocal imaging to routine histology. J Am Acad Dermatol 1999;40(5 Pt 1):708–13.

60. Astner S, González E, Cheung AC, et al. Non-invasive evaluation of the kinetics of allergic and irritant contact dermatitis. J Invest Dermatol 2005;124(2):351–9.

61. Astner S, Gonzalez E, Cheung A, et al. Pilot study on the sensitivity and specificity of in vivo reflectance confocal microscopy in the diagnosis of allergic contact dermatitis. J Am Acad Dermatol 2005;53(6): 986–92.

62. Astner S, González S, Gonzalez E. Noninvasive evaluation of allergic and irritant contact dermatitis by in vivo reflectance confocal microscopy. Dermatitis 2006;17(4):182–91.

63. Longo C, Segura S, Cesinaro AM, et al. An atypical Meyerson's naevus: a dermoscopic, confocal microscopic and immunohistochemical description of one case. J Eur Acad Dermatol Venereol 2007;21(3): 414–6.

64. Ardigò M, Longo C, Cristaudo A, et al. Evaluation of allergic vesicular reaction to patch test using in vivo confocal microscopy. Skin Res Technol 2012;18(1): 61–3.

65. Gonzalez S, Rajadhyaksha M, Rubenstein G, et al. Characterization of psoriasis in vivo by reflectance confocal microscopy. J Med 1999;30:337–56.

66. Ardigo M, Cota C, Berardesca E, et al. Concordance between in vivo reflectance confocal microscopy and histology in the evaluation of plaque psoriasis. J Eur Acad Dermatol Venereol 2009; 23(6):660–7.

67. Ardigò M, Maliszewski I, Cota C, et al. Preliminary evaluation of in vivo reflectance confocal microscopy features of discoid lupus erythematosus. Br J Dermatol 2007;156(6):1196–203.

68. Moscarella E, González S, Agozzino M, et al. Pilot study on reflectance confocal microscopy imaging of lichen planus: a real-time, non-invasive aid for clinical diagnosis. J Eur Acad Dermatol Venereol 2011 Sep 29. http://dx.doi.org/10.1111/j.1468-3083.2011.04279.x. [Epub ahead of print].

69. Ardigo M, Malizewsky I, Dell'anna ML, et al. Preliminary evaluation of vitiligo using in vivo reflectance confocal microscopy. J Eur Acad Dermatol Venereol 2007;21(10):1344–50.

70. Markus R, Huzaira M, Anderson RR, et al. A better potassium hydroxide preparation? In vivo diagnosis of tinea with confocal microscopy. Arch Dermatol 2001;137(8):1076–8.

71. Slutsky JB, Rabinovitz H, Grichnik JM, et al. Reflectance confocal microscopic features of dermatophytes, scabies, and demodex. Arch Dermatol 2011;147(8):1008.

72. Longo C, Pellacani G, Ricci C, et al. In vivo detection of Demodex folliculorum by means of confocal microscopy. Br J Dermatol 2012;166(3):690–2.

73. Longo C, Bassoli S, Monari P, et al. Reflectance-mode confocal microscopy for the in vivo detection of Sarcoptes scabiei. Arch Dermatol 2005;141(10): 1336.

74. Venturini M, Sala R, Semenza D, et al. Reflectance confocal microscopy for the in vivo detection of Treponema pallidum in skin lesions of secondary syphilis. J Am Acad Dermatol 2009;60(4):639–42.

75. Ulrich M, Krueger-Corcoran D, Roewert-Huber J, et al. Reflectance confocal microscopy for noninvasive monitoring of therapy and detection of subclinical actinic keratoses. Dermatology 2010;220(1):15–24.

76. Ahlgrimm-Siess V, Horn M, Koller S, et al. Monitoring efficacy of cryotherapy for superficial basal cell carcinomas with in vivo reflectance confocal microscopy: a preliminary study. J Dermatol Sci 2009; 53(1):60–4.

77. Nadiminti H, Scope A, Marghoob AA, et al. Use of reflectance confocal microscopy to monitor response of lentigo maligna to nonsurgical treatment. Dermatol Surg 2010;36(2):177–84.

78. Richtig E, Hofmann-Wellenhof R, Kopera D, et al. In vivo analysis of solar lentigines by reflectance confocal microscopy before and after Q-switched ruby laser treatment. Acta Derm Venereol 2011; 91(2):164–8.

79. Astner S, González S, Cuevas J, et al. Preliminary evaluation of benign vascular lesions using in vivo reflectance confocal microscopy. Dermatol Surg 2010;36(7):1099–110.

80. Bencini PL, Tourlaki A, Galimberti M, et al. Nonablative fractional photothermolysis for acne scars: clinical and in vivo microscopic documentation of treatment efficacy. Dermatol Therapy 2012, in press.

Dermatopathology Education
An Update

Molly A. Hinshaw, MD[a,b,c,]*

KEYWORDS

- Dermatopathology • Dermatology • Pathology • Education • History • Update

KEY POINTS

- The study of histology of the skin is more than 300 years old.
- Both dermatologists and pathologists have contributed to establishing and advancing dermatopathology.
- Graduate medical education requirements for dermatopathology are an evolving process achieved by contributions from Dermatology and Pathology leaders and respective Residency Review Committees within the Accreditation Council for Graduate Medical Education.

INTRODUCTION

Dermatopathology (DP) education is critical to the comprehensive training of dermatology and pathology residents and to the accurate diagnosis and management of cutaneous disease. What are the goals of DP education? How do we measure a trainee's or practitioner's DP knowledge and application of that knowledge for diagnosis and management of patients? How frequently should educational and assessment sessions occur? In what format should they be administered? And how should we continue to provide that education and measure how well it has been taught? Dermatopathology has seen tremendous growth, and its success depends on our ability to effectively educate future leaders, teachers, and researchers who will continue to advance the field.

This article focuses on DP education in the United States, although specific components, such as assessment of medical education and the future of DP education, are relevant to the larger DP community. It is hoped that this review will aid in discussions of direction and collaboration.

THE HISTORY OF DERMATOPATHOLOGY EDUCATION

The Origin of Dermatopathology and Dermatopathologists

The study of histology of the skin has a long documented history dating back to the 1600s. Discoveries first came from European physicians, with contributions since made by numerous notable pathologists and dermatologists from around the world. In 1792, Henry Seguin Jackson of London, England coined the term "dermatopathology" and in 1844 the German Julius Rosenbaum the term "dermatopathologists."[1] Formalized training in DP in the United States began in 1950 with the creation of the Osborne Fellowship at the Armed Forces Institute of Pathology (AFIP) directed by Dr Elson Helwig.[2]

The American Society of Dermatopathology and Board Certification in Dermatopathology

In 1963, the American Society of Dermatopathology (ASDP) was established. The idea for this new

The author has nothing to disclose.
Funding support: None.
[a] Dermpath Diagnostics, 12805 West Burleigh Road, Brookfield, WI 53005-3111, USA; [b] Department of Dermatology, University of Wisconsin School of Medicine and Public Health, Madison, WI, USA; [c] Department of Dermatology, Medical College of Wisconsin, 8701 Watertown Plank Road, Milwaukee, WI 53226
* Dermpath Diagnostics, 12805 West Burleigh Road, Brookfield, WI 53005-3111.
E-mail address: mhinshaw@dermpathdiagnostics.com

Dermatol Clin 30 (2012) 815–826
http://dx.doi.org/10.1016/j.det.2012.06.003
0733-8635/12/$ – see front matter © 2012 Published by Elsevier Inc.

derm.theclinics.com

society composed of pathologists and dermatologists came from the dermatopathologist Dr John Haserick of the Cleveland Clinic. In 1970, the ASDP approved a resolution to submit to their member boards (the American Board of Dermatology [ABD] and the American Board of Pathology [ABP]) a request for Subspecialization in Dermatopathology. Over the next 3 years negotiations between the ABD and the ABP continued, and in 1973 they agreed to a joint subspecialty certifying examination in DP, which was subsequently approved by the American Board of Medical Specialties (ABMS). The first DP certifying examination was held in 1974 in Washington, DC.[1] Initially, one was not required to have completed a DP fellowship to take the certifying examination. However, beginning in 1982, eligibility to take the DP certifying examination included the requirements that one must have completed an accredited graduate medical education (GME) program in dermatology or pathology residency, and DP fellowship of at least 1 year's duration.

The Practice of Dermatopathology

Maintaining subspecialty certification in DP is predicated on continued board certification in dermatology or pathology. In Europe and around the world, the practice of DP varies greatly between countries, between institutions, and even within a single institution. For example, in Germany both dermatologists and pathologists evaluate skin biopsies, whereas in Italy only pathologists are allowed to perform this specialized skill except in some academic institutions where dermatologists may also interpret skin biopsies.[3] In the United States, pathologists and dermatologists may interpret skin biopsies. In early American DP, individual medical specialty boards were responsible for certifying that a physician was qualified to practice their specialty. Today, residency and fellowship programs in the United States are accredited by the larger organization, the Accreditation Council for Graduate Medical Education (ACGME).

Accreditation Council for Graduate Medical Education and Dermatopathology Education

In 1981, the ACGME was created by the joint effort of the American Medical Association (AMA), the ABMS, the American Hospital Association (AHA), the Association of American Medical Colleges (AAMC), and the Council of Medical Specialty Societies (CMSS) because of a consensus within the medical community of the need for an independent accrediting organization for GME. Today, the ACGME is the sole organization that accredits educational programs for the medical profession.

In 1999, the ACGME broadened the scope of medical education from its primary focus of imparting medical knowledge when they endorsed the 6 core competencies (patient care, medical knowledge, practice-based learning and improvement, interpersonal and communication skills, professionalism, and systems-based practice). The ACGME and ABMS provided guidance for suggested best methods for measuring competency in each of these 6 areas. Little guidance was provided with respect to identifying, implementing, or measuring DP-specific core competencies. Specifically, in 2002 the guide to residency curricula and core competencies developed by the Association of Directors of Anatomic and Surgical Pathology excluded subspecialty areas with dedicated fellowships and board examinations (eg, DP).[4] To address the lack of DP-specific core competencies, one publication in 2006 provided some initial, measurable, competency-based objectives for GME programs to be considered when working to meet these ACGME requirements.[5]

The 6 core competencies were developed as part of the ACGME program termed The Outcomes Project. Now the ACGME has created the Milestone Project, and is working with Residency Review Committees (RRCs), specialty medical organizations, and specialty boards to detail specific skill and knowledge sets that residents must

---

Timeline of dermatopathology specialty and education milestones

1600s: First documented histologic descriptions of skin

1792: Henry Seguin Jackson coined the term "dermatopathology"

1844: Julius Rosenbaum coined the term "dermatopathologists"

1963: American Society of Dermatopathology established

1950: Armed Forces Institute of Pathology creates, and Dr Elson Helwig directs, first DP fellowship

1973: Subspecialty certifying examination in dermatopathology established (first administered 1974)

1981: Accreditation Council for Graduate Medical Education (ACGME) created

1999: ACGME endorses the 6 core competencies (created as part of The Outcomes Project)

2006: GME programs required to have implemented the 6 core competencies

Coming soon from the RRC within the ACGME: The Milestone Project

achieve by specific time points during training to progress toward mastery of the 6 competencies. Assessing achievement of those objectives and improving the evaluation process are challenging goals and they, like the objectives themselves, are in an evolving process targeted at public assurance of practice competency.

THE CURRENT STATE OF DERMATOPATHOLOGY EDUCATION IN GRADUATE MEDICAL EDUCATION
Residency Review Committee Requirements

Dermatopathology education is a critical component of a complete medical education for dermatology and pathology residents. The dermatology RRC stipulates that

> Residents will examine routinely stained histologic sections from the full spectrum of dermatologic disease. A significant portion of this exposure must occur in an active faculty-run sign-out setting...and training must include education relating to interpretation of direct immunofluorescence specimens, appropriate use and interpretation of immunohistochemistry (special stains, including immunoperoxidase) and electron microscopy.[6]

In the case of pathology, the DP education requirement is that residency programs provide pathology residents with "education in anatomic pathology that must include instruction in autopsy and surgical pathology, cytopathology, pediatric pathology, dermatopathology," and so forth. The ACGME requires at least semiannual evaluations of residents related to the 6 core competencies, and allows individual residency programs to create their own educational goals, teaching tools, and assessments.

Current Quantity and Components of Dermatopathology Education in Residency

Several studies have surveyed ACGME-approved residencies to document their approaches to DP education. In one study by Singh and colleagues,[7] the investigators surveyed anatomic and clinical pathology (n = 151; 59 responded; 39.1% response rate) as well as dermatology (n = 108; 51 responded; 47.2% response rate) residency programs via email, and asked how many hours of DP education were required of each resident in their program before matriculation (excluding elective time). The results of this study showed that pathology residencies averaged 216.5 hours of DP during a 4-year residency and that dermatology residencies averaged 570.4 hours of DP

education during a 3-year residency. In another survey study, investigators used the list serve of the Association of Professors of Dermatology (APD) to query dermatology residency programs as to their DP curriculum (n = 109 residency programs; 52 responded; 48% response rate). Results showed that, on average, 30% of dermatology residency education time was devoted to the study of DP.[8] This substantial amount of time devoted specifically to DP education speaks to the importance each specialty places on DP, particularly given the ever increasing educational demands on residents and residency programs.

When the gross quantity of DP-specific educational sessions is dissected, greater detail is observed as to the relative current use of various DP teaching tools. In the survey study of the APD membership previously mentioned, 38.5% of programs reported having 3 or more weeks of time on the DP service for postgraduate year (PGY)-2 residents, 59.6% for PGY-3 residents, and 69.2% for PGY-4 residents (**Table 1**).[8] In addition, 40.4% reported using a problem-based learning curriculum, 53.8% reported having a DP journal review, 71.2% have residents review biopsies that they obtain in clinic of whom 65.4% review them with a faculty member, and 19.2% reported using computer-based learning. This graduated experience in DP is the opposite of what some have recommended, including Ackerman.[9]

Dermatopathology Educators

A discussion of DP education would not be complete without considering resident access to dermatopathologists. Dermatopathology is best taught by a practicing dermatopathologist, preferably one with years of practice experience and interest and experience in teaching. The ACGME requires that a residency program have at least one board-certified dermatopathologist teaching DP and, in the case of the dermatology RRC, that a component of DP education occur during routine sign-out. If DP sign-out does not occur within the institution, residents may need to travel to an offsite location to attend sign-out sessions, thus potentially limiting access to material and correlation of clinical and pathologic features that are so important for learning DP.

The recent threat of reduced federal funding of DP fellowships could decrease the number of practicing dermatopathologists and, therefore, DP educators. During the 2010-2011 academic year, there were 54 ACGME-accredited DP fellowships approved to train 91 DP fellows.[10] In one survey study of DP fellows (n = 60), nearly one-third third (29%) entered fellowship intending to

Table 1
Summary of APD-derived data on DP education in dermatology residencies

Variable		Frequency	Percentage
No. of programs in sample by region	West	5	9.6
	Southwest	0	0
	South	3	5.8
	Midwest	18	34.6
	Northeast	18	34.6
	Southeast	8	15.4
Population size of community	<100,000	8	15.4
	100,000–500,000	8	15.4
	500,001–1,000,000	10	19.2
	>1,000,000	26	50
Programs training at different hospitals	Community hospital	21	40.4
	Veterans hospital	36	69.2
	Student health services	10	19.2
	University hospital and/or clinic	46	88.5
No. of residents	0–3	1	1.9
	4–8	14	26.9
	9–12	20	38.5
	≥13	17	32.7
No. of faculty who teach dermatopathology	1	4	7.7
	2	14	26.9
	3	13	25
	4	5	9.6
	>4	16	30.8
No. of faculty who teach dermatopathology and are board certified in dermatopathology and pathology	0	13	25
	1	15	28.8
	2	16	30.8
	3	2	3.8
	>3	6	11.5
No. of faculty who teach dermatopathology and are board certified in dermatopathology and dermatology	0	5	9.6
	1	16	30.8
	2	15	28.8
	3	7	13.5
	>3	9	17.3
No. of faculty who spend >50% in academic medicine	0	4	7.7
	1	17	32.7
	2	11	21.2
	3	9	17.3
	>3	11	21.2
Nonclinical hours/month for overall resident education	1–10	3	5.8
	11–19	8	15.4
	>19	41	78.8
Nonclinical hours/month for dermatopathology education	1–3	6	11.5
	4–6	20	38.5
	7–9	8	15.4
	10–12	9	17.3
	>12	9	17.3
Weeks in Dermatopathology Rotation by Postgraduate Year (PGY)			
PGY 1	0	49	94.2
	1–2	1	1.9
PGY 2	0	25	48.1
	1–2	5	9.6
	3–4	13	25
	>4	7	13.5

(continued on next page)

Table 1
(continued)

Variable		Frequency	Percentage
PGY 3	0	13	25
	1–2	6	11.5
	3–4	13	25
	>4	18	34.6
PGY 4	0	12	23.1
	1–2	2	3.8
	3–4	18	34.6
	>4	18	34.6
PGY 5	0	49	96.2
	>4	1	1.9
Microscope Time in Hours Led by Each Type of Teacher			
By board-certified dermatopathologist	1–2	7	13.5
	3–4	12	23.1
	>4	33	63.5
By board-certified dermatologist	0	41	78.8
	1–2	1	1.9
	3–4	3	5.8
	>4	7	13.5
By board-certified pathologist	0	43	82.7
	1–2	3	5.8
	3–4	1	1.9
	>4	5	9.6
By dermatopathology fellow	0	38	73.1
	1–2	6	11.5
	3–4	4	7.7
	>4	4	7.7
By residents	0	42	80.8
	1–2	4	7.7
	3–4	3	5.8
	>4	3	5.8
Programs using problem-based learning curriculum	Yes	21	40.4
	No	31	59.6
Programs using journal review	Yes	28	53.8
	No	24	46.2
Programs using computer-based learning	Yes	10	19.2
	No	42	80.8
Programs that have residents review their own slides that they obtained from patients in clinic	Yes	37	71.2
	No	15	28.8
If residents review their own slides that they obtained from patients in clinic, do they review the slides with faculty?	Yes	34	65.4
	No	18	34.6
Programs that promote attendance at DP board review program	Yes	15	28.8
	No	37	71.2
Attendance at DP board review program financially supported by residency program	Yes	13	25
	No	39	75
Set of teaching slides available for residents to review	Yes	47	90.4
	No	5	9.6

From Hinshaw MA, Hsu P, Lee LY, et al. The current state of dermatopathology education: a survey of the Association of Professors of Dermatology. J Cutan Pathol 2009;36(6):620–8; with permission.

pursue an academic career, and a greater number (34%) actually did choose academic careers while 60% entered private practice.[11] In the summer of 2011, in response to the decision to increase the federal debt limit, the Joint Select Committee on Deficit Reduction (the "Super Committee") was created and subsequently recommended to Congress that cuts to Medicare reimbursement of GME should be implemented as a component of federal spending reductions.[12] Specifically, the Simpson Bowles Commission recommended decreasing total GME funding by more than 50% ($60 billion over 10 years).[13]

Given these recent threats of reduced federal funding for GME, in October 2011 researchers with the ACGME published the results of a study they performed to assess the potential impact of various levels of reduced federal funding on residency and fellowship programs.[14] The study was an 18-question survey emailed to Designated Institutional Officials at each ACGME-accredited residency and fellowship program (n = 680; 306 responded; 45% response rate). Survey respondents reported that if federal funding of GME were reduced 50%, 82.3% of responding sponsors would slightly or significantly reduce the number of core residency positions, 76.2% would reduce the number of subspecialty fellowship positions, 14.0% would close all core residency programs, and 20.9% would close all subspecialty programs. These results highlight how critical federal funding is to the continuation of GME and DP education.

GOALS OF DERMATOPATHOLOGY EDUCATION

Defining goals for resident and fellow education is an intellectual challenge in the changing health care landscape in which we practice. Accomplished teachers of DP have been asking questions for years about the goals of education and the optimal ways to reach those goals. Is the program training a resident to correlate histologic findings with the clinical setting in order to optimize diagnosis and management? Is a residency program preparing a resident for fellowship should a resident choose to pursue one? Is a residency program training residents to read their own slides (a practice earned by board certification in pathology or dermatology, and one that has been commented on by some and not discussed further in this article[15])? What criteria do we use to judge competency and who judges it?[16]

There is no one optimal established method of teaching DP, and there are no universal goals for resident education in DP. Whereas it is known that by one measure, the median number of hours per month dedicated to DP education in dermatology residencies is 7, whether there is an optimal number of hours of DP-specific education during residency is unknown.[7] In contrast to residencies, the RRCs have more specifically defined the current composition of an accredited DP fellowship that must be completed before one is eligible for subcertification (1-year fellowship that includes 4 months exclusively for DP education and, for the remaining 8 months, 50% of each day as averaged over 1 week for education in clinical dermatology for pathologists or in anatomic pathology for dermatologists). Each program decides the complement of DP educational methods, that is, didactics, journal club, clinical-pathologic correlation conference, and daily sign-out.

Knowledge of histology of the skin improves dermatologists' diagnostic and management skills.[8] One reason why all dermatology residents must become competent in DP is that dermatologists routinely perform skin surgery. Appropriate surgical planning relies on numerous factors, including accurate histologic diagnosis and interpretation of the diagnosis in the context of the clinical setting. Mohs surgeons have a unique role that includes interpretation of frozen sections for melanocytic hyperplasia in the context of melanoma, follicular versus malignant basaloid epithelium, and squamous cell carcinoma versus benign reactive epithelial hyperplasia, to name a few.[17] Microscopic diagnosis is a skill learned over time with experience and guidance from colleagues and mentors. It should begin early and continue for the duration of one's career.

Results of 2 studies vary as to whether there is a relationship between the number of residents in a residency program and the amount of time each resident spends on DP. In one survey study of chief residents and program directors of ACGME-approved dermatology residencies during 2004 to 2005, the investigators reported that "there appeared to be no correlation between program size on the basis of number of residents and

---

Current dermatopathology education: key points

- The dermatology RRC stipulates that DP education must occur during faculty-run sign-out.[6]
- On average, 30% of dermatology residency education time is devoted to DP.[8]
- Debate exists as to the amount and timing of DP education during residency.
- Cuts to GME funding will substantially decrease residency and fellowship positions.

allocation of conference hours."[18] By contrast, a study of the APD membership in 2009 found that the greater the number of residents in a dermatology residency, the greater the number of weeks a resident spent on a DP rotation.[7] Specifically, for every additional resident in a program, the number of weeks on the DP service per resident increased by 0.79. In this same study, 6 residency programs reported that they did not have a DP rotation for residents during any year in training. These 6 programs tended to have fewer residents than those that did have a DP rotation. The investigators did not ask why a program lacked a DP rotation. Some potential explanations for these results are that time on the DP service may be viewed as a relatively more expendable method of DP education, that there is a lack of access to a dermatopathologist, or that there is difficulty in scheduling time on service when a dermatopathologist is signing out cases. Defining the goals of DP education and adhering to the curriculum created to achieve those goals provides the consistency in GME so important for trainees, regardless of the composition of their future career.

TEACHING TOOLS AND EVALUATION METHODS IN DERMATOPATHOLOGY EDUCATION

Several teaching methods are commonly currently used, although data as to the relative efficacy of one compared with another are lacking. Often a program will use a primary DP textbook, although multiple texts are used for resident education. Specifically, one survey study in late 2007 of residency program directors via the APD listserv documented the most frequently used and most preferred textbooks in dermatology residencies (**Figs. 1** and **2**).[8]

GME programs implement their own evaluation procedures and document resident performance at least twice yearly. As a means of guidance toward meeting this requirement, GME programs have asked the ACGME for examples of trainee evaluations. Evaluation methods have been proposed for DP-specific core competencies.[5] Of interest, one recent publication found that not all DP fellowship programs formally evaluate fellows, which is difficult to reconcile when the absence of these evaluations puts programs at risk of losing accreditation. Specifically, Freeman and colleagues[19] mailed a 6-page questionnaire to DP fellowship directors in ACGME-approved programs (n = 45; 24 responded; 53.5% response rate) in the United States (2006–2007). Six of the 24 DP programs (25%) reported that they did not formally evaluate fellows

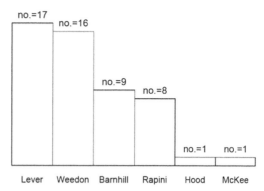

Most Used Textbook

Fig. 1. Lever and Weedon are the 2 most frequently used textbooks in dermatology residencies (*P* = .01). The programs were asked to list the textbook they used most for dermatopathology instruction. (*From* Hinshaw MA, Hsu P, Lee LY, et al. The current state of dermatopathology education: a survey of the Association of Professors of Dermatology. J Cutan Pathol 2009;36(6):620–8; with permission.)

at all. The evaluation process is seemingly an area for improvement in DP education.

CONTINUING MEDICAL EDUCATION IN DERMATOPATHOLOGY

Continuing medical education (CME) in DP begins at the completion of residency or DP fellowship and continues for one's professional lifetime. CME offerings have been reported by members

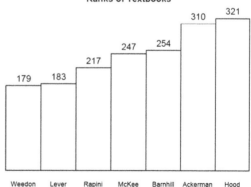

Ranks of Textbooks

Fig. 2. Cumulative textbook rank. Dermatology residencies were asked to rank textbooks in order of preference. For instance, 1 point was assigned if the book was used as their primary textbook. Therefore, the lower the number, the more the book was used in the program. Here Rapini and McKee, while not often used as primary texts, are often used as supplemental texts. (*From* Hinshaw MA, Hsu P, Lee LY, et al. The current state of dermatopathology education: a survey of the Association of Professors of Dermatology. J Cutan Pathol 2009;36(6):620–8; with permission.)

Teaching tools in dermatopathology

- Rotation on dermatopathology service with a dermatopathologist during sign-out
- Didactics at the microscope with a dermatopathologist
- Review of biopsies taken in clinic
- Grand rounds or clinical-pathologic case conference
- Book chapter review
- DP journal club
- Online slide libraries or courses
- Morbidity and mortality conference and specialty conferences (ie, tumor board)
- Local, regional, and national DP review courses
- Slide sets, including those created in each institution, slide-club sets, and industry-provided sets

to be the single most important benefit provided by the ASDP.[20] In 2011, the ASDP held its annual 4-day meeting during which 35 CME credits could have been earned per registered attendee. In 2012, the American Academy of Dermatology (AAD) will provide 24 DP-focused educational sessions (Forums, Focus Sessions, Self-Assessment Sessions, Courses) totaling 43.25 CME credits per registered attendee. In donating their time to teach at CME meetings, each expert in their field demonstrates their commitment to educating other professionals and to advancing DP.

Maintenance of Certification

The newly implemented Maintenance of Certification (MOC) program goes beyond CME. MOC is a 4-component program designed to assess the competence of physicians based on the 6 core competencies, and has been implemented by all 24 member boards of the ABMS including the ABD and the ABP (**Table 2**). Dermatologists who are board certified by the ABD and whose certification expires after 2006 must enter MOC. Dermatologists that certified in 1991 to 2005 enter MOC after successful completion of the recertification examination (time-limited certification). Those physicians board certified in DP before 2005 have a lifetime certification. Of note, a dermatologist with a lifetime certificate may choose not to pursue the MOC program without revocation of lifetime certification in dermatology; however, if that physician has a time-limited certificate in DP then they must successfully complete all elements of MOC to remain eligible for DP recertification. Pathologists board certified by the ABP before January 1, 2006 have non–time-limited certificates and are not required by the ABP to enroll in MOC, although all diplomats of the ABP are eligible to participate in the program. Anecdotally there may be other agencies that require participation in MOC, such as hospitals for privileging and

Table 2
Maintenance of certification in DP is predicated on MOC in dermatology or pathology

ABD	ABP
1. Evidence of Professional Standing: License attestation	1. Evidence of Professional Standing: License attestation Documentation of medical staff membership and hospital organization privileges
2. Evidence of Commitment to Lifelong Learning and Periodic Self-Assessment: Patient safety module CME attestation Periodic self-assessment of general knowledge	2. Evidence of Commitment to Lifelong Learning and Periodic Self-Assessment: CME attestation Periodic self-assessment of general knowledge
3. Evidence of Cognitive Expertise: Cognitive examination	3. Evidence of Cognitive Expertise: Cognitive examination
4. Evaluation of Performance in Practice: Patient communication survey Peer communication survey Practice assessment/Quality improvement	4. Evaluation of Performance in Practice: Peer attestations Laboratory accreditation, where applicable Participation by the diplomats laboratory in interlaboratory performance improvement and quality-assurance programs Participation by the diplomat in at least one performance improvement and quality-assurance program per year

payors for reimbursement, thus potentially making participation in MOC highly useful. Detailed information including specifics of CME requirements and answers to frequently asked questions can be found on the ABP and the ABD Web sites.

THE FUTURE OF DERMATOPATHOLOGY EDUCATION

Change is the future of DP education. As the extensive skill set required to practice the specialty of DP and the health care landscape become increasingly complex, so must we alter DP education. Some residency programs experience substantial barriers to DP education as a result of such changes. Current barriers range from access to dermatopathologists, limited space and microscopes for teaching, and the complex issue of outsourcing of tissue specimens (ie, teaching material sent to private laboratories) (**Box 1**).[7]

Box 1

APD DP education survey: barriers to dermatopathology education in dermatology residencies

Dermatopathology Specific

- Faculty left university to work for private laboratory
- Hospital contract for dermatopathology specimens was given to private laboratory
- Teaching slide sets lost
- Lack of text that includes most diagnoses while not being overly detailed
- Dermatopathology in Department of Pathology makes getting education difficult
- Laboratory is remote to where residents are located
- Low volume of specimens limited teaching material
- Limited space and microscopes for teaching

Dermatopathology Nonspecific

- Overall limited time of educators
- Overregulation by regulators such as ACGME makes teaching unappealing
- Limited time to teach all aspects of dermatology
- Financial (time out of clinic is loss of revenue)
- Overemphasis on teaching to pass the board examination

From Hinshaw MA, Hsu P, Lee LY, et al. The current state of dermatopathology education: a survey of the Association of Professors of Dermatology. J Cutan Pathol 2009;36(6):620–8; with permission.

The ACGME recognizes that the individual nature of each residency program makes their resources, needs, barriers, and solutions unique. In the future, the ACGME RRC will provide DP milestones (The Milestone Project) for programs to use in measuring trainee progression through residency (Erik J. Stratman, MD, Marshfield Clinic, Marshfield, WI, personal communication, January 2011). The ACGME is creating these milestones with input from leaders including those in the ABD and APD. Once milestones are defined, the challenge will be the need to interpret each milestone, then create valid and reliable tools to assess trainee performance against the milestones.

Duration of Dermatopathology Education

In the future, increasing the amount of time dedicated to DP education may be required to achieve our goals. American and European leaders in DP have either questioned the current length of DP education and/or have recommended that DP fellowships be of 2 years' duration.[1,16,21] Of interest, a recent family medicine publication describes one residency program's innovative curriculum overhaul in response to increasing health care demands.[22] Specifically, the Waukesha family medicine residency created a "Major" track (optional area of focused study decided on by the resident and approved by faculty after 19 months into residency, completed in 4 6-week blocks over the remainder of the 3-year residency) and a "Mastery" track (4-year residency during which the resident obtains a master's degree [MPH, MBA] from a sponsoring institution, or advanced obstetrics training). Related to Ackerman's long ago conceived consideration for longer DP training, one could conceive of such a "Major" in DP during residency in preparation for a DP fellowship. This publication and others comment on the importance of resident input into curriculum. Still others detail discrepancies between resident and faculty perceived needs for successful clinical practice.[23] In the future, we should consider setting minimum national standards for the duration and composition of DP education in residency. As the practice of DP and the health care environment in which we practice changes, so may our trainees benefit from more time for DP education.

Dermatopathology Teaching Tools

Whereas classic presentations of inflammatory and neoplastic conditions can be learned from a textbook or a slide set, the medical decision making involved in caring for patients via the practice of DP is best learned during sign-out.

Moreover, to facilitate clinical-pathologic correlation and DP learning, each program should have a mechanism in place for residents to routinely review the skin biopsies they obtain in the clinic.

One method of DP education thus far used in the curriculum by a minority of programs is computer-based learning.[7] In one study both dermatology and pathology residents in 14 residency programs reported that 23% were using virtual slide technology (high-resolution digital images of microscopic glass slides) while 71% were using Internet image libraries to learn DP.[24] Virtual microscopy has been used by the ABD for in-training and recertifying examinations and by the ABP for certifying and recertifying examinations.[25] Virtual microscopy has advantages as a teaching tool over conventional microscopy, including preservation of an image (tissue) and slide quality, as well as providing a ready source for sharing uncommon diagnoses that might not be available in every laboratory. In the future, computer-based learning including virtual microscopy and computerized algorithms may augment or replace components of current DP education.

A recent study aimed to measure the diagnostic accuracy and preferences of dermatology and pathology residents when using virtual microscopy versus traditional microscopy of glass slides (20 specimens: 10 inflammatory, 10 neoplastic).[24] Residents performed equally well whether using virtual or glass slides (mean [SD] correct for virtual vs glass, 5.48 [1.72] vs 5.57 [2.06]; $P = .70$). When asked their preferences, 79% favored using virtual microscopy as a learning aid while 44% favored using it in a testing situation (ie, board examination). In another study of the diagnostic accuracy of practitioners using virtual versus glass slides, 10 Nordic dermatopathologists and pathologists showed no statistical difference in diagnostic accuracy using either method, and most agreed that virtual microscopy was a useful tool for learning and testing.[25] As technology improves and experience and comfort with virtual microscopy grows, this resource will likely be used with greater frequency during residency and fellowship, and in CME.

Dermatopathology Assessment Tools

Assessment tools in DP education need to be developed and enhanced over time. Assessment of competency is a complicated process that begins with defining the construct being assessed. Performance of valid assessments is optimized when many short cases are scored by experienced evaluators using an assessment instrument with which they are comfortable.[26] One expanding area of medical education assessment (and teaching) of interest to DP education is simulation-based education.

Simulation-based education programs are experiential learning environments in which learners practice skills on models rather than on patients. Such programs can be used either for formative assessment (identifies deficiencies and motivates learning) or for summative assessment (judges competence as for practice readiness). To date, simulation laboratories have predominantly been used for procedural skills.[27] The successful practice of DP relies on use of established patterns and rules in the context of clinical judgment and experience. The interpretive nature of DP raises challenges for assessment. Specifically, procedural and surgical specialties are well served by cognitive-based tutoring systems (high enforcement; limits the number of acceptable actions at any step). As a diagnostic specialty, the competent practice of DP relies on histologic criteria and algorithms and on clinical experience and judgment, and thus lends itself to limited-enforcement tutoring (accepts a variety of steps to arrive at a diagnosis, and accommodates various student strategies). Simulation-based education in DP could occur at the microscope with mock cases. In addition, computer-based simulated DP cases are useful for assessment.

Computer-based simulations encompass more than the (very useful) slide libraries and online DP didactics that are currently widely available. One example of simulation-based DP education is SlideTutor. SlideTutor is a web-based system that uses limited-enforcement tutoring to teach and assess resident and practicing physician DP knowledge.[28] This novel program is a case-based system (thus far, limited numbers of inflammatory diseases and melanocytic cases have been developed) that teaches histopathologic diagnosis and report writing. It has been created to evaluate decision making based on algorithms, and ranks errors based on the degree to which they alter subsequent reasoning steps. This type of technology has the potential to overcome barriers to DP education and to fill a need for DP assessment.

Continuing Medical Education in Dermatopathology

CME in DP is important for practicing pathologists and dermatologists. For dermatologists, specialized care of patients with dermatologic concerns relies on the provider of that care having knowledge of histology of the skin; this holds true regardless of the practice composition of the dermatologists.[17]

The future of DP education: key points

- In the future, dermatopathology education will be guided by ACGME-provided milestones.

- Dermatology and pathology RRCs could set minimum standards for duration and composition of DP education.

- In a study published in 2009, computer-based learning was used by less than 20% of dermatology residency programs, and is an area of growth for teaching and assessment.[8]

- Simulation-based learning and assessment has the potential to advance DP education.

- DP leaders have questioned whether trainees should learn DP in more than one institution, and have suggested DP fellowship be expanded from 1 to 2 years' duration.

A related issue is the interpretation of skin biopsies by dermatologists and pathologists who are not board certified in DP. Once board certified in dermatology, a dermatologist may interpret skin biopsies. In practice they interpret a substantial number of biopsies for skin-related diseases. One study using claims data from the Medicare Current Beneficiary Survey from 1992 to 2000 evaluated the specialty of a physician (pathologist, dermatologist, or independent laboratory/group practice) submitting a claim for Current Procedural Terminology (CPT) code 88305 against the International Classification of Diseases, 9th Revision (ICD-9), Clinical Modification codes 078.x, 110.x-112.x, 172.x-173.x, 216.x, 238.2, 454.x, and 680.2-709.9.[29] These ICD-9 codes were chosen because they encompass the majority of codes used by physicians for skin-related disease. Results of the study showed that, for skin-related diagnoses, dermatologists performed 9.7 million (31.2%), pathologists performed 10.7 million (34.5%), and independent laboratories and group practices performed 10.2 million (32.8%) claims. Dermatologists and general pathologists are practicing DP. CME that includes DP-specific competencies must be part of career-long professional development.

SUMMARY

DP education is a critical component of dermatology and pathology residencies. Given the continually expanding body of knowledge that must be learned to practice DP, education leaders have questioned the optimal duration, methods, and assessments of DP education.

The goals of DP education for residents and DP fellows should continue to be considered and defined, because they guide curriculum development and learner assessment. In part because of the substantial changes in DP since formalized fellowship training began in 1950, some have advocated that DP fellowships be 2 years in duration. In addition, program directors could create ways for interested residents to gain more than the minimum DP education requirement before entering an accredited DP fellowship. Given existing barriers to DP education and interest in consistent assessments, more computer-based and simulation-based DP education tools should be developed.

Dermatopathologists will navigate the ACGME Milestone Project and its intent of documenting progression toward achievement of core competencies during and at the completion of training, and will continue to adapt and innovate just as those who have created and advanced this vibrant subspecialty have done over the past several hundred years since it was recognized as a unique and important area of study.

ACKNOWLEDGMENTS

The author sincerely thanks Drs William Aughenbaugh, Anita Gilliam, Erik Stratman, and Brian Swick for contributing their time and expertise in reviewing and providing thoughtful feedback on this article.

REFERENCES

1. Bhawan J. The evolution of dermatopathology—the American experience. Am J Dermatopathol 2006; 28(1):67–71.
2. Ackerman AB. Dermatopathology is for dermatologists and pathologists. Am J Dermatopathol 1983; 5(2):107–8.
3. Cerroni L, et al. Dermatopathology examination in Europe: a summary of 6 years of the European Board Certification. Am J Dermatopathol 2009; 31(8):803–5.
4. Connolly JL, Fletcher CD, Frable WJ, et al. Curriculum content and evaluation of resident competency in anatomic pathology: a proposal. Human Pathol 2003;34(11):1083–90.
5. Hinshaw MA, Stratman EJ. Core competencies in dermatopathology. J Cutan Pathol 2006;33(2):160–5.
6. ACGME website under Dermatology Program Requirements. Available at: http://www.acgme.org/ac Website/downloads/RRC_progReq/080dermatology_ 07012007.pdf. Accessed July 27, 2012.
7. Singh S, Grummer SE, Hancox JG, et al. The extent of dermatopathology education: a comparison of

pathology and dermatology. J Am Acad Dermatol 2005;53(4):694–7.

8. Hinshaw M, Hsu P, Lee LY, et al. The current state of dermatopathology education: a survey of the Association of Professors of Dermatology. J Cutan Pathol 2009;36(6):620–8.

9. Ackerman AB. Training residents in dermatopathology: why, when, where, and how. J Am Acad Dermatol 1990;22(6 Pt 1):1104–6.

10. ACGME website under ACGME Data Resource Book. Available at: http://www.acgme.org/acWebsite/dataBook/2010-2011_ACGME_Data_Resource_Book.pdf. Accessed July 27, 2012.

11. Goldenberg G, Patel MJ, Sangueza OP, et al. US dermatopathology fellows career survey: 2004-2005. J Cutan Pathol 2007;34(6):487–9.

12. Graduate medical education financing: focusing on educational priorities. Chapter 4. Medicare Payment Advisory Commission Report to Congress: aligning incentives. Washington, DC; 2010. p. 103–22. Available at: http://www.medpac.gov/chapters/Jun10_Ch04.pdf. Accessed July 27, 2012.

13. The moment of truth. Report of the National Commission on Fiscal Responsibility and Reform. Section 3.3.5. Reduce excess payments to hospitals for medical education. December 2010. p. 37. Available at: http://www.fiscalcommission.gov/sites/fiscalcommission.gov/files/documents/TheMomentofTruth12_1_2010.pdf. Accessed July 27, 2012.

14. Nasca TJ, Miller RS, Holt KD. The potential impact of reduction in Federal GME funding in the United States: a study of the estimates of designated institutional officials. The Accreditation Council for Graduate Medical Education. Chicago (IL). Available at: http://www.acgme.org/acWebsite/home/ImpactReductionFederalGMEFundingTJN.pdf. Accessed July 27, 2012.

15. Ackerman AB. Dermatologist not equal to dermatopathologist: no place in a profession for pretenders. J Am Acad Dermatol 2005;53(4):698–9.

16. Ackerman AB. Pedagogy in dermatopathology. Am J Dermatopathol 1982;4(3):197–8.

17. Ackerman AB. Dermatologic surgery cannot be practiced rationally without profound knowledge of cutaneous embryology, histology, and pathology. Dermatol Surg 1995;21(5):412–4.

18. Mehrabi D, Cruz PD Jr. Educational conferences in dermatology residency programs. J Am Acad Dermatol 2006;55(3):523–4.

19. Freeman SR, Nelson C, Lundahl K, et al. Similar deficiencies in procedural dermatology and dermatopathology fellow evaluation despite different periods of ACGME accreditation: results of a national survey. Dermatol Surg 2008;34(7):873–6 [discussion: 876–7].

20. Mahalingam M. Quality assurance and continuing medical education in dermatopathology—the ASDP way. J Cutan Pathol 2008;35(5):516–9.

21. Sterry W, European Dermatology Forum Guideline Committee. Guidelines: the management of dermatopathology. Eur J Dermatol 2006;16(5):476–8.

22. Mazzone M, Krasovich S, Fay D, et al. Implementing radical curriculum change in a family medicine residency: the majors and masteries program. Fam Med 2011;43(7):514–21.

23. Lagwinski N, Hunt JL. Fellowship trends of pathology residents. Arch Pathol Lab Med 2009; 133(9):1431–6.

24. Koch LH, Lampros JN, Delong LK, et al. Randomized comparison of virtual microscopy and traditional glass microscopy in diagnostic accuracy among dermatology and pathology residents. Hum Pathol 2009;40(5):662–7.

25. Mooney E, Hood AF, Lampros J, et al. Comparative diagnostic accuracy in virtual dermatopathology. Skin Res Technol 2011;17:251–5.

26. Schuwirth LW, van der Vleuten CP. Programmatic assessment and Kane's validity perspective. Med Educ 2012;46(1):38–48.

27. Bould MD, Naik VN, Hamstra SJ. Review article: new directions in medical education related to anesthesiology and perioperative medicine. Can J Anaesth 2012;59(2):136–50.

28. Payne VL, Medvedeva O, Legowski E, et al. Effect of a limited-enforcement intelligent tutoring system in dermatopathology on student errors, goals and solution paths. Artif Intell Med 2009; 47(3):175–97.

29. Hancox JG, Neville JA, Chen J, et al. Interpretation of dermatopathology specimens is within the standard of care of dermatology practice. Dermatol Surg 2005;31(3):306–9.

Index

Note: Page numbers of article titles are in **boldface** type.

A

Accreditation Council for Graduate Medical Education
and dermatopathology education, 816, 817
ACGME. See *Accreditation Council for Graduate Medical Education.*
Acquired elastotic hemangioma
and vascular neoplasms, 661
Actinic keratosis
and reflectance confocal microscopy, 807, 809
Actinic prurigo, 670
and polymorphous light eruption, 670
Acute hemorrhagic edema of infancy
immunofluorescence in, 788
AEC. See *Amino-9-ethylcarbozole.*
AFX. See *Atypical fibroxanthoma.*
AHEI. See *Hemorrhagic edema of infancy.*
AIDS
and new histopathologic variants of Kaposi sarcoma, 663, 664
AJCC. See *American Joint Committee on Cancer.*
Alefacept
adverse cutaneous reactions to, 702
Alemtuzumab
adverse cutaneous reactions to, 702
ALLP. See *Atypical lymphocytic lobular panniculitis.*
Alopecia
and anti-tumor necrosis factor-α therapy, 689, 690
areata, 687
in B cell lymphoma, 687
cellular proliferation in, 690
elastic tissue patterns in, 688, 689
ethnic variation in, 688
Langerhans cells in, 688
and lichen planopilaris, 685, 687, 688
and loose anagen hair syndrome, 690
lymphoma presenting as, 686, 687
in mycosis fungoides, 686
neutrophil-mediated, 686
overlap, 688
pattern, 690
progenitor cell populations in, 690
and reflectance confocal microscopy, 687
scarring, 686, 687
sectioning techniques, 685, 686
and selenium, 689
and telepathology, 689
traction, 688
and trichotillomania, 687

and tufting, 686
and vitamin D-resistant rickets, 692
Alopecia areata, 687
Alport syndrome
immunofluorescent mapping of, 791
American Joint Committee on Cancer
and advances in dermatopathology, 623–635
and guidelines for melanoma staging, 581–588
and staging for cutaneous squamous cell carcinoma, 627
and staging for Merkel cell carcinoma, 626
American Medical Association
and interpretation of histology specimens, 598, 599
American Society of Dermatopathology
and dermatopathology education, 815, 816
Amevive
adverse cutaneous reactions to, 702
Amino-9-ethylcarbozole
in immunohistochemistry, 567, 569, 570
ANCA. See *Antineutrophil cytoplasmic antibodies.*
Anti-P200 pemphigoid
and basement membrane zone, 768, 769
and direct immunofluorescence, 769
and light microscopy, 769
Anti-tumor necrosis factor-α
and alopecia, 689, 690
Antiendothelial cell antibodies
immunofluorescence detection of, 790
Antineutrophil cytoplasmic antibodies
and adverse cutaneous drug reactions, 707–711
Antiphospholipid antibody syndrome
and direct immunofluorescence, 789
pathogenesis of, 789, 790
Antiretroviral drugs
and immune reconstitution inflammatory syndrome, 744
Arteriovenous malformations
WT1 expression in, 657
Arteritis
lymphocytic thrombophilic, 673, 674
ASD. See *American Society of Dermatopathology.*
Atypical/dysplastic nevus
and medical malpractice, 606–608
Atypical fibroxanthoma
and CD10 expression, 645, 646
Atypical lentiginous melanocytic lesions
and medical malpractice, 606–608
Atypical lymphocytic lobular panniculitis

Dermatol Clin 30 (2012) 827–839
http://dx.doi.org/10.1016/S0733-8635(12)00132-5
0733-8635/12/$ – see front matter © 2012 Elsevier Inc. All rights reserved.

United States Postal Service

Statement of Ownership, Management, and Circulation
(All Periodicals Publications Except Requestor Publications)

1. Publication Title	2. Publication Number	3. Filing Date
Dermatologic Clinics of North America	0 0 0 - 7 0 0 5	9/14/12

4. Issue Frequency	5. Number of Issues Published Annually	6. Annual Subscription Price
Jan, Apr, Jul, Oct	4	$346.00

7. Complete Mailing Address of Known Office of Publication (*Not printer*) (*Street, city, county, state, and ZIP+4®*)

Elsevier Inc.
360 Park Avenue South
New York, NY 10010-1710

Contact Person: **Stephen R. Bushing**
Telephone (*Include area code*): 215-239-3688

8. Complete Mailing Address of Headquarters or General Business Office of Publisher (*Not printer*)

Elsevier Inc., 360 Park Avenue South, New York, NY 10010-1710

9. Full Names and Complete Mailing Addresses of Publisher, Editor, and Managing Editor (*Do not leave blank*)

Publisher (*Name and complete mailing address*)

Kim Murphy , Elsevier, Inc., 1600 John F. Kennedy Blvd. Suite 1800, Philadelphia, PA 19103-2899

Editor (*Name and complete mailing address*)

Stephanie Donley, Elsevier, Inc., 1600 John F. Kennedy Blvd. Suite 1800, Philadelphia, PA 19103-2899

Managing Editor (*Name and complete mailing address*)

Sarah Barth, Elsevier, Inc., 1600 John F. Kennedy Blvd. Suite 1800, Philadelphia, PA 19103-2899

10. Owner (*Do not leave blank. If the publication is owned by a corporation, give the name and address of the corporation immediately followed by the names and addresses of all stockholders owning or holding 1 percent or more of the total amount of stock. If not owned by a corporation, give the names and addresses of the individual owners. If owned by a partnership or other unincorporated firm, give its name and address as well as those of each individual owner. If the publication is published by a nonprofit organization, give its name and address.*)

Full Name	Complete Mailing Address
Wholly owned subsidiary of	1600 John F. Kennedy Blvd., Ste. 1800
Reed/Elsevier, US holdings	Philadelphia, PA 19103-2899

11. Known Bondholders, Mortgagees, and Other Security Holders Owning or Holding 1 Percent or More of Total Amount of Bonds, Mortgages, or Other Securities. If none, check box ☐ None

Full Name	Complete Mailing Address
N/A	

12. Tax Status (*For completion by nonprofit organizations authorized to mail at nonprofit rates*) (*Check one*)
The purpose, function, and nonprofit status of this organization and the exempt status for federal income tax purposes:
☐ Has Not Changed During Preceding 12 Months
☐ Has Changed During Preceding 12 Months (*Publisher must submit explanation of change with this statement*)

PS Form **3526**, September 2007 (Page 1 of 3 (Instructions Page 3)) PSN 7530-01-000-9931 PRIVACY NOTICE: See our Privacy policy in www.usps.com

---

13. Publication Title	14. Issue Date for Circulation Data Below
Dermatologic Clinics of North America	July 2012

15. Extent and Nature of Circulation			Average No. Copies Each Issue During Preceding 12 Months	No. Copies of Single Issue Published Nearest to Filing Date
a. Total Number of Copies (*Net press run*)			615	563
b. Paid Circulation (By Mail and Outside the Mail)	(1)	Mailed Outside-County Paid Subscriptions Stated on PS Form 3541. (*Include paid distribution above nominal rate, advertiser's proof copies, and exchange copies*)	233	207
	(2)	Mailed In-County Paid Subscriptions Stated on PS Form 3541 (*Include paid distribution above nominal rate, advertiser's proof copies, and exchange copies*)		
	(3)	Paid Distribution Outside the Mails Including Sales Through Dealers and Carriers, Street Vendors, Counter Sales, and Other Paid Distribution Outside USPS®	108	140
	(4)	Paid Distribution by Other Classes Mailed Through the USPS (e.g. First-Class Mail®)		
c. Total Paid Distribution (*Sum of 15b (1), (2), (3), and (4)*)			341	347
d. Free or Nominal Rate Distribution (By Mail and Outside the Mail)	(1)	Free or Nominal Rate Outside-County Copies Included on PS Form 3541	80	46
	(2)	Free or Nominal Rate In-County Copies Included on PS Form 3541		
	(3)	Free or Nominal Rate Copies Mailed at Other Classes Through the USPS (e.g. First-Class Mail)		
	(4)	Free or Nominal Rate Distribution Outside the Mail (Carriers or other means)		
e. Total Free or Nominal Rate Distribution (Sum of 15d (1), (2), (3) and (4))			80	46
f. Total Distribution (Sum of 15c and 15e)			421	393
g. Copies not Distributed (See instructions to publishers #4 (page #3))			194	170
h. Total (Sum of 15f and g)			615	563
i. Percent Paid (15c divided by 15f times 100)			81.00%	88.30%

16. Publication of Statement of Ownership

☐ If the publication is a general publication, publication of this statement is required. Will be printed in the **October** 2012 issue of this publication. — Publication not required

17. Signature and Title of Editor, Publisher, Business Manager, or Owner — Date

[signature] Stephen R. Bushing — Inventory/Distribution Coordinator — September 14, 2012

I certify that all information furnished on this form is true and complete. I understand that anyone who furnishes false or misleading information on this form or who omits material or information requested on the form may be subject to criminal sanctions (including fines and imprisonment) and/or civil sanctions (including civil penalties).

PS Form 3526, September 2007 (Page 2 of 3)

Moving?

Make sure your subscription moves with you!

To notify us of your new address, find your **Clinics Account Number** (located on your mailing label above your name), and contact customer service at:

Email: journalscustomerservice-usa@elsevier.com

800-654-2452 (subscribers in the U.S. & Canada)
314-447-8871 (subscribers outside of the U.S. & Canada)

Fax number: 314-447-8029

**Elsevier Health Sciences Division
Subscription Customer Service
3251 Riverport Lane
Maryland Heights, MO 63043**

*To ensure uninterrupted delivery of your subscription, please notify us at least 4 weeks in advance of move.

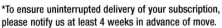

ELSEVIER

Printed and bound by CPI Group (UK) Ltd, Croydon, CR0 4YY

03/10/2024

01040352-0003